American Dietetic Association Guide to

Diabetes

Medical Nutrition Therapy and Education

Edited by

Tami A. Ross, RD, CDE,

Jackie L. Boucher, MS, RD, BC-ADM, CDE, and

Belinda S. O'Connell, MS, RD, CDE

Diabetes Care and Education Dietetic Practice Group

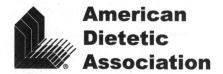

American Dietetic Association

Diana Faulhaber, Publisher
Kristen Short, Development Editor
Elizabeth Nishiura, Production Editor

10 9 8 7 6 5 4 3

Library of Congress Cataloging-in-Publication Data

American Dietetic Association guide to diabetes medical nutrition therapy and education/ by the Diabetes Care and Education Dietetic Practice Group; Tami Ross, Jackie Boucher, and Belinda O'Connell, editors.
    p. ; cm.
Includes bibliographical references and index.
ISBN 0-88091-333-9
1. Diabetes—Diet therapy. 2. Patient education.
[DNLM: 1. Diabetes Mellitus—diet therapy. 2. Nutrition Therapy—methods. 3. Patient Education. WK 818 A5115 2005] I. Title: Guide to diabetes medical nutrition therapy and education. II. Ross, Tami. III. Boucher, Jackie. IV. O'Connell, Belinda. V. American Dietetic Association. Diabetes Care and Education Dietetic Practice Group.

RC662.A435 2005
616.4'620654—dc22

2005001007

CONTENTS

Part 4   LIFE STAGES AND SPECIAL POPULATIONS

Part 5   NUTRITION EDUCATION: MEAL PLANNING

Part 6   NUTRITION EDUCATION FOR DIABETES COMORBIDITIES

APPENDIXES

FOREWORD

Interest in diabetes and its management has never been greater than it is today. However, the role of dietetics professionals in lessening the burden of diabetes for society and patients has not been fully recognized or realized. In the last 10 years, randomized control trials and observational studies of medical nutritional therapy (MNT) have demonstrated improved glycemic outcomes for individuals with type 1 and type 2 diabetes. The significance of these studies and the impact of MNT should not be underestimated. Evidence shows that MNT can reduce A1C levels as effectively as some pharmacologic interventions, and at far less cost. This information must be more effectively communicated to all persons with diabetes, to payers, and to other health care providers. Diabetes MNT works, and it saves money!

Unfortunately, the results of the NHANES III survey show that, overall, glycemic control in people with diabetes is declining in the United States. Most people with diabetes are not referred for diabetes MNT, and they never see a registered dietitian. More people with diabetes, as well as those at risk for developing diabetes, need to be able to access diabetes MNT services provided by registered dietitians.

As professionals, we are driven to develop and define processes that improve the quality and scope of the services we deliver. A noteworthy feature of this publication is information on the American Dietetic Association's Nutrition Care Process (NCP), which recognizes that

MNT has been redefined to include not only assessment and treatment, but also goal setting and evaluation. The NCP accurately describes the spectrum of nutrition care provided by dietetics professionals and outlines the consistent and specific steps that are to be used when delivering MNT. The first three chapters of this book clearly explain the NCP and its relationship to MNT, information that may be new for some professionals.

This book also covers diabetes self-management training (DSMT). DSMT provides overall guidance about the multiple aspects of diabetes self-management and glycemic control. It complements MNT by increasing diabetes-management knowledge and skills in persons with diabetes and by promoting behaviors of self-management.

People with diabetes are faced with the daily challenges of coordinating their foods, physical activity, blood glucose monitoring, and oral medications or insulin. Central to accomplishing these tasks is the ability to self-manage by recognizing blood glucose patterns, changing behaviors, and possibly self-adjusting medications. It is difficult to imagine that the average person with diabetes can accomplish complicated self-management tasks without assistance. All people with diabetes need the expertise and coaching of many health care professionals on a long-term basis. Diabetes MNT is only one component of diabetes care. Many registered dietitians are experienced providers of both diabetes MNT and DSMT. All dietetics professionals, whether they provide both services or not, need to support the team approach to managing diabetes as central to the care for people with diabetes.

This book establishes and enforces the nutrition component of the team approach to the treatment of diabetes. Most certainly, this cutting edge resource will be invaluable, not only for dietetics professionals, but also for other health care professionals involved in the care, treatment, and counseling of persons with diabetes. A greater understanding of the value and effectiveness of diabetes MNT by all health care providers will translate into increased referral to and use of diabetes MNT resources. This is a challenge for all of us, as well as an opportunity. Becoming skilled clinicians is not enough; we must continue to collect outcome data, publish and promote our effectiveness, and not rest until all people with diabetes have access to diabetes MNT and DSMT.

The American Dietetic Association Guide to Diabetes Medical Nutrition Therapy and Education reflects a strong commitment by the American Dietetic Association and the Diabetes Care and Education Dietetic Practice Group to increase professional knowledge about diabetes MNT in the management and care of persons with diabetes. Congratulations to all the authors of this publication, many of whom I have had the privilege to work with over the years. The diabetes and dietetics community are indebted to you for your time, effort, and willingness to share your expertise to move the profession forward and to improve the lives of people with diabetes.

MARY M. AUSTIN, MA, RD, CDE
President, American Association
of Diabetes Educators, 2004–2005
Past President, Diabetes Care and Education (DCE)
Dietetic Practice Group of ADA, 1996–1998

ACKNOWLEDGMENTS

The Diabetes Care and Education Dietetic Practice Group (DCE) wishes to thank the following individuals who contributed their valuable time to this guide:

DCE Editors
Tami A. Ross, RD, CDE
Jackie L. Boucher, MS, RD, BC-ADM, CDE
Belinda S. O'Connell, MS, RD, CDE

Guest Editors
Janine Freeman, RD, CDE
Patti Urbanski, MEd, RD, CDE
Jeffrey J. VanWormer, MS

DCE Committee Members
Janine Freeman, RD, CDE
Marion J. Franz, MS, RD, CDE

Chapter Authors
Marilynn S. Arnold, MS, RD, CDE
Jackie L. Boucher, MS, RD, BC-ADM, CDE
Tammy L. Brown, MPH, RD, BC-ADM, CDE
Carol Brunzell, RD, CDE
Linda M. Delahanty, MS, RD
Alison Evert, RD, CDE
Amy Fischl, MS, RD, BC-ADM, CDE
Marion J. Franz, MS, RD, CDE

Janine Freeman, RD, CDE
Gretchen A. Gates, RD
Patti Geil, MS, RD, FADA, CDE
Stephanie Gerken, MS, RD, CDE
Catherine M. Goeddeke-Merickel, MS, RD
Joyce Green Pastors, MS, RD, CDE
Heidi Gunderson, MS, RD, CDE
Cindy Halstenson, RD, CDE
Charlotte Hayes, MMSc, MS, RD, CDE
Joan M. Heins, MA, RD, CDE
Lois Hill, MS, RD, CSR
Lea Ann Holzmeister, RD, CDE
Megan Jahnes, RD
Wahida Karmally, DrPH, RD, CDE
Karmeen Kulkarni, MS, RD, BC-ADM, CDE
Sue McLaughlin, RD, CDE
Arlene Monk, RD, CDE
Belinda S. O'Connell, MS, RD, CDE
Diane Reader, RD, CDE
Janis Roszler, RD, CDE
Jan Kincaid Rystrom, MEd, RD, CDE
Patti Urbanski, MEd, RD, CDE
Jeffrey J. VanWormer, MS
Hope S. Warshaw, MMSc, RD, BC-ADM, CDE
Janelle Waslaski, RD, CDE
Madelyn L. Wheeler, MS, RD, FADA, CD, CDE
Judith Wylie-Rosett, EdD, RD

Foreword Author
Mary M. Austin, MA, RD, CDE

Reviewers
Ann Albright, PhD, RD
Gary Arsham, MD, PhD
Mary Austin, RD, MA, CDE
Julie Barboza, MS, RD, CSR, RN
Jill Crandall, MD
Kristine D'Angelo David, RD
Marion J. Franz, MS, RD, CDE
Janine Freeman, RD, CDE
Eve Gehling, MEd, RD, CDE
Patti Geil, MS, RD, FADA, CDE
Joy T. Hayes, MS, RD, CDE
Laura Hieronymus, MSEd, APRN, BC-ADM, CDE
Laurie Higgins, MS, RD, CDE

Deborah Hinnen, MN, RN, BC-ADM, CDE
Mariann Hutton, RD, CDE
Scott Jacober, DO
Tommy Johnson, PharmD, CDE
Maria Karalis, MBA, RD
Carolyn Leontos, MS, RD, CDE
Cathi Martin, RD, CSR
Melinda Marynuik, MEd, RD, FADA, CDE
Pam Michael, MBA, RD
Joe Nelson, MA
Philippa Norton, MEd, RD, CSR
Ellen Pritchett, RD, CPHQ
Gregg Simonson, PhD
Terri Ryan Turek, RD, CDE
Gail Underbakke, MS, RD
Patti Urbanski, MEd, RD, CDE

Part 1

Nutrition Care Process

Introduction to the Nutrition Care Process and Medical Nutrition Therapy for Persons With Diabetes

Marion J. Franz, MS, RD, CDE, and Arlene Monk, RD, CDE

CHAPTER OVERVIEW

- Medical nutrition therapy (MNT), although challenging for individuals with diabetes to implement, is an essential and integral component of the medical management of diabetes (1–5) and the prevention of type 2 diabetes (6,7).
- For MNT to be effective, it must be implemented in a standardized process. The Nutrition Care Process (NCP) defines a consistent structure and framework for the provision of nutrition care, including MNT (8).
- MNT is the clinical application of the NCP (8), which always involves a comprehensive assessment, individualized care, and the monitoring and evaluation of nutrition therapy interventions on diabetes treatment goals.
- Because of the complexity of nutrition issues, a registered dietitian (RD), knowledgeable and skilled in the process and content of diabetes management and education, should be the team member providing MNT (9,10).

THE ORIGINS OF MODERN NUTRITION CARE AND THERAPY FOR DIABETES

In 1994, the focus of nutrition therapy for diabetes changed dramatically (11,12). Before this time, the attempt was always to determine an ideal nutrition prescription that would apply to all persons with diabetes. Furthermore, the nutrition prescription, including a calorie level and percentages of macronutrients, was often recommended by a physician. A better method was to have the dietetics professional determine an assessment-based energy requirement for the individual with diabetes. Then, using a predetermined ideal percentage of carbohydrate, protein, and fat, a meal plan was developed. Implementation consisted of instructing patients on how to use this meal plan to make food choices. Although individualization was considered to be important, it is virtually impossible to individualize a nutrition prescription that dictates a specific number of calories and percentages of macronutrients. Not surprisingly, adherence to this approach by persons with diabetes was often unsuccessful. As a consequence of this approach, the dietetics professional was often isolated from other health care team members and had little input from and into the process of overall diabetes management.

In 1994, the American Diabetes Association "Nutrition Recommendations and Principles for People with Diabetes" recommended that the nutrition prescription be based on patient treatment goals, metabolic profile, and strategies known to improve metabolic abnormalities (11). Furthermore, the person with diabetes was to be an active member of the management team, and the nutrition prescription would reflect changes that the person with diabetes determined to be reasonable. This meant that predetermined nutrition prescriptions or "ADA diets" were no longer appropriate. Instead, the nutrition prescription was based on an assessment of changes the person with diabetes could incorporate into his or her lifestyle, and that would facilitate the accomplishment of treatment goals. This approach required the dietitian to be an active member of the health care team, with responsibilities to assess, implement, monitor, and evaluate diabetes treatment goals and to provide feedback on nutrition therapy interventions. This focus continues with the 2004 "Nutrition Principles and Recommendations in Diabetes" (10,13).

NUTRITION CARE PROCESS AND MEDICAL NUTRITION THERAPY: WHAT ARE THEY?

When MNT was first defined, its components included (*a*) a nutrition assessment of the nutritional status of the individual and (*b*) treatment, which included diet therapy, counseling, and the use of specialized nutrition supplements (14). However, because of the chronic nature of diabetes, the definition of diabetes MNT was expanded to include not only assessment and treatment but also goal setting and evaluation (15). More recently, MNT has been redefined as part of the 2001 Medicare MNT benefit legislation to be "nutritional diagnostic, therapy, and counseling services for the purpose of disease management, which are furnished by a registered dietitian or nutrition professional" (16). As a result of the change in definition, the American Dietetic Association has developed the NCP to more accurately describe the spectrum of nutrition care (eg, MNT or nutrition education) provided by dietetics professionals (8).

The NCP outlines the consistent and specific steps a dietetics professional would use when delivering MNT. The NCP is also to be used to guide nutrition education and other preventive nutrition care services. A key difference between MNT and other nutrition services using the NCP is that MNT always involves an in-depth, comprehensive assessment and individualized care, which differentiates it from other nutrition services. MNT is, therefore, the clinical application of the NCP. This means an individual can receive MNT for diabetes and receive nutrition education services or participate in a community-based weight loss program (17).

The NCP is visually represented in the Nutrition Care Model (see Figure 1.1). Central to providing care is the relationship between patient/client/group and dietetics professionals. The four steps of the NCP are illustrated next: (*a*) nutrition assessment; (*b*) nutrition diagnosis; (*c*) nutrition intervention; (*d*) nutrition monitoring and evaluation. The middle ring identifies the strengths and abilities that dietetics professionals bring to the process; the outer ring identifies some of the environmental factors that influence the process. Nutrition screening is a supportive system and not a step within the NCP; it is an identification step that provides access to the NCP. An outcomes management system evaluates the effectiveness and efficiency of the entire process; the fourth step of the NCP, "nutrition monitoring and evaluation," refers to the evaluation of the patient/client/group's progress in achieving outcomes. The major goal of outcomes management is to use the collected data to improve the quality of care that will be provided in the future.

Before the four steps of the NCP are further defined, the goals of nutrition therapy need to be articulated. It is critical to know the goals of MNT in order to implement the process of care needed to facilitate accomplishment of these goals.

GOALS OF MNT FOR PEOPLE WITH DIABETES

Nutrition care begins by identifying nutrition therapy goals. For persons with diabetes, the primary goals of MNT, as specified in the 2004 American Diabetes Association Position Statement "Nutrition Principles and Recommendations in Diabetes" (10), are as follows:

1. To achieve metabolic outcomes, including
   - blood glucose concentrations and hemoglobin A1C (A1C) levels as close to normal as is safely possible to prevent or reduce the risk for complications of diabetes.
   - lipid and lipoprotein profiles that reduce the risk for macrovascular disease.
   - blood pressure levels that reduce the risk for vascular disease.
2. To modify nutrient intake and lifestyle for the prevention and treatment of long-term complications of diabetes, such as cardiovascular disease, hypertension, nephropathy, and obesity.
3. To improve health and wellness through healthy food choices and physical activity.
4. To address individual nutrition needs, taking into consideration personal and cultural preferences and lifestyle, while respecting the individual's wishes and willingness to change.

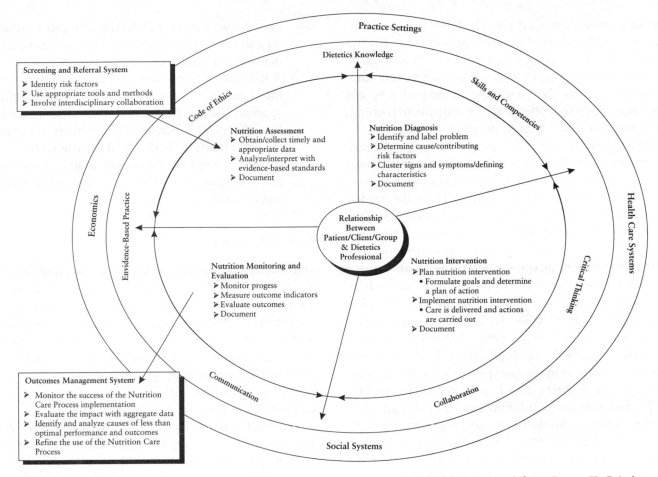

FIGURE 1.1. American Dietetic Association Nutrition Care Process and Model. Reprinted from Lacey K, Pritchett E. Nutrition care process and model: ADA adopts road map to quality care and outcomes. *J Am Diet Assoc.* 2003;103:1061–1072, with permission from the American Dietetic Association.

See Chapters 5, 6, and 15–17 to review MNT goals for specific populations.

NUTRITION PRACTICE GUIDELINES FOR DIABETES

The Diabetes Care and Education (DCE) Dietetic Practice Group and the American Dietetic Association (ADA) have written and validated by clinical trials nutrition practice guidelines (NPGs) for type 2 diabetes (1,18), type 1 diabetes (2,19), and gestational diabetes (20). NPGs recommend that patients with diabetes do the following:

- *Receive a referral to an RD.* For individuals newly diagnosed with type 1 or type 2 diabetes, the referral should occur within the first month after diagnosis. For a person newly diagnosed with gestational diabetes, the referral should occur within 1 week.

- *Have a series of visits with the RD.* Initially, a series of two to three visits is recommended, totaling approximately 2.5 to 3 hours. The time needed for the first visit is 60 to 90 minutes, with a minimum of 30- to 45-minute follow-up visits.

- *See the RD for follow-up care.* Additional visits are recommended if further education is needed, medications or insulin has been added to therapy, or regular contact is needed for weight management. Ongoing self-management training is recommended at 6-month to 1-year intervals.

As a result of validation by clinical testing, NPGs were developed into protocols (21,22). These protocols were used by the Centers for Medicare and Medicaid Services (CMS) in the National Coverage Determination Act, to delineate the duration and frequency of MNT for diabetes. Qualifying dietetics professionals enrolled as

Medicare providers must provide MNT in accordance with nationally accepted nutrition protocols for diabetes (type 2, type 1, and gestational diabetes). In addition to this part B coverage for MNT, Medicare beneficiaries with diabetes may also be eligible for the part B benefit that provides for diabetes self-management training, including diabetes nutrition education.

Initially and throughout the nutrition care process, the person with diabetes and the health care team must have established rapport if the nutrition care process is to be successful. The knowledge and skills needed to implement nutrition recommendations and self-management cannot be acquired in one session, and MNT must be an ongoing component of diabetes care. For patients whose diabetes is newly diagnosed, a staged approach to education and implementation works best, with the initial sessions focusing on basic food/eating and physical activity skills. Additional information and skills are added after the patient has had time to adjust to the diagnosis of diabetes. Topics and skills are numerous and vary according to the patient's needs, desires, and type of diabetes. MNT is implemented individually, and nutrition education can be implemented in groups. Groups should be composed of fewer than 10 patients, and all should understand and speak the same language. Patients with diabetes who will benefit from individual sessions include those who require an interpreter, who need a very simplified approach or have learning barriers, who have complications that require specific nutrition recommendations, whose therapy is being intensified, or who are using an insulin pump. For all patients with diabetes, ongoing education and support are essential.

THE PROCESS OF PROVIDING MNT AND NUTRITION EDUCATION

The following steps are necessary to assist persons with diabetes in acquiring and maintaining the knowledge, skills, attitudes, behaviors, and commitment to successfully meet the challenges of daily diabetes self-management:

1. An assessment of the individual's food and diabetes self-management knowledge and skills. This involves obtaining appropriate data, and analyzing and interpreting the data based on evidence-based standards.
2. A nutrition diagnosis that identifies and labels the problem. The nutrition diagnosis includes the domain and description, class name and description, category name and description, and nutrition diagnostic label, which includes modifiers and defining characteristics.
3. A nutrition intervention that involves both planning and implementing a food/meal planning approach; also, educational materials that match the individual's needs, and identification and negotiation of individually designed lifestyle goals.
4. Nutrition monitoring and evaluation that involves monitoring progress and measuring and evaluating outcome indicators.

Step 1: Assessment

Data from the referral source (or the individual's medical record) and information from the individual with diabetes are necessary before beginning self-management education and goal-setting. By collecting as much of these data as possible before the first session, implementation can begin more efficiently. A questionnaire to be completed by the individual with diabetes before the counseling session can be used to collect data that were unavailable from the referral source.

Minimum referral data include age, diagnosis of diabetes and other pertinent medical history, reason for referral and expected outcomes, laboratory data (A1C, cholesterol fractionation, and renal function if applicable), blood pressure, diabetes therapy/duration/level of control, and clearance for exercise. Other assessment considerations are the patient's goals, knowledge, skill level, attitude and motivation, support systems, cultural influences, readiness to learn and change behaviors, barriers to learning, literacy level, and psychosocial and economic issues.

Anthropometric measures include weight, height (for adults at initial visit and for children at every visit), and body mass index (BMI). Social history measures are occupation, hours worked at school or away from home, living situation, and financial issues. A diabetes history includes previous diabetes and nutrition education; use of blood glucose monitoring; diabetes problems or concerns, such as hypoglycemia, hyperglycemia, or fear of insulin; and medications taken.

A food and nutrition history can begin by reviewing a 24-hour recall or a typical day's intake, and includes meal and snack eating times; exercise routine, including type, amount, and time of exercise; travel frequency; usual sleep habits; alcohol use; weight history and weight goals; and vitamin and mineral supplement use and herbal supplement use. In reviewing the 24-hour recall, cultural and religious habits/practices and financial/economic barriers must also be considered. The assessment should be done as efficiently as possible, so most of the consult time can be spent on the intervention.

Successful nutrition therapy is a continuous process of assessment, problem solving, adjustment, and readjustment. Each session begins with an assessment of what direction and information the patient identifies will be helpful for him or her. Success at or barriers to meeting behavioral goals identified in the previous sessions are reviewed. At each session, clinical outcome data are collected and evaluated. Food and blood glucose monitoring records are compared with the initial food plan, to assess whether the food plan was feasible for the patient to implement and to determine whether medical goals are being met. Measuring and evaluating outcomes of MNT are important; however, it is essential that this information be used to change medical therapy if target glucose goals are not being achieved.

Step 2: Nutrition Diagnosis

The nutrition diagnosis identifies and labels a nutrition problem that dietetics professionals are responsible for treating independently (8). At the end of the assessment step, data are clustered, analyzed, and synthesized. Nutrition diagnosis should not be confused with medical diagnosis, which in this case would be diabetes mellitus. A medical diagnosis does not change as long as the disease or condition exists, whereas a nutrition diagnosis changes as the individual with diabetes changes nutrition-related issues that impact on the nutrition diagnosis. For example, an individual may have the medical diagnosis of type 2 diabetes; however, after performing a nutrition assessment, the dietetics professional may diagnose one or more nutrition problems, such as "inconsistent carbohydrate intake," "inappropriate intake of food fats," or "not ready for diet/lifestyle changes." Analyzing assessment data and naming the nutrition diagnosis (or diagnoses) provide a link to selecting appropriate interventions, setting realistic and measurable outcomes, and measuring progress in attaining these expected outcomes.

Step 3: Nutrition Interventions

Initial education focuses on basic self-management skills, and prioritizing nutrition guidelines and recommendations is important. Additional topics and in-depth information can be addressed after the individual has had time to adjust to the diagnosis of diabetes. Topics are numerous and vary according to the type of diabetes and the personal characteristics and needs of the individual with diabetes.

The session begins by asking for questions and concerns that the individual has with regard to food and meal planning. An appropriate food/meal planning approach is selected, and strategies for behavior changes that enhance motivation and adherence to necessary lifestyle strategies are identified. A number of food/meal planning approaches are available (see Chapter 18). None of the food/meal planning approaches have been shown to be more effective than any other, and the approach selected depends on the individual's stage of learning and his or her needs.

Short-term behavior goals related to lifestyle changes (ie, food, physical activity, and self-monitoring of blood glucose) are determined with the individual with diabetes at the close of the session. Common self-management behavioral goals are consistent carbohydrate servings for meals and snacks, regular physical activity, correct medication doses (if needed), and monitoring blood glucose as needed. Goals must be specific, written in behavioral language, and realistic for the patient. Achievement of goals is an outcome of MNT intervention and should be evaluated at the start of every return visit.

The session should end on a positive note. Key points and goals are summarized, and appreciation expressed for the individual's participation. Before the individual leaves the initial session, future goals and an appointment for a follow-up session are determined. In making plans for follow-up, ask the individual to keep a 3-day (or weekly) food record with blood glucose data. At follow-up sessions, these records can be compared with the food plan, to assess whether the initial food plan was feasible for the individual to implement and whether medical goals are being met.

Step 4: Nutrition Monitoring and Evaluation

Monitoring refers to the review and measurement of predetermined outcome measures for the individual with diabetes. Evaluation is the comparison of current findings with previous status, intervention goals, or a reference standard (8). For persons with diabetes or at risk for diabetes, A1C or glucose concentrations, lipid levels, blood pressure, progression from impaired glucose tolerance to diabetes, a healthy baby, weight maintenance or loss, quality of life, and satisfaction with care provided are examples of outcome measures. However, just collecting data is not enough—it must be evaluated, used to develop individualized treatment goals, and if goals are not met, used to change both nutrition and medical therapy. This requires the dietetics professional to communicate MNT outcomes to the entire health care team.

Documentation

All steps include documentation, which is an ongoing process that supports all steps in the NCP (8). Documentation of each visit is essential for coordination of care and reimbursement and should include the name and identification information for the individual with diabetes, date of MNT visit and amount of time spent with the individual, reason for visit, diagnosis, laboratory test results and current medications, others present during MNT, and the physician's referral for MNT (if billing Medicare).

Summaries of the nutrition assessment (or the individual's progress and successful behavior changes if it is a follow-up visit), nutrition diagnosis and problem list, interventions provided (food/meal plan and educational topics covered), short- and long-term goals, the dietetics professional's assessment of the individual's acceptance and understanding, anticipated adherence, and additional skills or information needed are other areas that require documentation. Planning for follow-up for eval-

uation, continued self-management education, and ongoing care are essential and are included in the documentation.

EXPECTED OUTCOMES AND EVALUATION OF OUTCOMES

In today's medical environment, just completing an assessment; implementing an intervention using NPGs; and collecting, monitoring, and evaluating outcomes is not enough. Dietetics professionals must also know the expected outcomes from their interventions, when to evaluate these outcomes, and what are appropriate actions to take after the evaluation. At the individual level, outcomes are used to improve quality of nutrition care and to integrate nutrition care into the medical management of diabetes. This requires that systems of care and communications include the dietetics professional as an active participant in the disease management or prevention team. Furthermore, outcomes from representative populations can be aggregated and used to demonstrate effectiveness of MNT and the role of dietetics professionals at local and national levels. Outcomes can also be reported to patients/clients/groups, referring providers, colleagues, and payers. Table 1.1

TABLE 1.1   Effectiveness of Medical Nutrition Therapy for Diabetes

Endpoint	Expected Outcome	When to Evaluate
Glycemic Control		
A1C	1%–2% unit (15%-22% overall) decrease	6 wk and 3 mo
Plasma glucose (fasting)	50–100 mg/dL decrease	
Lipids		
LDL cholesterol	18–25 mg/dL (12%–16%) decrease	6 wk; if goals are not achieved, MNT should be intensified and evaluated again in 6 wk
Total cholesterol	24–32 mg/dL (10%–13%) decrease	
Triglycerides	15–17 mg/dL (8%) decrease	
HDL cholesterol • No exercise • With exercise	• 3 mg/dL (7%) decrease • No decrease	
Hypertension (in hypertensive patients)	5 mm Hg decrease in systolic and 2 mm Hg decrease in diastolic	Measured at every medical visit

Abbreviations: HDL, high-density lipoproteins; LDL, low-density lipoproteins.
Source: Adapted with permission from Pastors JG, Franz MJ, Warshaw H, Daly A, Arnold M. How effective is medical nutrition therapy in diabetes care? *J Am Diet Assoc.* 2003;103:827–831.

summarizes expected outcomes from MNT on glycemia, lipids, and blood pressure (23).

Randomized controlled trials and observational studies of MNT for diabetes have demonstrated improved glycemic outcomes of an approximate 1% to 2% unit decrease in A1C (an overall decrease from baseline of 15% to 22%) (23,24). In individuals with newly diagnosed type 2 diabetes, intensive nutrition therapy provided by dietitians decreased A1C levels by approximately 2% (1,3); in patients with an average duration of type 2 diabetes of 4 years, A1C levels decreased by approximately 1% (1). In individuals with type 1 diabetes, intensive therapy provided by dietitians decreased A1C by approximately 1% (2,4).

Nutrition therapy for diabetes has the greatest impact early in the course of type 2 diabetes, either at diagnosis or for prevention, but it continues to be effective at any time during the disease process. Type 2 diabetes is a progressive disease, and as beta-cell function decreases, blood-glucose-lowering medication(s) need to be combined with MNT to achieve blood glucose goals. The outcomes from MNT on A1C will be evident by 6 weeks to 3 months (1,2) and are similar to those from oral diabetes medications. Between 6 weeks and 3 months after the initial session, the dietetics professional should determine whether the individual is making progress toward his or her individualized glucose goals. If no progress is evident, the individual with diabetes and the dietetics professional should reassess and consider possible lifestyle changes. However, if the individual has lost weight with no improvement in glycemia, if the individual is doing well with lifestyle and further lifestyle interventions are unlikely to improve glycemia, and if the individual has done all that he or she can or is willing to do, and the blood glucose concentration and A1C percentage have not shown a downward trend, a change in medical therapy (medications) should be recommended to the referring health care provider in order for the patient to achieve glycemic goals.

In persons with type 1 diabetes, the DAFNE (dose adjusted for normal eating) study, in which dietitians educated individuals with type 1 diabetes on how to adjust their mealtime insulin doses based on the planned carbohydrate content of their meals (insulin-to-carbohydrate ratios), reported a 1% unit improvement in A1C, which was maintained for 12 months (4). Subjects were able to greatly improve their dietary freedom without increases in weight, lipid levels, incidents of severe hypoglycemia, or a clinically significant increase in insulin dose. General well-being and treatment satisfaction also were significantly improved, despite an increase in the number of insulin injections and blood-glucose-monitoring tests.

With regard to lipids in persons with diabetes, the first priority is to lower low-density lipoprotein (LDL) cholesterol to a target goal of less than 100 mg/dL (9). Maximal MNT for lipids has been shown to typically reduce LDL cholesterol by 15 to 25 mg/dL (25,26). The American Diabetes Association recommends that if the LDL cholesterol exceeds the goal by more than 25 mg/dL, pharmacological therapy may be started at the same time as nutrition therapy for high-risk patients (ie, individuals with diabetes with prior myocardial infarction and/or other cardiovascular risk factors) (27). In other individuals with diabetes, nutrition therapy may be evaluated at the 6-week interval, with consideration of pharmacological therapy between 3 and 6 months.

Lowering sodium intake to 2,400 mg/day is associated with a decline in systolic blood pressure of 6 mm Hg and in diastolic blood pressure of 2 mm Hg in hypertensive individuals, and of 3 mm Hg systolic and 1 mm Hg diastolic in normotensive patients (28). Although there are wide variations in blood pressure responses, the lower the sodium intake, the greater is the lowering of blood pressure (29). Responses to sodium restriction may be greater in individuals who are "salt sensitive," a characteristic of many individuals with diabetes. Furthermore, data from clinical trials have shown that a weight loss of 4.5 kg (10 lb) can be as effective as first-level drugs in controlling blood pressure (30). The Dietary Approaches to Stop Hypertension (DASH) trial reported that a low-fat diet that includes fruits, vegetables, and low-fat dairy products also effectively lowers blood pressure (31). The American Diabetes Association recommends that blood pressure be monitored at every medical visit (9).

STANDARDS OF PRACTICE AND STANDARDS OF PROFESSIONAL PERFORMANCE

The American Dietetic Association defines dietetics as "the integration and application of principles derived from the sciences of food, nutrition, management, communication and biological, physiological, behavioral and social sciences to achieve and maintain optimal human health," with flexible scope of practice boundaries to capture the breadth of the profession (32). Dietetics practice is differentiated according to the dietetics professional's educational preparation and level of practice, and is further defined by the role of the dietetics professional and the work setting.

RDs demonstrate their competence to provide diabetes care based on their education, training, and competency maintained through the RD credential, and assume responsibility for maintaining skills and competencies specific to diabetes care if they work with this population. The dietetics professional uses the *Professional Development Portfolio (PDP)* to demonstrate the process of self-assessment, planning, improvement, and commitment to lifelong learning (33). Dietetics professionals who choose to develop expertise in diabetes care can also demonstrate this specialized knowledge base by obtaining additional certification beyond the RD credential. The current certifications available to RDs in diabetes care are the Certified Diabetes Educator (CDE), a specialty certification, and the Board Certified-Advanced Diabetes Management (BC-ADM), an advanced practice certification.

The American Dietetic Association recently approved new core Standards of Practice in Nutrition Care and updated Standards of Professional Performance, which are designed as blueprints to accommodate the development of specialty and advanced-level practice standards for registered dietitians (34). Under the guidance of the ADA Quality Management Committee, DCE has developed new Standards of Practice and Standards of Professional Performance for Registered Dietitians in Diabetes Care (35) to replace an outdated document, *Scope of Practice for Qualified Dietetics Professionals in Diabetes Care and Education,* which was published in 2000 (36). The Standards are reflective of new insights about the main purpose for standards of practice and standards of professional performance, which is to serve as a guide for the evaluation and improvement of practice that all RDs will use to demonstrate competence in diabetes care. Thus, these new standards are written in a step-wise format, which describes each standard in the document by first noting the measurement criteria for a generalist RD working with patients with diabetes, followed by the additional measurement criteria for an RD at the specialty level of practice, and finally the additional measurement criteria for an RD in advanced practice. This measurement criteria approach creates an outcomes-based framework.

These RD standards of practice and standards of professional performance in diabetes care are core requirements that RDs must demonstrate to practice at specialty and advanced practice levels. RDs with the appropriate hours of practice who also meet the additional requirement of the credentialing boards for the CDE or BC-ADM certifications can choose to obtain the CDE or BC-ADM credentials (37).

This approach to standards recognizes the independent provider status for RDs resulting from the Medicare MNT statute that became effective January 1, 2001. Independent provider status recognizes the RD credential as indicating an individual is qualified to provide and be reimbursed directly for MNT services (16). These standards acknowledge the flexibility of an RD to demonstrate competence to provide diabetes services, with or without the additional specialty or advanced certification. The standards are also reflective of the Nutrition Care Process and Model.

SUMMARY

Managing diabetes is a team effort. Dietetics professionals, nurses, physicians, behavioral counselors, and other health care providers contribute their expertise to the development of therapeutic plans that allow individuals with diabetes to achieve the best metabolic control and quality of life possible. The goals of MNT are to provide individuals with diabetes with the knowledge, skills, and motivations to incorporate lifestyle management into their daily lives.

REFERENCES

1. Franz MJ, Monk A, Barry B, McClain K, Weaver T, Cooper N, Upham P, Bergenstal R, Mazze RS. Effectiveness of medical nutrition therapy provided by dietitians in the management of non-insulin-dependent diabetes mellitus: a randomized, controlled clinical trial. *J Am Diet Assoc.* 1995;95:1009–1017.

2. Kulkarni K, Castle G, Gregory R, Holmes A, Leontos C, Power M, Snetselaar L, Splett P, Wylie-Rosett J. Nutrition practice guidelines for type 1 diabetes mellitus positively affect dietitian practices and patient outcomes. The diabetes care and education dietetic practice group. *J Am Diet Assoc.* 1998;98:62–70.

3. UK Prospective Diabetes Study Group: Response of fasting plasma glucose to diet therapy in newly presenting type II diabetic patients, UKPDS 7. *Metabolism.* 1990;39:905–912.

4. DAFNE Study Group. Training in flexible, intensive insulin management to enable dietary freedom in people with type 1 diabetes: dose adjustment for normal eating (DAFNE) randomised controlled trial. *BMJ.* 2002;325:746–752.

5. Delahanty LM, Halford BH. The role of diet behaviors in achieving improved glycemic control in intensively treated

patients in the Diabetes Control and Complications Trial. *Diabetes Care.* 1993;16:1453–1458.

6. Wylie-Rosett J, Delahanty L. An integral role of the dietitian: implications of the Diabetes Prevention Program. *J Am Diet Assoc.* 2002;102:1065–1068.

7. Lindstrom J, Louheranta A, Mannelin M, Rastas M, Salminen V, Eriksson J, Usitupa M, Tuomilehto J for the Finnish Diabetes Prevention Study Group. The Finnish Diabetes Prevention Study (DPS): lifestyle intervention and 3-year results on diet and physical activity. *Diabetes Care.* 2003;26:3230–3236.

8. Lacey K, Pritchett E. Nutrition care process and model: ADA adopts road map to quality care and outcomes management. *J Am Diet Assoc.* 2003;103:1061–1072.

9. American Diabetes Association. Standards of medical care in diabetes. *Diabetes Care.* 2005;28(suppl 1):S4–S36.

10. American Diabetes Association. Nutrition principles and recommendations in diabetes (position statement). *Diabetes Care.* 2004(suppl 1);27:S36–S46.

11. American Diabetes Association. Nutrition recommendations and principles for people with diabetes mellitus (position statement). *Diabetes Care.* 1994;17:519–522.

12. Franz MJ, Horton ES, Bantle JP, Beebe CA, Brunzell JD, Coulston AM, Henry RR, Hoogwerf BJ, Stacpoole PW. Nutrition principles for the management of diabetes and related complications. *Diabetes Care.* 1994;17:490–518.

13. Franz MJ, Bantle JP, Beebe CA, Brunzell JD, Chiasson J-L, Garg A, Holzmeister LA, Hoogwerf BJ, Mayer-Davis E, Mooradian AD, Purnell JQ, Wheeler M. Evidence-based nutrition principles and recommendations for the treatment and prevention of diabetes and related complications. *Diabetes Care.* 2002;25:148–198.

14. ADA's definition for nutrition screening and nutrition assessment. *J Am Diet Assoc.* 1994;94:838–839.

15. Tinker LF, Heins JM, Holler HJ. Commentary and translation: 1994 nutrition recommendations for diabetes. Diabetes Care and Education, a Practice Group of the American Dietetic Association. *J Am Diet Assoc.* 1994;94:507–511.

16. Final MNT Regulations. CMS-1169-FC. Federal Register, November 1, 2001. Department of Health and Human Service. 42 CFR Parts: 405, 410, 411, 414, and 415. Available at: http://cms.hhs.bov/physicians/pfs/cms1169fc.asp. Accessed June 27, 2003.

17. Medicare Coverage Policy Decision: Duration and Frequency of the Medical Nutrition Therapy (MNT) Benefit (no. CAG-00097N). Available at: http://cms.hhs.gov/ncdr/memo.asp?id=53. Accessed June 2, 2003.

18. Monk A, Barry B, McClain K, Weaver T, Cooper M, Franz MJ: Practice guidelines for medical nutrition therapy provided by dietitians for persons with non-insulin-dependent diabetes mellitus. International Diabetes Center. *J Am Diet Assoc.* 1995;95:999–1006.

19. Kulkarni K, Castle G, Gregory R, Holmes A, Leontos C, Powers MA, Snetselaar L, Splett PL, Wylie-Rosett J for the Diabetes Care and Education Dietetic Practice Group of the American Dietetic Association. Nutrition practice guidelines for type 1 diabetes: an overview of content and application. *Diabetes Spectrum.* 1997;10:248–256.

20. Reader D, Sipe M. Key components of care for women with gestational diabetes. *Diabetes Spectrum.* 2001;14:188–191.

21. *American Dietetic Association Medical Nutrition Therapy Evidence-Based Guides for Practice: Nutrition Practice Guidelines for Type 1 and Type 2 Diabetes* [CD-ROM]. Chicago, Ill: American Dietetic Association; 2001.

22. *American Dietetic Association Medical Nutrition Therapy Evidence-Based Guides for Practice: Nutrition Practice Guidelines for Gestational Diabetes Mellitus* [CD-ROM]. Chicago, Ill: American Dietetic Association; 2001.

23. Pastors JG, Franz MJ, Warshaw H, Daly A, Arnold M. How effective is medical nutrition therapy in diabetes care? *J Am Diet Assoc.* 2003;103:827–831.

24. Pastors JG, Warshaw H, Daly A, Franz M, Kulkarni K. The evidence for the effectiveness of medical nutrition therapy in diabetes management. *Diabetes Care.* 2002;25:608–613.

25. Grundy SM, Balady GJ, Criqui MH, Fletcher G, Greenland P, Kiratzka LF, Houston-Miller N, Kris-Etherton P, Krumholz HM, LaRosa J, Ockene IS, Pearson TA, Reed J, Smith SC, Washington R. When to start cholesterol-lowering therapy in patients with coronary heart disease. A statement for healthcare professionals from the American Heart Association Task Force on Risk Reduction. *Circulation.* 1997;95:1683–1685.

26. Yu-Poth S, Zhao G, Etherton T, Naglak M, Jonnalagadda S, Kris-Etherton PM: Effects of the National Cholesterol Education Program's Step I and Step II dietary intervention programs on cardiovascular disease risk factors: a meta-analysis. *Am J Clin Nutr.* 1999;69:632–646.

27. American Diabetes Association. Management of dyslipidemia in adults with diabetes (position statement). *Diabetes Care.* 2001;25(suppl 1):S74–S77.

28. Cutler JA, Follmann D, Allender PS: Randomized trials of sodium restriction: an overview. *Am J Clin Nutr.* 1997; 65(suppl 1):643S–651S.

29. Sacks FM, Svetkey LP, Vollmer WM, Appel LJ, Bray GA, Harsha D, Obarzanek E, Conlin PR, Miller ER, Simons-Morton DG, Karanja N, Lin P-H. Effects on blood pressure of reduced dietary sodium and the Dietary Approaches to Stop Hypertension (DASH) diet. DASH-Sodium Collaborative Research Group. *New Engl J Med.* 2001; 344:3–10.

30. Staessen J, Fagard R, Liunen P, Amery A. Body weight, sodium intake, and blood pressure. *J Hypertens.* 1989;7(suppl):S19–S23.

31. Appel LJ, Moore TJ, Obarzanek E, Vollmer VW, Svetkey LP, Sacks FM, Bray GA, Vogt TM, Cutler JA, Windhauser MM, Lin PH, Karanja N. A clinical trial of the effects of dietary patterns on blood pressure. DASH Collaborative Research Group. *N Engl J Med.* 1997;336:1117–1124.

32. O'Sullivan-Maillet J, Skates J, Pritchett E. American Dietetic Association: scope of dietetics practice framework. *J Am Diet Assoc.* 2005;105 (in press).

33. Weddle DO. The professional development portfolio process: setting goals for credentialing. *J Am Diet Assoc.* 2002;102:1439–1444.

34. Kieselhorst K, Skates J, Pritchett E. American Dietetic Association's Standards of Practice in Nutrition Care and the Updated Standards of Professional Performance. *J Am Diet Assoc.* 2005;105(in press).

35. Kulkarni K, Boucher JL, Daly A, Shwide-Slavin C, Silvers BT, O'Sullivan-Maillet J, Pritchett E. American Dietetic Association: Standards of Practice and Standards of Professional Performance for Registered Dietitians (Generalist, Specialty, and Advanced) in Diabetes Care. *J Am Diet Assoc.* 2005;105 (in press).

36. Diabetes Care and Education Dietetic Practice Group. Scope of practice for qualified dietetics professionals in diabetes care and education. *J Am Diet Assoc.* 2000; 100:1205–1207.

37. Daly A, Kulkarni K, Boucher J. The new credential: advanced diabetes management. *J Am Diet Assoc.* 2001; 101:940–943.

2

Reimbursement for Medical Nutrition Therapy and Diabetes Self-Management Training

Patti Urbanski, MEd, RD, CDE

CHAPTER OVERVIEW

- Payers include private payers, public payers, Medicaid, other state government programs, and Medicare.
- Medicare is a federal program administered by the Centers for Medicare and Medicaid Services (CMS). Medicare benefits are divided into Part A (hospital insurance) and Part B (medical insurance) services. Part B Medicare covers medically necessary doctors' services provided in a variety of medical settings.
- Medicare reimburses for diabetes self-management training (DSMT). Medicare also reimburses for medical nutrition therapy (MNT) provided to individuals with diabetes and chronic renal insufficiency.
- Registered dietitians (RDs) and nutrition professionals must become Medicare providers to bill Medicare for MNT. As Medicare providers, RDs must follow Medicare billing practices and comply with Medicare rules.

PAYER OVERVIEW

A payer is an insurance company, third-party administrator, self-funded employer, managed care organization, or federal health benefit program, such as Medicare or Medicaid, that reimburses health care claims. Other federal health programs include the Veterans Administration, Indian Health Service, federal employee health plans, and military health plans. Federal health benefits programs are often referred to as public payers, whereas private payers mainly consist of insurance companies, third-party administrators, self-funded employer plans, and managed care organizations. Private and public payers are discussed in the following sections.

PRIVATE PAYERS

Benefits under private payers vary considerably and therefore are not described in detail in this chapter. In addition, benefits vary from one plan to another offered by the same private payer. Participants in private payer plans may find that they need to obtain medical services from in-network providers to have the service reimbursed, or that certain services are not covered by the benefit plan. Private payers may limit the amount of service reimbursed (such as 3 hours of MNT services per calendar year) and may require a copayment for services or dictate that a deductible first be met before particular services are paid by the payer. A patient with private insurance should contact the private payer to obtain details about coverage for diabetes services, such as MNT and DSMT services, before receiving the services.

As of 2003, 46 states plus the District of Columbia had enacted state laws that require health insurance policies and managed-care plans to provide coverage for diabetes education and supplies (1). Private payers, also known as commercial payers, are subject to the laws in the state in which the policy is sold or delivered. However, because of the Employment Retirement Insurance Security Act, employer self-funded or self-insured plans are regulated by the US Department of Labor and do not have to offer benefits that are required by state mandate laws. Approximately half the insurance plans in each state are employer self-funded or self-insured plans (2). Therefore, those plans are exempt from the state laws requiring insurance reimbursement for diabetes education and supplies.

PUBLIC PAYERS

Public payers include federal and state programs that target particular segments of the population. These groups include the elderly, disabled, certain low-income groups, veterans, and Native Americans.

Medicaid

Medicaid is a federal and state joint health care plan for specific groups of low-income individuals, families with children, and people who are aged, blind, or disabled. Medicaid became law in 1965 under Title XIX of the Social Security Act. Medicaid is administered at the state level, and benefits vary from state to state. Each state establishes its own eligibility standards, determines the type, amount, duration, and scope of services offered, and sets the rate of payment for services (3). MNT services are often not covered by Medicaid.

State Children's Health Insurance Program

The State Children's Health Insurance Program is a federal program administered at the state level. State governments are invited to develop a program to serve low-income uninsured children who are residents within the state (4).

Veteran and Military Programs

The Veterans Administration provides medical care, long-term care, and support services to veterans who served in the active military, have served in specific wars, have a service-related disability, suffer from environmental exposure to contaminants, or are identified as low-income. Care is provided free of charge to some veterans,

whereas other veterans receive medical care with a co-insurance payment (5).

Tricare is a health care program that provides coverage for active duty and retired members of military service, their families, and their survivors. Services are provided in medical facilities of all branches of the military and networks of civilian health care professionals (6).

Indian Health Service

The Indian Health Service provides health care to American Indians and Alaska Natives in federally recognized tribes. Services are provided free of charge (7).

Bureau of Primary Health Care

The Bureau of Primary Health Care provides health care services to underserved and vulnerable people with financial, geographic, or cultural barriers to accessing health care. Facilities are designated as a federally qualified health center (FQHC) or rural health center (RHC), and services are provided on a sliding-scale fee schedule (8,9).

Federal Employees Health Benefit Program

The Federal Employees Health Benefit Program provides health care coverage for federal workers, retirees, and their dependents. This program contracts with hundreds of health care plans operating across the country. The program establishes minimum benefits that each plan must cover, including diabetes education, equipment, and supplies. Benefits provided by federal government health insurance plans are not subject to state coverage mandates (10).

Medicare

Medicare is a federal program administered by CMS, which was formerly called the Health Care Finance Administration (HCFA). Medicare provides health coverage for individuals 65 years and older, persons younger than 65 years who are permanently disabled, and individuals with end-stage renal disease. To qualify for Medicare, individuals must have paid Medicare taxes while working. Individuals who did not pay Medicare taxes during their working years may still be able to purchase Medicare coverage. Medicare benefits are divided into Part A (hospital insurance) and Part B (medical insurance) services (11).

All Medicare participants (also called beneficiaries) qualify for Part A. Most beneficiaries do not pay a monthly premium for Part A coverage. Part A covers inpatient hospital, inpatient care in a skilled nursing facility after a covered hospital stay, home care, and hospice services. Beneficiaries must pay deductibles and co-insurance (or copayments) for services covered by Part A.

Part B Medicare covers medically necessary doctors' services provided in a variety of medical settings, outpatient hospital care, ambulance service in limited cases, some diagnostic tests, and some other medical services that Part A does not cover, such as physical therapy, occupational therapy services, and some home health care services. Part B also helps pay for some supplies when they are medically necessary, such as blood glucose testing supplies. Payment for DSMT and MNT services falls under Part B. Part B is an elective program. Beneficiaries may enroll in Part B any time during a 7-month period that begins 3 months before the beneficiary turns 65 years old. The monthly premium for Part B is $78.20 in 2005 (12). For beneficiaries who do not choose to participate in Part B when they first turn 65, the monthly premium cost may increase by 10% for each 12-month period that the person qualified for Part B coverage but did not enroll for this coverage (12). Like Medicare Part A, beneficiaries must pay deductibles and copayments for Part B services.

Within the Medicare program, beneficiaries have a choice of health plans in which they may enroll. The original Medicare plan, also sometimes called fee-for-service, is available nationwide. This plan has higher total out-of-pocket costs than some other options. This option offers no extra benefits but has the widest doctor choice of any type of plan. The second group of options within Medicare is called Medicare + Choice (Medicare plus Choice), previously known as Medicare Part C. The Medicare + Choice plans, including managed care plans, such as health management organizations (HMOs), preferred provider organizations (PPOs), and private fee-for-service plans, provides care under contract to Medicare. These plans may not be available in all parts of the United States (13).

The managed care plan within Medicare + Choice has lower total out-of-pocket costs and may include some extra benefits, such as prescription drug coverage, eye examinations, hearing aids, and routine physical examinations. Beneficiaries must usually see doctors, specialists, and health care providers within the managed care plan. A Medicare managed care plan must provide the same services that a beneficiary would be eligible to receive from Medicare if he or she was not a managed care plan enrollee (13).

Private fee-for-service plans may include extra benefits, such as health care coverage for foreign travel or extra days in the hospital. Because they may choose any doctor or specialist who accepts the plan's payment, beneficiaries usually have a wide selection of doctors. The out-of-pocket costs for private fee-for-service plans are usually medium to high (13).

Medigap Insurance

Some private payers offer supplemental insurance policies to Medicare beneficiaries to cover some of the out-of-pocket costs of Medicare. Medigap policies may cover such things as the annual Medicare deductible, copayments, and prescription drug costs.

Medicare Administration

CMS contracts with private insurance companies to administer the Medicare Part B program, including provider enrollment and claims processing activities. Fiscal intermediaries are contracted by CMS to administer Part A services, and in some circumstances to process Part B hospital-based claims. Claims processing for Part B professional services, such as physician office visits, MNT, and DSMT services, are administered by local Medicare carriers. Claims for Medicare MNT services are generally sent to the local carrier; however, as of April 1, 2003, MNT services can be billed to fiscal intermediaries when performed in a hospital outpatient setting (14). Typically, most clinic-based services are billed to a local carrier. There are currently 21 different local carriers that maintain offices throughout the United States (15).

Part B durable medical equipment and supplies, such as diabetes blood glucose testing supplies, are paid by four regional Durable Medical Equipment Regional Carriers (DMERCs). A listing of fiscal intermediaries, local carriers, and DMERCs by geographic location is available online from CMS (16).

Medicare Regulation

Congress is one of the entities that makes decisions and passes laws that affect the Medicare program. Other groups involved are the Department of Health and Human Services, Office of the Inspector General, Peer Review Organization, Social Security Agency, and CMS. CMS is responsible for developing the regulations to implement these laws. For laws that establish Medicare benefits, such as the Medicare MNT benefit, CMS develops a first draft of regulations for the new benefit and publishes this draft in the Federal Register as a proposed rule. The public is then invited to send in comments concerning the proposed rule. After a designated commentary period, CMS reviews all letters received and publishes the final rules. CMS also publishes program memorandums for the fiscal intermediaries, local carriers, and DMERCs. These memorandums explain the details of the regulations and give the intermediaries, carriers, and DMERCs instructions about how to implement the regulations. In some cases, the intermediaries or carriers may be given authority to decide how to implement the regulations. Therefore, exact details about how the rules are followed may vary from one carrier or intermediary to the next one. This information is frequently included in the carrier's Local Medical Review Policies.

CMS hires Peer Review Organizations (PROs) to review the medical necessity and quality of care provided to Medicare beneficiaries. PROs are charged with ensuring that Medicare services are provided effectively and economically to beneficiaries. PROs perform review functions, such as audits of programs and facilities providing Medicare services, to prevent unnecessary utilization of care and to ensure efficiency and quality of care (17).

PAYER MIX IN THE UNITED STATES

The payer mix in each practice setting may determine how billing systems are designed. According to the Centers for Medicare and Medicaid Services, the payer mix for 2000 in the United States broke down as follows (18):

- 34% private insurance
- 17% Medicare
- 15% Medicaid and SCHIP
- 15% out-of-pocket
- 12% other public, which includes workers' compensation, public health activity, Department of Defense, Department of Veteran Affairs, Indian Health Service, and state and local government hospital subsidy and school health
- 6% other private, which includes industrial in-plant, privately funded construction, and nonpatient revenues, including philanthropy

Multiple Payers

People sometimes have more than one health insurance policy. This may occur because of insurance coverage from the person's employer as well as coverage from a spouse's employer. Medicare beneficiaries may also have health insurance through a spouse, or may also have Medigap insurance. When a person has coverage from more than one health insurance policy, one insurance provider is considered the primary payer and the other provider is considered the secondary payer. The primary payer is billed first, and then the secondary payer considers payment of the remaining expenses after the primary payer has paid the amount they cover (19).

When a Medicare beneficiary also has private insurance from a spouse, it is recommended that the Medicare intermediary or carrier be contacted to determine which payer is the primary payer. In general, if the beneficiary is age 65 or older and the non-Medicare health plan is provided by an employer with 20 or more employees, the group health plan is the primary payer. If the beneficiary is younger than 65 years and disabled, and the group health plan is provided by an employer with fewer than 100 employees, Medicare is generally the primary payer. For patients with more than one policy from private payers, it is best to contact the payers to determine which payer will be considered the primary payer (19).

When a Medicare beneficiary also has Medigap insurance, the Medigap policy is a supplemental policy that fills the gaps and covers charges that Medicare does not cover, such as deductibles and copayments. Medicare beneficiaries and providers can call the Medicare Coordination of Benefits Contractor (800/999-1118) with questions about Medicare, who pays first, or how the client's coverage works with Medicare (19).

DIABETES SELF-MANAGEMENT TRAINING

Medicare Reimbursement

Effective February 27, 2001, Medicare reimburses for DSMT services (20). To qualify for DSMT, Medicare beneficiaries must have a fasting glucose level greater than or equal to 126 mg/dL on two different occasions, or a 2-hour postglucose challenge greater than or equal to 200 mg/dL on two different occasions, or a random glucose test greater than 200 mg/dL and symptoms of uncontrolled diabetes (21). Diabetes training programs must follow rules for DSMT reimbursement published

BOX 2.1

Summary of Centers for Medicare and Medicaid Services Program Regulations for Diabetes Self-Management Training

- Diabetes Self-Management Training (DSMT) program must be approved by an accreditation organization approved by Centers for Medicare and Medicaid (CMS). Currently, the American Diabetes Association and the Indian Health Service are the only organizations able to approve DSMT programs for Medicare reimbursement.
- DSMT program must meet standards specified in the National Standards for Diabetes Self-Management Education.
- DSMT must be provided in a group setting, unless no group training is available within 2 months of the date that training is ordered, or the beneficiary's physician documents special needs in the beneficiary's medical record. These special needs include severe vision, hearing, or language limitations, or other special conditions, identified by the treating physician or nonphysician provider, that will hinder effective participation in a group learning setting.
- Of the 10 hours of initial training, 1 hour may be used for an individual assessment, to determine the beneficiary's training needs.
- The initial 10 hours of training must be provided within a 12-month period.
- During subsequent years, 2 hours of follow-up DSMT are covered per beneficiary year by Medicare Part B. This follow-up DSMT may be provided as either group or individual training.

Source: Data are from references 22 and 23.

---

by CMS to receive payment from Medicare for DSMT services (see Box 2.1) (22,23).

DSMT must be ordered by a physician or qualified nonphysician practitioner who is treating the beneficiary's diabetes. The training orders must include a plan of care, established by the physician or qualified nonphysician practitioner, that outlines the content, number of sessions, frequency, and duration of the training. Examples of DSMT physician order forms are available from the American Association of Diabetes Educators (24).

The physician plan of care must include a statement that the physician or qualified nonphysician practitioner is managing the beneficiary's diabetes and that the DSMT described in the plan of care is needed to provide the beneficiary with the skills and knowledge necessary to help manage the beneficiary's diabetes (22).

Medicare covers up to 10 hours of initial DSMT for qualifying beneficiaries, and up to 2 hours per year in subsequent years (20). Nutrition is one of the 15 topics included in DSMT, as defined by the CMS final rules for DSMT (20).

In a hospital setting, DSMT may be billed on a CMS-1450 (also known as a UB-92) billing form and sent to the hospital's fiscal intermediary, or on a CMS-1500 billing form and sent to a local carrier. In a private practice or physician clinic setting, DSMT is usually billed on a CMS-1500 form and sent to the local carrier. All DSMT is billed in 30-minute increments. Specific Healthcare Common Procedure Coding System (HCPCS) codes have been developed for DSMT. See Table 2.1 for a description of these billing codes (20,22).

An RD who is also a Medicare provider for MNT may choose to establish an approved DSMT program and bill Medicare for all DSMT services provided using the RD's Medicare Provider Identification Number (PIN) (25). The RD should consider the tax and personal liability risks involved with this type of business decision. If the

TABLE 2.1 HCPCS Codes for Diabetes Self-Management Training

Code	Description
G0108	Diabetes outpatient self-management training services, individual, per 30 minutes
G0109	Diabetes outpatient self-management training services, group session (two or more), per 30 minutes

Source: Data are from references 20 and 22. HCPCS codes, descriptions, and material only are copyright © 1999, American Medical Association. All rights reserved.

RD's Medicare MNT PIN is linked to his or her Social Security number (SSN), the RD is assuming personal liability for the DSMT program, and the program's income would be reported to the Internal Revenue Service under the RD's SSN. The RD may choose to set up a limited liability partnership (LLP), incorporation, or some other type of business arrangement. A business adviser and lawyer can assist with these decisions.

Private Payer Reimbursement

Private payers may cover DSMT, but the specifications of coverage may vary. Covered services are typically outlined in a document provided by the health care plan to each plan participant. Participants may also contact their insurance company for specifics concerning coverage of DSMT, including limitations of coverage, applicable deductibles, and/or copayments.

MEDICAL NUTRITION THERAPY (MNT)

Medicare Reimbursement

Effective January 1, 2002, Medicare reimburses for MNT provided to patients with diabetes, chronic renal insufficiency, or postrenal transplant (26). Beneficiaries must have a fasting glucose level greater than or equal to 126 mg/dL to meet the diagnostic criterion of diabetes. Gestational diabetes is defined as any degree of glucose intolerance with onset or first recognition during pregnancy. Chronic renal insufficiency is defined as the stage of renal disease associated with a decrease in renal function not severe enough to require hemodialysis or renal transplantation, and a glomerular filtration rate of 13 to 50 mL/min/1.73m^2 (26). Beneficiaries qualify for MNT up to 36 months after kidney transplant (27).

A referral from the beneficiary's treating physician must be provided for MNT to be reimbursed by Medicare (26). The referral must include the beneficiary's diagnosis related to the covered MNT benefit, must indicate the medical necessity for MNT, and must include the doctor's Unique Physician Identification Number (UPIN) (27). The referral must be dated and signed by the physician. A physician referral covers one episode of care, which is defined as the initial 3 hours of MNT in the first year, or 2 hours of MNT in subsequent years (27). An episode of care must fall within 1 calendar year (28). For example, if an initial MNT referral is received on December 1, a new referral for a subsequent episode of care would be required on January 1 of the next year, even if the benefi-

ciary has not yet received the full 3 hours of initial MNT. It should also be noted that a referral for MNT must come from the treating physician, whereas a referral for DSMT may come from a physician or qualified nonphysician provider, such as a nurse practitioner or physician's assistant (26). Examples of MNT order forms are available from the American Dietetic Association Web site (29).

Beneficiaries who receive 3 hours of MNT in 1 year may receive additional hours of MNT in the same year if the physician determines that further MNT is medically necessary because of a change in diagnosis, medical condition, or treatment plan (27). The physician needs to write a new referral for this new episode of care (27).

Registered Dietitian Enrollment in Medicare

To bill Medicare for MNT, a qualified RD or nutrition professional must obtain a PIN from Medicare (27). CMS has defined qualifications that RDs must meet to become a Medicare provider (see Box 2.2) (26).

To enroll as a Medicare provider and receive a PIN, CMS Form 855I must be completed. RDs who work in a hospital outpatient or clinic setting where the billing office staff will be billing Medicare on their behalf will need to complete a CMS Form 855R. This form allows the nutrition professional to reassign Medicare payment

---

BOX 2.2

Qualified Medical Nutrition Therapy Providers

- Dietitian or nutritionist licensed or certified by a state as of December 21, 2000.
- Dietitians or nutritionists not state licensed or certified by December 21, 2000, must have:
  - bachelor's or higher degree in nutrition or dietetics from an accredited college or university.
  - completed at least 900 hours of supervised dietetics practice.
  - licensure or certification by the state in which the services are performed.
- In states that do not license or certify nutrition professionals, an individual who is recognized as a registered dietitian by the Commission on Dietetic Registration or who meets the college degree and supervised dietetics practice requirements is considered to have met this state licensure requirement.

Source: Data are from reference 26.

for MNT services to the RD's workplace. Finally, RDs who work in a group practice of RDs who provide MNT services must complete a CMS Form 855B, to obtain a PIN for the RD group practice. The process of applying for a PIN includes sending documentation, such as proof of state licensure and/or verification of RD status. Information about enrolling in Medicare as a provider and obtaining a PIN can be obtained from the Medicare carrier in the RD's geographic location or from the American Dietetic Association (30). It is important for an RD working in a clinic or hospital setting to protect his or her PIN and to be sure that the billing office personnel are using the PIN appropriately.

Medicare Billing

Medicare MNT billing is done on a CMS-1500 form in a physician's office, private practice, and some hospital outpatient settings. Detailed instructions for completing a CMS-1500 billing form are available at ADA's Web site (31). CMS-1500 billing forms are submitted to local carriers.

Effective January 1, 2003, billing for Medicare MNT from the hospital outpatient setting may be completed on a CMS-1450 (also known as a UB-92) form (14). On the CMS-1450, the revenue code 942 ("education and training") is listed in space FL 42. The MNT billing code is listed in space FL 43, and the definition of the billing code in space FL 44. If a CMS-1450 bill is used, the bill is submitted to the hospital's fiscal intermediary.

On all billing forms, the Current Procedural Terminology (CPT) or HCPCS codes specifically designated for MNT should be used (see Table 2.2) (14,26). Individual MNT is billed in 15-minute units, whereas group MNT is billed in 30-minute units. Medicare will reimburse for a beneficiary to see both a physician for medical care and a RD for MNT on the same day. However, Medicare will not pay for DSMT and MNT services provided on the same day (27).

Diagnosis codes must also be included on either a CMS-1450 or CMS-1500 billing form, to support the medical necessity of services provided. Diagnosis codes are also known as ICD-9-CM codes, which stands for International Classification of Diseases, 9th edition, Clinical Modification. These codes are developed by the World Health Organization and are revised approximately every 10 years. CMS publishes annual updates of the ICD-9-CM codes. Because diagnosing is not considered to be within the scope of practice for RDs, diagnosis codes must be provided by the referring physician.

TABLE 2.2 Current Procedural Terminology (CPT) and Healthcare Common Procedure Coding System (HCPCS) Billing Codes for Medical Nutrition Therapy (MNT)

Code	Description
CPT	
CPT 97802	MNT, initial assessment and intervention, individual, face-to face with the patient, each 15 minutes
CPT 97803	MNT reassessments and intervention, individual, face-to-face with the patient, each 15 minutes
CPT 97804	Group, two or more individuals, each 30 minutes
HCPCS	
G0270	MNT reassessment and subsequent intervention(s) after second referral in same year for change in diagnosis, medical condition, or treatment regimen (including additional hours needed for renal disease), individual, face to face with the patient, each 15 minutes
G0271	MNT reassessment and subsequent intervention(s) after second referral in same year for change in diagnosis, medical condition, or treatment regimen (including additional hours needed for renal disease), group (two or more individuals), face-to-face with the patient, each 30 minutes

Source: CPT codes are from reference 26. HCPCS codes are from reference 14. CPT and HCPCS codes, descriptions, and material only are copyright © 2000 and 2002 (respectively), American Medical Association. All rights reserved.

Medicare Reimbursement Rates

The Medicare allowed reimbursement rates are adjusted annually by CMS, determined by congressional budget decisions. Medicare pays the lesser of the actual charge for the MNT services or 85% of the physician fee schedule (26). The Medicare carrier reimburses 80% of this approved amount after the beneficiary has reached his or her annual Medicare deductible ($110 in 2005) (12). The beneficiary is responsible to pay the remaining 20%. This 20% copayment may be covered by a secondary payer, such as a Medigap policy. The payment amount for

MNT codes can be found on the Medicare local carriers' Web page, which can be accessed through the CMS Web site (32) or the ADA's members-only site (33). Note that the rates listed are physician rates, which must be reduced by 15% for RDs and nutrition professionals.

When an RD decides to become a Medicare provider and receives a Medicare provider number, the RD must "accept assignment." This means that the RD will accept the payment rate for MNT as set by CMS. The RD may not collect any additional money, other than the beneficiary's 20% copayment from either the beneficiary or any supplemental insurance policy the beneficiary may have.

Nutrition Protocols

The final rules for the Medicare MNT benefit specify that nationally recognized treatment protocols must be used for MNT (34). Using protocols ensures that all RDs provide MNT using a consistent structure and process of care, including nutrition assessment, nutrition diagnosis, nutrition intervention, and then nutrition monitoring and evaluation. The American Dietetic Association and members of the Diabetes Care and Education Dietetic Practice Group have developed MNT evidence-based guides for practice and protocols for type 1, type 2, and gestational diabetes (35,36). The guides for practice are based on evidence from research studies and are organized into worksheets and other templates for application in practice. The protocols are also designed to aid in the collection of outcome data.

RDs need to remember that, when providing MNT within all the rules and guidelines of Medicare, the provision of MNT services is only one application of the nutrition care process (NCP) developed by the American Dietetic Association (37). The NCP articulates the consistent and specific steps a dietetics professional uses when delivering MNT, including the four steps of nutrition assessment, nutrition diagnosis, nutrition intervention, and nutrition monitoring and evaluation.

ADDITIONAL MEDICARE CONSIDERATIONS

Opting Out

An RD who decides not to become a Medicare provider and therefore not to accept the MNT payment rates from Medicare for the two covered diagnoses has two options. One option is for the RD to refer all Medicare beneficiaries who are referred for diabetes or renal MNT to an RD who is a Medicare provider. A second option for the RD is to opt out and not participate in the Medicare program. Opting out of Medicare is a formalized agreement between the health care provider and CMS that requires an affidavit from the health care provider, and the practitioner is bound to the 2-year agreement, even if the practitioner's place of employment changes during the 2-year opt-out period. RDs who are considering opting out of Medicare are strongly encouraged to consult the *Federal Register* (34) for details about the opting out process, to fully consider all the details and ramifications of this option. Other articles have also examined the issues of opting out of Medicare (38). Once an RD has formally opted out of Medicare, he or she must enter into a contract for services with each Medicare patient with diabetes or kidney disease. In the opt-out situation, neither the RD nor the Medicare beneficiary is able to submit claims to Medicare.

Advance Beneficiary Notices

An Advance Beneficiary Notice (ABN) is a written notice used by Medicare providers and suppliers to notify Medicare beneficiaries that the beneficiary will be responsible for payment of services and supplies not paid by Medicare. An ABN is used only for Medicare-covered services when there is uncertainty about whether the service will be reimbursed by Medicare. An ABN must be signed before a service is provided to the beneficiary. The ABN must state that Medicare will probably deny payment for the service or supply, the reason that the provider expects Medicare to deny payment, and that the beneficiary is responsible for payment if Medicare denies payment. The ABN must also describe the service and include the beneficiary's name, billing account number, Medicare number, signature, and the date. According to the Medicare Carriers Manual, having ABNs signed for all services is not an acceptable practice (39). RDs should have beneficiaries sign an ABN if there is a possibility that the beneficiary has already received MNT services for diabetes or renal disease reimbursed by Medicare earlier in the year, or in cases when a physician has ordered follow-up MNT during the same year that Medicare has already paid for MNT services. In this second case, the carrier may determine that follow-up MNT was not medically necessary and may deny payment of the claim. CMS requires use of its standardized ABN form, available from the CMS Web site (40).

Medicare Secondary Payer Forms

To make sure the appropriate payer is billed, it is important to identify situations where Medicare is the secondary payer rather than the primary payer. This should occur before MNT services are provided. Many hospitals and clinics use a Medicare Secondary Payer screening form, to determine whether Medicare is the primary or secondary payer. Further information concerning this process is available from CMS (41).

Modifiers

Modifiers are special designators that add to the description of a billing code. Use of modifiers can ensure that services are reimbursed appropriately. Modifiers are listed directly after the CPT or HCPCS code on the billing form. The modifier "GA" is used when a provider expects denial for payment and an ABN has been signed by the beneficiary (42). If Medicare denies payment for the MNT services and the "GA" modifier has been used, the provider is able to bill the beneficiary for the services that Medicare did not pay.

A "GY" modifier is used when a service is statutorily excluded or does not meet the definitions of a Medicare benefit (42). Patients with a secondary insurance may first need to have a denial for payment from Medicare, in order for the secondary insurance to reimburse for services. For example, a diagnosis of hyperlipidemia is not covered under the Medicare MNT benefit, and the "GY" modifier could be used to obtain a Medicare denial of payment, in order to get payment from a secondary insurance policy. This type of situation—where a payment determination is needed by a secondary insurance—is called a "no-pay" or "demand bill." An ABN is not necessary in this situation.

A "GZ" modifier is used when a service is expected to be denied, because it was not reasonable or necessary and the RD did not obtain a signed ABN from the patient (42). Modifier "25" is used if billing for DSMT and physician services on the same day, if the physician's PIN will be used for billing both the medical care and DSMT services. The "25" modifier is placed after the Evaluation and Management billing code used by the physician. Further details about modifiers can be obtained from hospital and clinic billing offices.

Federally Qualified Health Centers (FQHCs) and Rural Health Centers (RHCs)

The final Medicare MNT benefit rules specify that MNT services for diabetes and renal disease may not be provided in FQHCs and RHCs (26). The government reimburses for nutrition education/nutrition services that are bundled or included among the other services provided at these facilities. Therefore, billing for MNT services for diabetes or renal disease as part of the Medicare MNT benefit is not allowed in facilities with these designations.

"Incident to" Billing

Under Medicare rules, certain services provided by nonphysicians may be covered under a concept referred to as "incident to" a physician's service. These incident to services are furnished as an integral but incidental part of the physician's services in the course of the diagnosis or treatment of an injury or illness. CMS stipulates that the physician must provide direct supervision to nonphysicians providing "incident to" services. In years before Medicare reimbursement for MNT, some RDs may have provided MNT services subsequent to physician services and may have billed these services "incident to" the physician's services using physician CPT codes. RDs should be aware that the final Medicare MNT benefit rules for diabetes and renal disease state that these services should not be billed incident to physician services (26). In addition, DSMT is not billed incident to; rather, the entity that has established the DSMT program (such as the physician, RD, or hospital) bills the Medicare carrier or fiscal intermediary using his/her PIN.

Medicare Compliance

RDs must be sure that the MNT and DSMT services they are providing to Medicare beneficiaries comply with Medicare rules. Because the RD's PIN number is listed on the Medicare billing form when billing for MNT, and may also be used on the Medicare billing form for DSMT, the professional will be held responsible if Medicare rules are not followed. A good working relationship with the clinic or hospital billing officers will help RDs to understand the facility's billing processes and will ensure appropriate use of the RD's Medicare PIN. An internal audit system, to evaluate the MNT and

DSMT referrals, documentation, and billing systems, allows nutrition professionals to be sure that their MNT and DSMT services are in compliance with Medicare rules and regulations. In addition, RDs working in a clinic or hospital setting can work with the facility compliance officer, who can assist with making sure Medicare rules are being followed. Further compliance information can be obtained by American Dietetic Association members from the ADA Web site (43).

RDs in private practice should consider the compliance implications of contracting with an external company to oversee billing procedures for the RD's practice. In addition, RDs must be sure that their business practices are in compliance with the Health Insurance Portability and Accountability Act (HIPAA) regulations. Details about these regulations and sample forms and documents to comply with HIPAA regulations are available for members of the American Dietetic Association from the ADA Web site (44).

BILLING PRIVATE PAYERS FOR MNT SERVICES

As with DSMT, some private payers reimburse for MNT and some do not. If MNT is a covered service, private payers have the right to determine how they want MNT services billed. Some private payers are now using the CPT MNT codes, whereas others may want MNT services billed using Evaluation and Management (E and M) CPT codes, which are the billing codes often used by physicians. Using E and M codes to bill for MNT services may make tracking MNT services within a hospital or clinic difficult, and may affect utilization reviews and the ability to demonstrate cost savings of providing MNT.

Private payers require the use of diagnosis codes that define the diagnosis or condition to the highest level of specificity, and procedural codes that most clearly define the service provided. Some private payers may require the RD to become enrolled as a provider in their plan or network. The contract established between the RD and the plan generally specifies payment amount, services provided, billing codes, and service limits. It is advisable to contact each private payer, to determine if the RD can become a plan provider and how MNT services should be billed. Details about covered services are usually outlined in a document provided by the insurance company to each plan participant, but patients may also want to check with their insurance company concerning limitations of coverage before receiving MNT.

SUMMARY

MNT reimbursement is a process that involves many rules and an understanding of how both Medicare and private payer systems work. RDs must be prepared to stay abreast of changes in the reimbursement rules and to develop systems to ensure that the reimbursement guidelines and regulations are being followed.

REFERENCES

1. American Diabetes Association. Maintaining state-regulated health insurance for diabetes. Available at: http://www.diabetes.org/advocacy-and-legalresources/state-legislation/healthinsurance.jsp. Accessed September 26, 2004.

2. Kaiser Family Foundation and Health Research and Educational Trust. Employer health benefits 2004 summary of findings. Available at: http://www.kff.org/insurance/7148/sections/ehbs04–10-7.cfm. Accessed September 26, 2004.

3. Centers for Medicare and Medicaid Services. Medicaid: a brief summary. Available at: http://www.cms.hhs.gov/publications/overview-medicare-medicaid/default4.asp. Accessed September 26, 2004.

4. Centers for Medicare and Medicaid Services. State Children's Health Insurance Program (SCHIP): site for consumers' information. Available at: http://www.cms.hhs.gov/schip/consumers_default.asp. Accessed September 26, 2004.

5. Department of Veterans Affairs. A guide to VA health care. Available at: http://www1.va.gov/elig/docs/Benefits_Guide_v4.pdf. Accessed September 26, 2004.

6. Military Health System/Tricare Web site. A look at Tricare. Available at: http://www.tricare.osd.mil/tricarehandbook/results.cfm?tn=1&cn=5. Accessed September 26, 2004.

7. US Department of Health and Human Services Indian Health Service. Indian Health Service fact sheet. Available at: http://www.ihs.gov/PublicInfo/PublicAffairs/Welcome_Info/ThisFacts.asp. Accessed September 26, 2004.

8. Rural Assistance Center. Federally qualified health centers. Available at: http://www.raconline.org/info_guides/clinics/fqhc.php. Accessed September 26, 2004.

9. Rural Assistance Center. Rural health clinics. Available at: http://www.raconline.org/info_guides/clinics/rhc.php. Accessed September 26, 2004.

10. Office of Personnel Management, Federal Government's Human Resources Agency. The FEHB program. Available at: http://www.opm.gov/insure/health/about/fehb.asp. Accessed September 26, 2004.

11. Medicare Eligibility Tool. Available at: http://www. medicare.gov/MedicareEligibility/Home.asp?dest=NAV |Home|GeneralEnrollment#TabTop. Accessed September 26, 2004.

12. Medicare Questions. Available at: http://medicare. custhelp.com/cgibin/medicare.cfg/php/enduser/std_ adp.php?p_faqid=1560&p_created=1095443945. Accessed September 26, 2004.

13. Medicare Plan Choices. Available at: http://www. medicare.gov/Choices/Overview.asp. Accessed September 26, 2004.

14. Medical nutrition therapy (MNT) services for beneficiaries with diabetes or renal disease—policy change. Centers for Medicare and Medicaid Services Program Memorandum. Transmittal: A-02-0115. November 1, 2002. Change request 2402. Available at: http://cms.hhs.gov/manuals/ pm_trans?A02115.pdf. Accessed October 12, 2004.

15. American Dietetic Association. State carrier information. Available at: http://www.eatright.org/Member/ PolicyInitiatives/83_statecarriers.cfm. Accessed September 26, 2004.

16. Centers for Medicare and Medicaid Services. Intermediary-carrier directory. Available at: http://www.cms.hhs. gov/contacts/incardir.asp#1. Accessed October 12, 2004.

17. Centers for Medicare and Medicaid Services. Peer review organization manual: Part 1—background and responsibilities. Available at: http://www.cms.hhs.gov/ manuals/19_pro/pr01.asp#_1_4. Accessed September 26, 2004.

18. Centers for Medicare and Medicaid Services. U.S. health care system. Available at: http://www.cms.hhs.gov/ charts/default.asp. Accessed June 18, 2004.

19. American Dietetic Association. Medicare and other insurance. Available at: http://www.eatright.org/Member/ PolicyInitiatives/83_otherins.cfm. Accessed October 12, 2004.

20. Medicare program, expanded coverage for outpatient diabetes self-management training and diabetes outcome measurements; final rule and notice. 65 *Federal Register* 83130–83154 (2000) (codified at 42 CFR 410,414,424, 480,498).

21. Medicare program, revisions to payment policies under the physician fee schedule for calendar year 2004; final rule and notice. 68 *Federal Register* (2003) (codified at 42 CFR 410,414). Available at: http://www.cms.hhs.gov/ regulations/pfs/2004fc/default.asp? Accessed October 13, 2004.

22. CMS manual system publication 100-02. Medicare benefit policy. Transmittal 13. May 28, 2004. Change request 3185. Available at: http://www.cms.hhs.gov/manuals/ pm_trans/R13BP.pdf. Accessed October 13, 2004.

23. Mensing C, Boucher J, Cypress M, Weinger K, Mulcahy K, Barta P, Hosey G, Kopher W, Lasichak A, Lamb B, Mangan M, Norman J, Tanja J, Yauk L, Wisdom K, Adams C. National standards for diabetes self-management education. *Diabetes Care.* 2000;23:682–689.

24. American Association of Diabetes Educators and Roche Diagnostics Corporation. *AADE Reimbursement Primer.* Chicago, Ill: American Association of Diabetes Educators; 2000.

25. Centers for Medicare and Medicaid Services. Payment to registered dietitians for diabetes outpatient self-management training (DSMT) services. Transmittal B-02-062. October 4, 2002. Change request 2386. Available at: http://www.cms.hhs.gov/manuals/pm_trans/b02062. pdf. Accessed October 13, 2004.

26. Medicare program: revisions to payment policies and five-year review of and adjustments to the relative value units under the physician fee schedule for calendar year 2002; final rule. 66 *Federal Register* 55246–55332 (2001) (codified at 42 CFR 405).

27. Additional clarification for medical nutrition therapy (MNT) services. CMS Program Memorandum Intermediaries/Carriers. Transmittal AB-02-059. May 1, 2002. Change request 2142. Available at: http://www.cms. hhs.gov/manuals/pm_trans/AB02059.pdf. Accessed October 12, 2004.

28. Clarification regarding non-physician practitioners billing on behalf of a diabetes outpatient self management training services (DSMT) program and common working file edits for DSMT and medical nutrition therapy (MNT). CMS Program Memorandum Intermediaries/Carriers. Transmittal AB-02-151. October 25, 2002. Change request 2372. Available at: http://www.cms.hhs.gov/ manuals/pm_trans/AB02151.pdf. Accessed October 12, 2004.

29. American Dietetic Association. Sample physician referral form for MNT RD services. Available at: http://www. eatright.org/Member/Files/physrefform.doc. Accessed October 14, 2004.

30. American Dietetic Association. Frequently asked questions—Medicare general enrollment. Available at: http://www.eatright.org/Member/PolicyInitiatives/83_ genenroll2.cfm?CFID=4488271&CFTOKEN=47439623. Accessed October 13, 2004.

31. American Dietetic Association. Sample completed CMS 1500 claim form. Available at: http://www.eatright.org/ Member/PolicyInitiatives/83_hcfaform.cfm. Accessed October 12, 2004.

32. Centers for Medicare and Medicaid Services. Medicare Fee-for-Service Provider/Supplier Enrollment Web site. Available at: http://www.cms.hhs.gov/providers/enrollment/ contacts/default.asp. Accessed October 26, 2004.

33. American Dietetic Association. 2004 Physician Fee Schedule. Available at: http://www.eatright.org/Member/PolicyInitiatives/83_18434.cfm. Accessed October 26, 2004.

34. Medicare Program; Revisions to Payment Policies and Adjustments to the Relative Value Units Under the Physician Fee Schedule for Calendar Year 1999. 63 *Federal Register* 58812-58860, 58901-5890542 (1998) (codified at 42 CFR 405).

35. American Dietetic Association. *American Dietetic Association Medical Nutrition Therapy Evidence-Based Guides for Practice: Nutrition Practice Guidelines for Type 1 and Type 2 Diabetes Mellitus* (CD-ROM). Chicago, Ill: American Dietetic Association; 2001.

36. American Dietetic Association. *American Dietetic Association Medical Nutrition Therapy Evidence-Based Guides for Practice: Nutrition Practice Guidelines for Gestational Diabetes Mellitus* (CD-ROM). Chicago, Ill: American Dietetic Association; 2001.

37. Lacey K, Pritchett E. Nutrition care process and model: ADA adopts road map to quality care and outcomes management. *J Am Diet Assoc.* 2003;103:1061–1072.

38. Infante MC, Michael P, Pritchett E. Opting out of Medicare: a serious business decision. *J Am Diet Assoc.* 2002;102:1061–1062.

39. Centers for Medicare and Medicaid Services. Medicare Claims Processing Manual, 40.3, Advance beneficiary notice standards. Available at: http://www.cms.hhs.gov/manuals/104_claims/clm104c30.pdf. Accessed October 12, 2004.

40. Centers for Medicare and Medicaid Services. Advance Beneficiary Notice [ABN], form CMS-R-131. Available at: http://www.cms.hhs.gov/medicare/bni/CMSR1312.pdf. Accessed October 12, 2004.

41. Centers for Medicare and Medicaid Services. Medicare coordination of benefits: Medicare secondary payer and you. Available at: http://www.cms.hhs.gov/medicare/cob/msp/msp_detail.asp. Accessed October 13, 2004.

42. Coding for non-covered services and services not reasonable and necessary. Centers for Medicare and Medicaid Services Program Memorandum Carriers. Transmittal B-01-58. September 25, 2001. Change request 1820. Available at: http://www.cms.hhs.gov/manuals/pm_trans/b0158.pdf. Accessed October 13, 2004.

43. American Dietetic Association. Medicare compliance program backgrounder. Available at: http://www.eatright.org/Member/PolicyInitiatives/83_compbckgrnd.cfm. Accessed October 13, 2004.

44. American Dietetic Association. Privacy (HIPAA—Health Insurance Privacy and Portability Act) information. Available at: http://www.eatright.org/Member/PolicyInitiatives/83_10636.cfm. Accessed October 13, 2004.

ADDITIONAL RESOURCES

American Diabetes Association Education Recognition Program. American Diabetes Association Web site. Available at: the: http://www.diabetes.org/home.jsp. Accessed October 26, 2004.

CMS Quarterly Provider Update (electronic updates of recent CMS regulations and instructions). Available at: http://www.cms.hhs.gov/providerupdate/main.asp. Accessed August 25, 2004.

The Guide to Reimbursement. Chicago, Ill: American Association of Diabetes Educators; 2003.

Litt AS, Mitchell FB. *American Dietetic Association Guide to Private Practice.* Chicago, Ill: American Dietetic Association; 2004.

Medicare MNT Benefit Provider Information. 2nd ed. Chicago, Ill: American Dietetic Association; 2005.

The Medicare MNT Provider (newsletter). Available by subscription from the American Dietetic Association (http://www.eatright.org).

Medicare MNT Part B Coverage and MNT Billing Guidelines. Available at: http://www.eatright.org/Member/PolicyInitiatives/83_16153.cfm. Accessed October 26, 2004.

Money Matters in MNT: Increasing Reimbursement Success in All Practice Settings, the Complete Guide. Palos Heights, Ill: Mary Ann Hodorowicz Consulting, LLC; 2000.

Nutrition Entrepreneur's Guide to Reimbursement Success. 2nd ed. Chicago, Ill: American Dietetic Association; 1999.

On the Pulse. (E-mail newsletter published by the American Dietetic Association's Policy Initiatives and Advocacy Group. Send subscription requests to pulse@eatright.org.)

Physician Information Resources for Medicare Web site (general provider information). Available at: http://www.cms.hhs.gov/physicians/default.asp?. Accessed August 25, 2004.

Universal Diabetes Referral Form for Medicare MNT and Medicare DSMT. (The American Dietetic Association and the American Association of Diabetes Educators [AADE] have collaborated to create this form. The project responds to the American Health Quality Association and Medicare Quality Improvement Organizations' interest in increasing Medicare beneficiaries' access to diabetes services. Feedback from CMS was critical to the form's final development. The referral form includes only the key referral information required to meet Medicare regulatory requirements for referral to MNT and DSMT services. It has been streamlined to one page, to make it easy for physicians and qualified nonphysician practitioners to complete it. The form will be available on the Web sites of ADA [http://www.eatright.org] and AADE [http://www.aadenet.org]).

A Web-Based Resource: Part B Medicare Benefits for MNT Diabetes and Renal Disease. (A joint project of the Diabetes Care and Education Dietetic Practice Group [http://www.dce.org], the American Diabetes Association [http://www.diabetes.org], the American Association of Diabetes Educators [http://www.aadenet.org], and the American Dietetic Association [http://www.eatright.org]. Members of these organizations may access six articles concerning DSMT and MNT reimbursement at the organizations' Web sites.)

3

Introduction to Counseling and Behavior Change

Linda M. Delahanty, MS, RD, and Joan M. Heins, MA, RD, CDE

CHAPTER OVERVIEW

- Psychosocial and behavioral determinants may influence the ability of individuals with diabetes to change, affecting achievement of their diabetes self-management treatment goals.
- The task of the dietetics professional is to identify motivation and willingness to change, to facilitate change by increasing the self-efficacy of individuals with diabetes while promoting autonomy, and to support individuals as they make changes to manage their diabetes.
- Behavior change is important, but understanding key educational principles is also important. How individuals learn, their literacy level, and other factors such as age, all affect their ability to comprehend information critical to managing their diabetes.
- Together, the dietetics professional and the individual with diabetes can develop a realistic, achievable diabetes self-management plan.

OVERVIEW OF STAGES OF CHANGE

One of the assessment areas that dietetics professionals need to address before implementing an intervention approach is stage of change. The stage-of-change model was developed by Prochaska and colleagues and can be used as an overall guiding framework to assess a person's motivation, or readiness, to change a specific behavior (1). The stage-of-change model theorizes that the process of behavior change involves a progression through five stages: precontemplation, contemplation, preparation, action, and maintenance (see Table 3.1) (2). People do not always progress through the stages in a linear fashion. They can enter or exit different stages in the model at any point and can recycle through the stages by relapsing and repeating stage progressions (1,3).

STAGES OF CHANGE AND NUTRITION COUNSELING

When dietetics professionals provide nutrition education and counseling, they typically use behavior therapy on several target behaviors. Behavior therapy is best suited for people in the preparation, action, or maintenance stage of change and not for people in the earlier stages (precontemplation or contemplation). People who are in precontemplation or contemplation may be resistant, angry, or ambivalent to change and therefore need more emphasis on cognitive therapy. Cognitive therapy targets thoughts and beliefs with counseling strategies designed to raise awareness, and it explores feelings, concerns, and perceived barriers to change. Individuals with diabetes who are in the preparation stage may benefit from a combination of some cognitive therapy and some behavior therapy.

TABLE 3.1 Counseling Strategies Based on Stages of Change

Stage	Definition	Client Characteristics	Counseling Strategies
Precontemplation	No intention of changing behavior in the next 6 months	• May be unaware a problem exists • Sees no reason to change • Not interested in discussing change • Feels unable to change	• Raise self-awareness of their behavior • Discuss health concern and implications • Show how client's behavior affects others • Encourage client to discuss his/her feelings
Contemplation	Thinking about changing within the next 6 months	• Has limited knowledge of the problem • Weighing the pros/cons of change • Has no sense of urgency • Waiting to get motivated	• Discuss concerns, beliefs, and barriers • Show client that the pros outweigh the cons • Clarify/discuss ambivalence to change • Suggest resources for further information
Preparation	Planning to change within the next 30 days	• Is motivated and ready to change • Not sure how to get started • May have tried small changes • Could slip back to ambivalence	• Help develop doable action steps • Teach specific "how to" skills • Foster self-efficacy • Provide resources to foster change
Action	Has made changes within the last 6 months	• Efforts to change are noticeable • Believes change is possible • Has modified environment for success • Wants feedback and reinforcement	• Help evaluate progress and teach new skills • Reinforce decision to change and support • Help client add positive cues • Discuss and distinguish lapse vs relapse
Maintenance	Has made established changes for at least 6 months	• Change has become part of routine • Trying not to slip back to old habits • Confident about maintaining change • Dealing with high-risk situations	• Offer suggestion to maintain change • Continue teaching relapse prevention • Remind client of his/her overall progress • Help build supportive environment

Source: Adapted from Table 1 and Table 2 in Gehling E. Changing us or changing them? *Newsflash* (newsletter of the Diabetes Care and Education practice group of the American Dietetic Association). 1999;20:31–33, with permission from HealthPartners, Center for Health Promotion. Copyright © 1999, HealthPartners, Center for Health Promotion. All Rights Reserved.

Although ready to make changes, such individuals can easily become ambivalent and revert back to the contemplation stage if they feel overwhelmed or lack confidence.

Figure 3.1 (4) illustrates how nutrition therapy can integrate the stage-of-change model into the counseling approach. This decision tree involves four important steps.

Step 1: Establish and Maintain Rapport

To establish and maintain rapport with an individual with diabetes, the dietetics professional should use appropriate body language and attentive listening.

Step 2: Clarify Agenda and Goals

The counselor should clarify the agenda by asking each individual open-ended questions, such as "How can I help you?" or "What are your goals for today's session?" The individual's stated goals for the session may be different from clinical care goals based on standards of care. For example, an individual may say, "I would like to lose 20 pounds," or "I feel best when my blood glucose is around 200 [mg/dL]." Although the individual's blood glucose goal is not consistent with current blood glucose recommendations, focusing on areas where he or she is ready and willing to make changes may help the individual achieve a goal and at the same time improve his or her blood glucose control.

Step 3: Assess Stage of Change and Determine Therapy Options

A person may be in the preparation or action stage for losing weight (ready for behavior therapy—how and what to change) but may be in the contemplation stage for other self-care behaviors, such as self-monitoring of blood glucose (in which case the counseling focus should be placed on cognitive therapy—why to change).

Step 4: Provide Therapy Options

Behavior Therapy Focus

When a person is ready for behavior therapy, the dietetics professional could select a meal planning approach designed to help the individual lose weight and proceed to explain what and how to change. In this process, the meal planning and behavioral counseling strategies are

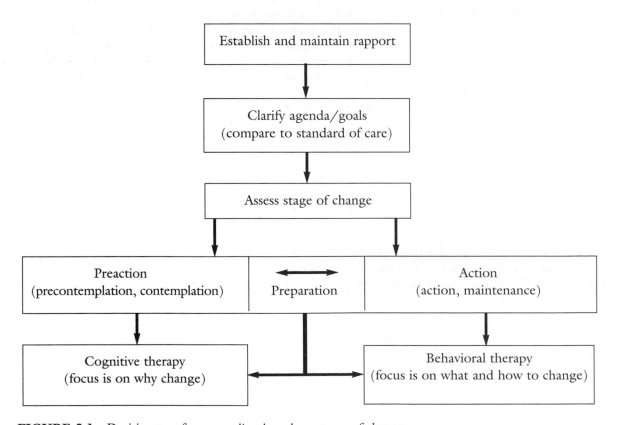

FIGURE 3.1 Decision tree for counseling based on stages of change.

tailored to the individual, and the dietetics professional and individual with diabetes will continue to build rapport and proceed to set goals and a plan for follow-up to reassess progress.

Cognitive Therapy Focus

On the other hand, if the individual does not appear ready to make changes in how often or when to test his or her blood glucose, the counseling process to approach for this issue should emphasize cognitive therapy. The dietetics professional may use the cognitive therapy techniques described in Table 3.1 (2).

As dietetics professionals provide nutrition education and counseling, it is critical that they assess each individual's stage of change for each relevant self-care behavior in relation to a standard, or goal, for the behavior that will produce beneficial results. For example, for most individuals with type 1 diabetes, it is recommended that they perform self-monitoring of blood glucose 3 or more times per day (5). The objective is to help individuals with type 1 diabetes achieve this level of self-monitoring. Incremental goals, however, are sometimes required to achieve this standard.

CONSCIOUSNESS RAISING: A COUNSELING APPROACH FOR PRECONTEMPLATORS

For individuals in the precontemplation stage for a particular behavior, the first step is to ask open-ended questions and raise their awareness. Dietetics professionals should ask questions to assess whether lack of knowledge, skills/resources to change, competing priorities, or distorted health beliefs are potential explanations (4). It is important for the dietetics professional to use paraphrasing and reflective listening to enhance rapport and to make sure that the individual understands the factors that contribute to being in the precontemplation stage. The dietetics professional can then use the counseling strategy of consciousness raising to address motivation. The following steps can be used to help raise consciousness:

1. Identify the medical problem or concern.
2. Review the individual's laboratory tests related to his or her condition and show how these results compare to normal values.
3. Review the impact of food choices, activity level, and other self-care behaviors on diabetes and laboratory tests, to clarify any misunderstandings.

4. Use visual aids to enhance the message (eg, test tubes of fat, 1-lb or 5-lb fat models, convenient size of blood glucose meter, brochures).
5. Elicit feedback and evaluate the individual's verbal and nonverbal responses to counseling.

If the underlying problem is lack of knowledge, skills, or resources to change, then the consciousness-raising approach can often help move the individual forward through the stages within one session. If competing priorities or distorted health beliefs are driving the lack of readiness, however, it is less likely that the individual will progress as quickly. The following case scenario demonstrates the use of consciousness raising to move an individual out of precontemplation.

COUNSELOR: How can I help you? What are your goals for today's session?

CLIENT (arms crossed): I don't know. I'm here because my doctor said I should come to see you.

COUNSELOR: What was your last A1C result?

CLIENT: The same as always, between 8.5% and 9.0%.

COUNSELOR: What is your A1C goal?

CLIENT: Not sure.

COUNSELOR: Typically the goal for A1C is to achieve and maintain a level less than 7%, which is equivalent to an average blood glucose of 150 mg/dL or less. This is because such a level is associated with fewer complications from diabetes over the long term. The A1C level that you have is associated with about a 60% greater likelihood of developing complications from diabetes. What are your thoughts about that?

CLIENT (arms uncrossed and leaning forward): Well, I don't want to develop complications for diabetes, so I guess I should talk about how I can lower my A1C.

MOTIVATIONAL INTERVIEWING: A COUNSELING APPROACH FOR CONTEMPLATORS

Individuals in the contemplation stage for any self-care behaviors related to diabetes management likely view the pros and cons of the change as about equal (with the cons being slightly greater than the pros). The dietetics professional will need to focus the session on asking questions that can help to identify the individual's concerns, beliefs, and perceived barriers toward change.

Once the dietetics professional has gained a better understanding of the individual's ambivalence about changing the behavior, he or she may be able to help the individual reframe the change in more positive terms through motivational interviewing (4). Two counseling strategies that could be used in this case are decisional balance and exploring importance and confidence (6).

Counseling Strategy 1: Decisional Balance

To assess decisional balance, the dietetics professional needs to (*a*) explore the advantages of not changing (ie, staying the same); (*b*) explore the disadvantages of not changing; and (c) summarize by paraphrasing. Decisional balance can be used to explore eating behaviors, exercise behaviors, and self-monitoring of blood glucose, as well as medication taking or record keeping related to food, exercise, or blood glucose readings (4,6). In the following case example, the decisional balance is used to consider reducing energy intake and losing weight as possible means to improve the blood glucose level.

Step 1: Explore the Advantages of Changing

COUNSELOR: What are some of the positive aspects of not eating fewer calories to lose weight?

CLIENT: I can eat what I want.

COUNSELOR: What else is good about it?

CLIENT: I don't have to feel deprived of food, and I don't have to risk failing at weight loss again.

COUNSELOR: What else?

CLIENT: Those are the main things.

Step 2: Explore the Disadvantages of Changing

COUNSELOR: What are some of the not-so-good things about continuing with your current food choices and maintaining your current weight?

CLIENT: My clothes don't fit well. I need more diabetes medications at this weight. I feel sluggish.

COUNSELOR: Anything else?

CLIENT: I'll probably need more and more diabetes medications, and that could get expensive.

COUNSELOR: Any other disadvantages?

CLIENT: I might get diabetes complications like my parents, and then I won't be healthy enough to enjoy doing things with my family.

COUNSELOR: Anything else?

CLIENT: Not right now.

Step 3: Summarize

COUNSELOR: It sounds like you enjoy your food and that eating what you want is less stressful. I also get the sense that you are concerned that you might feel deprived if you try to eat fewer calories and possibly feel like a failure if you don't succeed in losing weight. On the other hand, it sounds as if there are some disadvantages to your current way of eating and your present weight—your clothes don't fit well, you feel sluggish, and you need more diabetes medications at this weight.

CLIENT: That's right.

COUNSELOR: How do you feel about this right now? What would you like to do about this?

CLIENT: I'm not sure.

COUNSELOR: It is important to enjoy your food and to not feel deprived or stressed about your food choices. However, if we could come up with some ideas together to help you eat fewer calories and lose weight that work for you and won't make you feel deprived, would you be interested?

Counseling Strategy 2: Exploring Importance and Confidence

An individual's belief that change is important and his or her confidence that she can make a change also influence the decision to change (6). Dietetics professionals can use the counseling approach of exploring importance and confidence to elicit information from individuals about their degree of motivation, their level of self-efficacy, barriers to change, and potential solutions (4,6). This process can help the dietetics professional to facilitate a dialogue with individuals who are ambivalent and in the contemplation stage.

Step 1: Assess Importance

COUNSELOR: Based on our discussion so far, I'm not really sure how you feel about eating fewer calories to lose weight. I'd like to ask you a few questions to help me understand how you feel. On a scale of 0 to 10, with 10 being most important and 0 being not important at all, how important is it for you right now to eat fewer calories to lose weight?

CLIENT: Probably a 5 or a 6.

Step 2: Assess Confidence

COUNSELOR: On a scale of 0 to 10, with 10 being the highest confidence and 0 being no confidence at all, how confident are you right now that you could eat fewer calories to lose weight?

CLIENT: Probably a 7.

Step 3: Evaluate Ratings for Importance and Confidence

If the individual gives a low rating (< 3) to the importance of making a change, or if importance is rated lower than or equal to the rating for confidence, then counseling should focus on discussing importance first. However, if the individual gives importance a high rating and indicates a low level of confidence (< 3), then counseling should focus on improving confidence first. If the individual gives low ratings (< 3) to both importance and confidence, then counseling should focus on the individual's feelings about further participation in the session. (In the previous dialogue, the dietetics professional would explore importance first.)

Step 4: Explore Importance

When exploring importance and confidence, the counselor should ask why ratings are not lower, to assess the advantages of behavior change. Next the counselor should ask why the ratings are not higher, to assess barriers to or disadvantages of behavior change. Asking what it would take to increase rating by 3 to 4 points may elicit possible solutions.

COUNSELOR: You rated the importance of eating fewer calories to lose weight as a 5 or a 6, so that sounds like it is somewhat important to you. Why didn't you give it a 1 or a 2?

CLIENT: Because I know that my diabetes would probably be better controlled and that I could probably reduce my medications if I lost weight.

COUNSELOR: Why is that important to you?

CLIENT: Because I really don't want to get diabetes complications like my mother did. She lost her toes and her eyesight to diabetes.

COUNSELOR: So eating fewer calories to lose weight is somewhat important to you right now because you would like to have better control of your diabetes and avoid complications like your mother had. You also think that you would feel better if you lost weight. So why didn't you rate the importance an 8 or a 9?

CLIENT: Because it takes a lot of work to lose weight and I have found that when I lose weight, I end up gaining the weight back. I'm also just trying to

enjoy the present and when I feel stressed, eating is one of the ways that I relax.

COUNSELOR: It sounds like you have been able to successfully lose weight in the past and it took a lot of effort on your part and that the hard part was keeping the weight off. It sounds like you tend to eat when you are stressed and that you associate enjoyment of food with relaxation. So what would have to happen to move your rating to an 8 or a 9?

CLIENT: I would need to find other ways to cope with stress so that I would not be so reliant on food to cope. I would also need to find a way to get long-term help with keeping the weight off once I lose it so that I would feel that if I invest the effort to lose weight then it is not for nothing.

Step 5: Summarize

In this step, the counselor paraphrases the client's statements about importance.

Step 6: Explore Confidence

COUNSELOR: It also sounds like you feel fairly confident that you could lose weight right now if you really wanted to. What made you rate your confidence a 7 and not a 1 or a 2?

CLIENT: I have lost weight before, and I know what to do to lose weight. I just haven't been able to keep the weight off.

COUNSELOR: Tell me more about that.

CLIENT: I was successful with Weight Watchers and have also used fat-gram counting to lose weight. It is easier in the beginning when I see more weight loss on the scale, but when the weight loss starts to slow down, I get discouraged and tend to lose focus.

COUNSELOR: So, it sounds like you know what to do to lose weight and have been successful several times, and that it's keeping the weight off that it difficult for you. Are there any other reasons why you wouldn't rate your confidence a 9 or a 10?

CLIENT: No, it is mainly my track record of regaining weight every time I lose it.

COUNSELOR: So what would it take to increase your confidence rating to a 9 or a 10?

CLIENT: I would need to view weight loss as a long-term process and not just a short-term effort. I probably also would need to value weight maintenance and find other reinforcements that will keep me focused.

COUNSELOR: What do you think would help reinforce your efforts?

CLIENT: Probably focusing on improvements in my blood tests such as my A1C and cholesterol levels, and maybe focusing on the new clothes that I can buy and wear.

Step 7: Summarize

In this step, the counselor paraphrases the client's statements about confidence.

GOAL SETTING—A COUNSELING APPROACH FOR THE PREPARATION STAGE

Miller and Rollnick (4) suggest that there are six counseling elements to effective interventions that promote motivation for change. These are summarized in the FRAMES model (Box 3.1) (4). The FRAMES approach can be particularly useful when counseling individuals who are in the preaction stages of change (precontemplation and contemplation), but it can also be useful for individuals in the preparation stage of change.

Individuals in the preparation stage are ready to receive specific guidance and support around diabetes care. Dietetics professionals can use the FRAMES approach to guide individuals toward specific action plans and begin the process of goal setting. Together, the dietetics professional and the individual with diabetes can formulate goals that are specific, measurable, achievable, positive, and short-term. In addition, it is important to anticipate any potential barriers to success and discuss strategies to deal with them to increase the likelihood that the individual will achieve his or her goals. The dietetics professional can also continue using importance and confidence scales periodically, to check in on each individual's motivation throughout the change process. If individuals feel that the goals are not achievable, then it is possible that they could revert back to contemplation and not return for a follow-up session.

SELF-MANAGEMENT SKILLS TRAINING: A COUNSELING APPROACH FOR THE ACTION STAGE

Individuals in the action stage have started making changes to improve diabetes care and need positive reinforcement and support to strengthen and build on their

BOX 3.1

FRAMES Model for Motivational Counseling

Feedback. Clearly discuss the individual's current health status based on a thorough assessment. This would include a review of laboratory test results and how they compare with target levels as defined by clinical standards of care and a review of the roles of nutrition, exercise, self-monitoring of blood glucose, and other self-care habits in relation to diabetes care goals.

Responsibility. Focus on the fact that it is the individual's responsibility to change.

Advice. Provide clear advice to the individual about recommendations for change.

Menu. Offer the individual a menu of options to try to achieve a specific goal or recommendation, to enhance the sense of personal choice and responsibility.

Empathy. Use attentive listening skills to show warmth, respect, understanding, caring, and support.

Self-efficacy. Reinforce the individual's self-efficacy, hope, and optimism, by focusing on past successes, small wins, and positive steps in the direction of desired behavioral outcomes. Research has demonstrated that the counselor's belief in the individual's ability to change behavior is a significant determinant of positive outcomes.

Source: Data are from reference 5.

success. Some of the behavioral counseling strategies that can be used in this stage involve teaching self-monitoring and stimulus control.

Self-monitoring

When individuals with diabetes keep records of food choices, activity, oral diabetes medications or insulin, and blood glucose tests, they can start to see the effects of these variables on blood glucose patterns. Throughout this process, individuals can work with the dietetics professional to learn how to adjust oral diabetes medications or insulin dosages in response to patterns of hyperglycemia or hypoglycemia and accommodate changes in food choices or physical activity.

Stimulus Control

Another behavioral strategy that dietetics professionals can use to help individuals is to rearrange their environment for success. Individuals can learn to minimize exposure to undesirable foods by following a shopping list that includes only healthy food choices and by removing problem foods from their environment. Individuals can also learn to add positive cues to their environment, to increase the likelihood of achieving exercise goals (eg, keeping exercise shoes and clothes visible and within reach when returning home from work).

PROBLEM SOLVING AND COPING STRATEGIES: COUNSELING APPROACHES FOR MAINTENANCE

Individuals in the maintenance stage have changed their behavior for at least 6 months. At this point, dietetics professionals can help individuals learn problem-solving skills and coping strategies designed to help manage lapses and prevent relapse. When individuals identify barriers that interfere with their success in achieving diabetes self-management goals, dietetics professionals can teach them the following steps to the problem-solving approach:

1. Describe the problem.
2. Brainstorm options to address it.
3. Pick an option to try.
4. Make a positive action plan/goal.
5. Anticipate and plan to handle roadblocks.
6. Identify ways to make success more likely.
7. Try the plan and see how it goes.

As individuals practice the problem-solving approach, they increase their skills and self-efficacy in dealing with barriers to successful diabetes self-management (7).

In addition to problem solving around barriers, individuals must also learn how to prevent relapse (8). It is important that dietetics professionals remind individuals that lapses are normal and to be expected, and then coach them to (a) deal effectively with lapses when they occur, and (b) identify their own personal high-risk situations that increase the likelihood of a lapse. Dietetics professionals can help individuals with diabetes cope with lapses so that they can prevent a relapse. The following steps are useful to prevent lapses:

1. Anticipate and identify high-risk situations.
2. Use the problem-solving approach to create a plan to deal with the situation.

3. Evaluate the effectiveness of the plan.

If a lapse occurs, individuals need to learn to deal with their cognitive reaction to the lapse and try to evaluate whether their self-talk is reasonable, as well as to counter any negative self-talk statements with positive ones. Individuals must also remember to try to stay focused on overall progress and on the benefits to be gained from continuing to focus on diabetes self-management.

OTHER TOOLS AND TECHNIQUES FOR COUNSELING

Tools

There are a wide variety of tools available to help facilitate behavioral counseling for nutrition therapy; many of them are described in the chapters on meal planning strategies (see Chapters 18 to 20). One tool, described by Gehling (9), was developed for evaluating education materials and matching them to an individual's stage of change. In addition to print materials, dietetics professionals have used food models, food labels, and a variety of creative visual aids to teach principles of portion control, label reading, and other essential skills. Adults may come to a counseling session with limited experience in cooking or meal preparation. Eating out and ordering in are the norms in many households, with food preparation limited to popping a packaged food in the microwave. Increasingly, dietetics professionals are challenged to develop meal-planning tools for individuals who cannot or will not cook.

Techniques

Just as people learn in different ways, nutrition education and counseling can be conducted in more than one way. Individual counseling for medical nutrition therapy (MNT) is the model reimbursed by Medicare (see Chapter 2) and outlined in most nutrition practice guidelines. Individual counseling sessions maximize the process of MNT (see Chapters 1 and 6). Group counseling is the model reimbursed by Medicare for diabetes self-management training (DSMT). A review of the effectiveness of DSMT found mixed results for interventions that focused on knowledge, skills, and lifestyle. Group classes were generally more effective than individual counseling for lifestyle behavior changes (10). A combination of individual counseling and group education is used in some clinical settings. Distance counseling by phone or computer is relatively new to the practice of dietetics. Although departing from traditional face-to-face counseling, distance counseling provides a more economically viable alternative to fiscally strapped health systems, as well as to individuals with limited time for office visits. Given the limited body of literature, it is difficult to speculate on the efficacy of this approach. Some large-scale clinical trials (eg, Diabetes Control and Complications Trial, Diabetes Prevention Program), however, suggest that a combined approach involving individual counseling and follow-up phone contact is effective for preventing and managing diabetes (11,12).

EDUCATION

Dietetics professionals who provide nutrition education and counseling are both educators and counselors. Individuals with diabetes must first understand the connection between their lifestyle behaviors and key outcomes related to diabetes self-management (eg, glucose control, improved lipid levels, and controlled blood pressure). More specifically related to nutrition therapy, individuals with diabetes also need to be educated on the fundamentals of their meal plan and need to be trained in the skills required to implement it on a daily basis. Individuals in different stages of change will be more receptive to one learning strategy than to another. For example, individuals in the contemplation stage will need teaching techniques directed toward the cognitive process of learning, whereas those in action will need

techniques that develop behavioral skills. No matter what the stage, however, individuals differ in how they learn. An understanding of the learning process allows dietetics professionals to select tools and techniques that will maximize the effect of the counseling session.

How People Learn

People learn in various ways (see Table 3.2) (13).The educational literature describes learning in terms of areas or domains (14,15). Each domain includes several hierarchical levels that can be targeted and used to set educational goals. For example, the cognitive domain spans from basic knowledge to comprehension, application, analysis, synthesis, and ultimately to evaluation. In working with an individual who is able to verbalize the fundamentals of carbohydrate counting but has difficulty applying them to daily eating, the dietetics professional could set a cognitive goal to advance learning to the level of application.

People differ in the ways they prefer to learn. These differences, or learner styles, capture both the cognitive processes of learning and the influences of the learning environment. Osterman identified several characteristics that differentiate four styles of learning (Table 3.2) (13). Dietetics professionals use this model to identify an individual's preferred learning style. Some people ("thinkers") will carefully read everything that you give them, whereas others ("sensors") only want to know what they need to eat. When asked, some people ("feel-

TABLE 3.2   How People Learn

Domains of Learning

Domain	Process	Outcome
Cognitive	Factual information	Knowledge
Affective	Pros and cons	Attitude
Psychomotor	Demonstration	Skills

Learner Style

Style	Looks for	Learns by	Best Method	Likes to Ask
Feeler	Meaning	Listening	Discussion	Why?
Thinker	Facts	Thinking	Lecture	What?
Sensor	Applications	Problem solving	Demonstration	How?
Intuitor	Alternatives	Trial and error	Self-discovery	If?

Source: Data are from reference 11.

ers") may tell you that they like to discuss options before deciding on a meal plan, whereas others ("intuitors") say they prefer to try one out first.

Other Factors That Influence Learning

In addition to domain and style, learning is influenced by a variety of other factors.

Age

Children learn what is presented to them. Adults select what they are willing to learn. Experts on adult learning describe learning in terms of (*a*) a need to know, (*b*) performance-centered learning, and (*c*) experiential learning that emphasizes the importance of active involvement (16). In counseling adults, dietetics professionals must reconcile the often competing demands of prescribing a therapeutic plan and addressing what the individual wants to discuss. A diagnosis of diabetes does not automatically trigger a need to know in adults. The stage-of-change approach (1) offers dietetics professionals a way to communicate the nutrition prescription in a manner that maximizes the individual's willingness to learn.

Literacy

Ability to read, reading level, and comprehension also should be included in an assessment of literacy. To assess an individual's ability and comprehension, the health professional should ask the individual to read a simple nutrition tool, then ask what the information means. There are a variety of methods for evaluating the reading grade level of print materials. The Committee on Health Literacy of the American Medical Association recommends that health education materials be written at a 6th-grade level or lower (17). However, multiple-syllable words, such as carbohydrate, calorie, and cholesterol, give many excellent nutrition tools a reading level higher than 6th grade. These tools can be used in nutrition education and counseling, if time and attention are given to clarifying complex words.

Culture

Health beliefs, rules for communication, and language vary across cultures. With the changing demographics in the United States, dietetics professionals are counseling an increasingly diverse clientele. The *Ethnic and Regional Food Practice Series* (published by the American Dietetic Association) provides an overview of traditions and beliefs that influence the eating patterns of people from various cultures (18). Although this series of books does not include all ethnicities, it does provide some background on issues that differ by culture and allows dietetics professionals to develop sensitivity to the variations that influence learning. It is important to recognize that cultural competency in nutrition counseling requires more than tailored teaching materials. Culturally competent dietetics professionals use their awareness of cultural differences to adapt their counseling techniques to each individual.

SUMMARY

Lifestyle behavior change is a fundamental component of diabetes management. Dietetics professionals working with individuals with diabetes need to learn to use various counseling and education techniques to promote and support long-term behavior change. The stages of change, motivational interviewing, and other behavioral theories and strategies can be used to address and focus on the core components of diabetes self-management education.

REFERENCES

1. Prochaska JO, Velicier WF, Rossi JS, Goldstein MG, Marcus BH, Rakowski W, Fiore C, Harlow LL, Redding CA, Rosenbloom D, Rossi SR. Stages of change and decisional balance for 12 problem behaviors. *Health Psychol.* 1994; 13:39–46.
2. Gehling E. Changing us or changing them? *Newsflash* (newsletter of the Diabetes Care and Education practice group of the American Dietetic Association). 1999; 20:31–33.
3. Prochaska JO, DiClemente CC, Norcross JC. In search of how people change: applications to addictive behaviors. *Diabetes Spectrum* 1993;6:25–33.
4. Miller WR, Rollnick S. *Motivational Interviewing: Preparing People for Change.* 2nd ed. New York: Guilford Press; 2002.
5. American Diabetes Association. Standards of medical care in diabetes (position statement). *Diabetes Care.* 2004; 27(suppl 1):S15–S35.
6. Heins JM, Delahanty L. Tools and techniques to facilitate eating behavior change. In: Coultson AM, Rock CL, Monsen ER, eds. *Nutrition in the Prevention and Treatment of Disease.* San Diego, Calif: Academic Press; 2001:105–122.
7. D'Zurilla TJ, Nezu A. Social problem solving in adults. In: Kendall PC, ed. *Advances in Cognitive-Behavioral Research and Therapy.* New York: Academic Press; 1982:201–274.

8. Marlatt GA, Gordon JR. *Relapse Prevention: Maintenance Strategies in the Treatment of Addictive Behaviors.* New York: Guilford Press; 1985.

9. Gehling E. Stage-matching your client education materials. *Newsflash* (newsletter of the Diabetes Care and Education practice group of the American Dietetic Association). 2002;23:23–26.

10. Norris SL, Engelgau MM, Narayan KM. Effectiveness of self-management training in type 2 diabetes: a systematic review of randomized controlled trials. *Diabetes Care.* 2001;24:561–587.

11. Diabetes Control and Complications Trial Research Group. Nutrition interventions for intensive therapy in the Diabetes Control and Complications Trial. *J Am Diet Assoc.* 1993;93:768–772.

12. Diabetes Prevention Program Research Group. The Diabetes Prevention Program (DPP): description of lifestyle intervention. *Diabetes Care.* 2002;25:2165–2171.

13. Osterman DN. The feedback lecture: matching teaching and learning styles. *J Am Diet Assoc.* 1984;84:1221–1222.

14. Mager RF. *Preparing Instructional Objectives.* Belmont, Calif: Fearon; 1975.

15. Houston C, Haire-Joshu D. Application of health behavior models. In: Haire-Joshu D, ed. *Management of Diabetes Mellitus: Perspectives Across the Lifespan.* Saint Louis, Mo: Mosby-Year Book; 1995.

16. Knowles M. *The Adult Learner: A Neglected Species.* Houston, Tex: Gulf Publishing; 1985.

17. Health literacy: report of the Council on Scientific Affairs. Ad hoc Committee on Health Literacy for the Council on Scientific Affairs, American Medical Association. *JAMA.* 1999;281:552–557.

18. *Ethnic and Regional Food Practices.* Chicago, Ill: American Dietetic Association; 1989–1999.

ADDITIONAL RESOURCES

Motivational Interviewing. Available at: http://www.motivationalinterview.org. Accessed December 20, 2004.

Prochaska JO, Norcross JC, DiClemente CC. *Changing for Good.* New York, NY: William Morrow & Co; 1995.

Rollnick S, Mason P, Butler C. *Health Behavior Change: A Guide for Practitioners.* London, England: Churchill Livingstone; 1999.

Ruggerio L. Helping people with diabetes change behavior: from theory to practice. *Diabetes Spectrum.* 2000; 13:125–132.

Part 2

Diabetes Classification, Diagnosis, and Prevention

4

Diabetes Classification, Pathophysiology, and Diagnosis

Belinda S. O'Connell, MS, RD, CDE

CHAPTER OVERVIEW

- *Diabetes* is the term used to describe a group of endocrine disorders characterized by elevated blood glucose level.
- Diabetes is often considered simply a disease of glucose metabolism when, in fact, it results from dysregulation of a complex combination of hormonal and metabolic processes affecting carbohydrate, lipid, and protein metabolism, and a range of organ systems including the circulatory and nervous systems.
- By recognizing the underlying disease pathologies of diabetes, dietetics professionals can better understand the interactions of food, activity, and pharmacologic treatments in the management of diabetes, and the disease's associated acute and chronic complications.

PREVALENCE AND COSTS OF DIABETES

Diabetes is a rapidly increasing public health concern in the United States. Future diabetes prevalence rates are expected to increase dramatically as demographic characteristics, including aging, changes in race composition, obesity, and lifestyle of the United States population, change. Approximately 18.2 million people, or 6.3% of the population, have diabetes, and another 41 million people have prediabetes (1). It has been estimated that the prevalence of diagnosed diabetes will increase by 165%, from 11 million in 2000 to 29 million by 2050 (2).

Of the 18.2 million people with diabetes, nearly one third (5.2 million people) remain undiagnosed (1). Undiagnosed diabetes is a concern because it is known that complications of diabetes often begin long before diagnosis, and because early treatment can decrease morbidity and mortality associated with diabetes (1,3,4).

The large number of Americans with diabetes and prediabetes represents a significant social and economic burden (1). Diabetes was the sixth leading cause of death in the United States in 2000 (1). People with diabetes have increased rates of heart disease, stroke, high blood pressure, kidney disease, and nontraumatic lower-limb amputation. Diabetes is the leading cause of new cases of blindness (1), results in damage to the nervous system, and has potentially life-threatening acute complications.

The economic costs of diabetes run into the billions. A study undertaken by the American Diabetes Association estimated direct health care costs and indirect costs due to increased disability and mortality to be $132 billion in 2002 (2). The costs will continue to increase as the number of people with diabetes increases.

Although the future potential cost of diabetes is staggering, recent research in the areas of diabetes prevention and diabetes treatment provides hope that, with increased early diagnosis and aggressive intervention, the human and economic costs of diabetes can be managed (3–5).

FUEL METABOLISM IN DIABETIC AND NONDIABETIC STATES

In normal metabolism, blood glucose level is regulated by the opposing and coordinated action of anabolic (fed-state) and counterregulatory (fasted-state) hormones. The coordination of these hormones is essential in maintaining glucose and lipid homeostasis, and disruption in the action and regulation of these hormones in diabetes results in chronic hyperglycemia and increased rates of dyslipidemia. For a summary of the metabolic effects of fed and fasted states, see Table 4.1.

Diabetes has been referred to as a state of accelerated fasting where the lack of insulin, due to either an absolute deficiency or insulin resistance, results in the following:

- Decreased peripheral glucose uptake
- Unopposed action of counterregulatory hormones
- Increased hepatic glucose production
- Increased lipolysis
- Dyslipidemias

When the absence of insulin and the increase in counterregulatory hormones are extreme and prolonged, accumulation of ketone bodies and osmotic diuresis can lead to acidosis; loss of anions such as sodium, potassium, and bicarbonate; dehydration; and diabetic ketoacidosis (DKA).

CLASSIFICATION OF DIABETES

Diabetes is defined by the presence of hyperglycemia as a result of impaired or absent insulin secretion, decreased insulin action, or a combination of both. It can be divided into several distinct subtypes based on genetics, presenting symptoms, and the underlying disease pathology (6). In 1997, the 1979 National Diabetes Data Group classification scheme was revised to focus on underlying disease etiopathologies. It eliminated the terms "insulin-dependent diabetes mellitus" and "non-insulin-dependent diabetes mellitus," and designated type 1 and type 2 diabetes with arabic numerals rather than roman numerals (6). Categories of diabetes and impaired glucose tolerance include type 1 diabetes, type 2 diabetes, gestational diabetes, prediabetes, and other less common types of diabetes (6).

Type 1 Diabetes

Type 1 diabetes, previously referred to as "juvenile diabetes" or "insulin-dependent diabetes mellitus," is characterized by autoimmune destruction of pancreatic beta cells, insulin deficiency, and the requirement of exogenous insulin for survival (1). Type 1 diabetes affects 5% to 10% of people with diabetes. Onset is generally before

TABLE 4.1 Summary of Normal Metabolism

	Fed State	Fasted State
Key regulatory hormone	Insulin	Glucagon
Metabolic effects	• Increased insulin release from pancreatic beta cells • Increased circulating insulin levels • Decreased glucagon and counterregulatory hormone levels • Metabolic shift toward anabolic processes, such as glucose, amino acid, and triglyceride transport and storage	• Decreased insulin release from pancreatic beta cells • Decreased circulating insulin levels • Increased levels of counterregulatory hormones, such as glucagon • Metabolic shift toward catabolic processes, such as breakdown of glucose stored in glycogen (glycogenolysis), hepatic glucose synthesis (gluconeogenesis), protein breakdown, and lipolysis
End result	• Decreased blood glucose level	• Increased blood glucose level, increased free fatty acid levels, and, under extreme conditions, synthesis of ketones by the liver

age 30 years, although development of type 1 diabetes can occur in older individuals.

Both genetic and environmental factors contribute to the development of type 1 diabetes. People with a first-degree relative with type 1 diabetes have an increased risk of developing the disease (7).

A genetic predisposition for type 1 diabetes is conferred by the presence of specific histocompatability locus antigens (HLAs), although many people with genetic risk factors do not develop the disease (7). In people with a genetic predisposition toward type 1 diabetes, exposure to an environmental trigger, such as viral infection, initiates an autoimmune response resulting in inflammation and destruction of the beta cells of the pancreas (8).

Between 85% and 95% of individuals with type 1 diabetes have islet cell autoantibodies, insulin autoantibodies, glutamic acid decarboxylase (GAD) antibodies, or other immune response markers at diagnosis (6). Fifty percent of relatives of people with type 1 diabetes, who themselves have high levels of islet cell autoantibodies, develop diabetes within 5 years (8). People with type 1 diabetes also have increased incidence of other autoimmune diseases, such as pernicious anemia, celiac disease, and Graves disease (6).

The autoimmune process underlying type 1 diabetes is generally present for some time before hyperglycemia occurs (8). Type 1 diabetes is characterized by the rapid development of the following classic symptoms of diabetes:

- Polyuria
- Polydipsia
- Polyphagia
- Weight loss
- Ketoacidosis (in some cases)

Type 2 Diabetes

The most prevalent form of diabetes is type 2 diabetes, previously referred to as "adult-onset" or "non–insulin-dependent" diabetes. In type 2 diabetes, initial insulin resistance generally predates the development of hyperglycemia, which becomes apparent only when the pancreas is no longer able to produce sufficient insulin to compensate for decreased peripheral tissue sensitivity (6).

Type 2 diabetes affects 16 million to 17 million people in the United States and accounts for 90% to 95% of cases of diabetes (1). Type 2 diabetes has a greater genetic linkage than is found in type 1 (7). In offspring of people with diabetes, risk of type 2 is 15% and risk of developing impaired glucose tolerance is 30% (7).

Because symptoms are generally less pronounced than in type 1 diabetes, diagnosis of type 2 diabetes often occurs years after the initial development of glucose intolerance. The time lag between disease onset and diagnosis is a concern, because early, effective blood glucose management can decrease the incidence of microvascular and macrovascular complications, which are frequently present at diagnosis. The development of type 2 diabetes results from abnormalities in both the action of insulin (insulin resistance) and insulin secretion.

Insulin Secretion Abnormalities

One defect in insulin metabolism in type 2 diabetes is impaired insulin secretion. Early abnormalities in insulin release in type 2 diabetes include impaired early-phase insulin release and a protracted late-phase insulin release (9). As type 2 progresses, a decline in the ability of the beta cell to synthesize insulin results in significant insulin deficiency (6). Chronic hyperglycemia and increased free fatty acids also contribute to the deficient beta cell response. This is often referred to as glucose toxicity (10).

Insulin Action Abnormalities

Insulin resistance is a central component of type 2 diabetes and prediabetes, as well as the metabolic syndrome. Decreased insulin sensitivity occurs in target tissues, such as adipose, muscle, and liver (6). Causes of insulin resistance include the following (11):

- Increased levels of free fatty acids, which inhibit glucose uptake into muscle tissue
- Increased levels of cytokines, which inhibit translocation of glucose transporters to the cell surface in response to insulin
- Defects in a group of nuclear receptors that regulate genes involved in adipogenesis and insulin action (peroxisomal proliferator-activated receptor [PPAR])
- Decreased insulin receptor number and activation, due to chronic exposure to insulin or other causes
- Postreceptor defects in insulin-mediated signal transduction pathways

Risk Factors

Factors that influence insulin sensitivity, such as age, low physical activity level, obesity, and ethnicity, are

BOX 4.1

Major Risk Factors for Type 2 Diabetes

Age ≥ 45 years

Overweight (BMI ≥ 25 kg/m^2) (may vary with ethnicity)

Family history of diabetes (ie, parents or siblings)

Habitual physical inactivity

Race/ethnicity (ie, African-American, Latino, Native American, Asian-American, Pacific Island ethnicities)

Previously identified IFG or IGT

History of GDM or delivery of baby weighing > 9 lb

Hypertension (≥ 140/90 mm Hg in adults)

HDL cholesterol < 35 mg/dL and/or a triglyceride level > 250 mg/dL

Polycystic ovary syndrome

History of vascular disease

Have other clinical conditions associated with insulin resistance (eg, acanthosis nigricans)

Abbreviations: BMI, body mass index; GDM, gestational diabetes mellitus; HDL, high-density lipoprotein; IFG, impaired fasting glucose; IGT, impaired glucose tolerance.

Source: Adapted with permission from American Diabetes Association. Clinical practice recommendations 2005: standards of medical care in diabetes. *Diabetes Care.* 2005;28(suppl 1):S4–S36. Copyright © 2005 American Diabetes Association.

associated with risk of type 2 diabetes (12). Risk factors for type 2 diabetes are summarized in Box 4.1 (13).

Therapy Options

The choice of therapy for management of type 2 diabetes varies with the natural history of the disease. Medical nutrition therapy (MNT) is the cornerstone of diabetes management throughout all stages of type 2 diabetes, as well as in prediabetes. MNT resulting in a 5% to 10% loss of body weight and increased physical activity can delay or prevent the development of diabetes in people with impaired glucose tolerance (5). MNT is often an effective monotherapy early in the disease process when there is still reserve insulin secretory capacity. In later stages of type 2 diabetes, as pancreatic beta cell function declines, MNT often needs to be combined with one or more oral diabetes agents or with insulin for effective blood glucose control.

Note: The need for oral diabetes medications, or for insulin, should not be interpreted as a behavioral failure of lifestyle change—simply a result of disease progression.

Prediabetes

A blood glucose level greater than normal but less than those required for the diagnosis of diabetes is strongly associated with an increased incidence of diabetes and may also increase the risk of cardiovascular disease (12,14). This intermediate stage between normal blood glucose and diabetes is now referred to as "prediabetes." Individuals with prediabetes include the following:

- People with impaired glucose tolerance (IGT) (75-g glucose 2-hour oral glucose tolerance test value of 140 to 199 mg/dL)
- People with impaired fasting glucose (IFG) (fasting blood glucose value of 100 to 125 mg/dL) (13).

Recent research, discussed in greater depth in Chapter 5, indicates that diabetes can be prevented or delayed in these high-risk individuals and that therapeutic lifestyle change is an essential component of these preventive strategies (5).

Other Conditions of Insulin Resistance

Insulin resistance is characteristic of type 2 diabetes, but it can occur alone or associated with other independent conditions, such as hypertension, metabolic syndrome, and polycystic ovary syndrome (PCOS) (15,16).

Metabolic Syndrome

Metabolic syndrome is a separate condition but shares some characteristics of type 2 diabetes, most notably insulin resistance. Metabolic syndrome is also referred to as the insulin resistance syndrome, syndrome X, dysmetabolic syndrome, and Reaven's syndrome, after Gerald Reaven, who first described the condition. It is estimated that 47 million people in the United States and 80% of individuals with type 2 diabetes have metabolic syndrome (17,18).

Metabolic syndrome is characterized by abdominal obesity, insulin resistance, hyperglycemia, dyslipidemia

TABLE 4.2 Diagnosis of Metabolic Syndrome

Risk Factor	NCEP ATP III Criteria*	WHO Criteria†
Abdominal obesity	Men: Waist circumference > 102 cm (> 40 in) Women: Waist circumference > 88 cm (> 35 in)	Men: Waist-to-hip ratio > 0.9 or BMI > 30 Women: Waist-to-hip ratio > 0.85 or BMI > 30
Triglycerides, mg/dL	≥ 150	> 150
High-density lipoprotein cholesterol, mg/dL	Men: < 40 Women: < 50	Men: < 35 Women: < 39
Blood pressure, mm Hg	≥ 130/≥ 85	> 140/90
Fasting glucose, mg/dL	≥ 110	
Insulin resistance		Defined as the highest quartile of the $HOMA_{IR}$ index
Microalbumin		Urinary excretion rate > 20 µg/min or alb/cr > 30 µg/mg creatinine

Abbreviations: BMI, body mass index; $HOMA_{IR}$, homeostasis model assessment of insulin resistance; NCEP ATP III, National Cholesterol Education Program Adult Treatment Panel III; WHO, World Health Organization.
*Presence of any three of these conditions.
† Presence of glucose intolerance, impaired glucose tolerance, or diabetes, and/or insulin resistance and two or more other components.
Source: Data are from references 15 and 16.

(elevated triglycerides, small dense low-density lipoproteins, and low high-density lipoprotein cholesterol levels), hypertension, and increased thrombotic risk (15,16). Table 4.2 summarizes the clinical conditions used to diagnose metabolic syndrome (15,16).

Polycystic Ovary Syndrome

PCOS is an endocrine disorder characterized by increased androgen production, disordered gonadotrophin secretion, insulin resistance, and chronic anovulation. Insulin sensitivity is decreased 35% to 40% in women with PCOS, independent of obesity. Women with PCOS are at risk for impaired glucose tolerance and type 2 diabetes, and undiagnosed diabetes is sevenfold greater in women with PCOS than in other premenopausal women in the United States (19).

Gestational Diabetes

Gestational diabetes (GDM) is defined as glucose intolerance that is first diagnosed during pregnancy (1,20). Approximately 7% of all pregnancies are complicated with GDM (20). Women with clinical characteristics consistent with high risk of GDM are those with marked obesity, a personal history of GDM, glycosuria, or a strong family history of diabetes (13,20). Women who have had GDM have a 20% to 50% chance of developing diabetes in the next 5 to 10 years (1).

During the second and third trimesters of pregnancy, several metabolic changes occur to ensure the availability of fuel for the growing fetus. Increased production of hormones, such as human placental lactogen, by the placenta results in insulin resistance. Under normal conditions, insulin production increases significantly to compensate for its decreased effectiveness, and blood glucose level remains within the normal range. Gestational diabetes develops in women who have an inadequate compensatory beta cell response (21).

DIAGNOSIS OF DIABETES

As shown in Table 4.3 (6), diabetes can be diagnosed in one of three ways. Confirmation on a separate day is recommended in the absence of unequivocal hyperglycemia. Use of an A1C measurement is not currently recommended as a method for diagnosing diabetes (6).

TABLE 4.3 Criteria for Diagnosis of Glucose Intolerance and Diabetes

Condition	Diagnostic Criteria
Impaired fasting glucose	Fasting plasma glucose 100–125 mg/dL*
Impaired glucose tolerance	2-hour postglucose load 140–199 mg/dL
Diabetes (Diagnosis by one of these three methods and confirmed on a separate occasion in the absence of unequivocal hyperglycemia.)	• Symptoms of diabetes and a casual plasma glucose ≥ 200 mg/dL[†] • Fasting* plasma glucose ≥ 126 mg/dL • 2-hour postglucose load ≥ 200 mg/dL during OGTT[‡]

*Fasting is defined as no energy intake for 8 hours.
†Casual is defined as any time of day without regard to time of last meal. The classic symptoms of diabetes include polyuria, polydipsia, and unexplained weight loss.
‡Oral glucose tolerance test (OGTT) performed using WHO criteria and 75 g anhydrous glucose dissolved in water.
Source: Data are from reference 6.

Diagnostic criteria have been established for an intermediate category of glucose intolerance where blood glucose level is greater than normal but below the thresholds established for diabetes. These are impaired fasting glucose and impaired glucose tolerance, depending on the diagnostic method (6).

Gestational diabetes should be diagnosed using a 3-hour, 100-g oral glucose tolerance test (OGTT). The diagnosis can be made using a 75-g glucose load, but that test is not as well validated for detection of at-risk infants or mothers as the 100-g OGTT. Table 4.4 summarizes the blood glucose values that indicate GDM (6,13,20).

TABLE 4.4 Diagnostic Criteria for Gestational Diabetes Using 100-g Oral Glucose Tolerance Test*

	Glucose Level, mg/dL
Fasting	≥ 95
1-hour	≥ 180
2-hour	≥ 155
3-hour	≥ 140

*Meeting or exceeding 2 or more of the venous plasma values listed in the table indicates gestational diabetes mellitus. This test should be done in the morning after an overnight fast of 8 to 14 hours.
Source: Adapted with permission from American Diabetes Association. Clinical practice recommendations 2005: standards of medical care in diabetes. 2005;28(Suppl 1):S4–S36. Copyright © 2005 American Diabetes Association.

SCREENING FOR DIABETES

Prediabetes and Type 2 Diabetes

The American Diabetes Association recommends opportunistic screening of high-risk individuals for diabetes because early diagnosis and appropriate treatment of diabetes have been shown to decrease the development of chronic complications (3,4,6).

Screening for diabetes in asymptomatic individuals should be considered at age 45 years and older, or before 45 years of age in individuals who are overweight (BMI ≥ 25) or have additional risk factors for diabetes. Box 4.1 summarizes the major risk factors for type 2 diabetes (13) and Box 4.2 summarizes screening criteria (13).

The fasting plasma glucose test (FPG) is the recommended clinical screening test (13,22). Community screening for type 2 diabetes is not recommended at this time because of a lack of evidence as to its benefit and cost effectiveness (13,22). Screening guidelines for type 2 diabetes in asymptomatic adults, children, and adolescents are summarized in Box 4.2 (13).

Type 1 Diabetes

Widespread screening for type 1 diabetes is not recommended because of its low incidence, the generally short time period between onset of symptoms and diagnosis, and a lack of consensus as to appropriate cutoff values for immune marker assays, or the appropriate response to a positive test (22).

Gestational Diabetes

Current screening guidelines for GDM recommend selective screening of women with average or increased risk, rather than universal screening of all pregnant women (13,20). Screening by glucose challenge should be conducted between the 24th and 28th weeks of gestation. This involves a two-step approach, using an initial 1-hour, 50-g oral glucose tolerance test, followed by a diagnostic oral glucose tolerance test in women with 1-hour values equal to or greater than 140 mg/dL. Table 4.4 summarizes the blood glucose values that indicate GDM (13).

Women at low risk for the development of GDM do not need to undergo screening by glucose challenge (13,20). This includes women who meet *all* the follow-ing criteria: younger than 25 years of age and of normal body weight, no family history of diabetes, no history of abnormal glucose tolerance or poor obstetric outcome, and not a member of an ethnic group with increased rates of diabetes (13,20).

High-risk individuals should be tested as early as possible. Women with a blood glucose level meeting the diagnostic criteria for diabetes (see Table 4.3), and confirmed on a second occasion in the absence of unequivocal hyperglycemia, do not need to undergo screening via glucose challenge (13).

THERAPEUTIC GOALS

Blood Glucose

There is now significant evidence that achieving intensive glycemic control (A1C < 7%) can decrease or delay the development of complications in both type 1 and type 2 diabetes (3,4). It is estimated that there is a relative risk reduction of 15% to 30% for each 1% decrease in A1C (13).

Elevated postprandial blood glucose level is common in type 2 diabetes and has been hypothesized to play a unique role in the development of complications, particularly cardiovascular disease (14,23). The American Diabetes Association postprandial blood glucose goal is less than 180 mg/dL 1 to 2 hours after the beginning of the meal (13,23). The American College of Endocrinology (ACE) recommends that the 2-hour postprandial blood glucose level be 140 mg/dL or lower (14).

Table 4.5 summarizes current glycemic goals for adults (14,20,24). Blood glucose goals should be individualized based on the abilities and characteristics of the person with diabetes. Higher targets may be appropriate in young children, older persons, people with increased risk of hypoglycemia, and those with significant comorbidities. Lower targets are recommended in pregnancy.

Targets for glycemic control when individuals with diabetes are hospitalized are also different. Goals for blood glucose levels are as follows (13):

- *Critically ill patients:* blood glucose level should be kept as close to 110 mg/dL as possible and generally less than 180 mg/dL.
- *Noncritically ill patients:* premeal blood glucose should be kept as close to 90–130 mg/dL as possible given the clinical situation, and a postprandial blood glucose level should be less than 180 mg/dL.

TABLE 4.5 American Diabetes Association Glycemic Goals for Adults

	Goals for Men and Nonpregnant Women	Preconception Goals for Women
A1C*	< 7.0%	< 1% above the upper limits of normal
Preprandial plasma glucose, mg/dL*	90–130	80–110
Postprandial plasma glucose, mg/dL*	< 180 (1–2 hours after start of meal)	< 155 (2 hours after start of meal)

*The American College of Endocrinology and the American Association of Clinical Endocrinologists Consensus Panel (14) recommends a goal A1C of < 6.5%, fasting plasma and preprandial blood glucose levels < 110 mg/dL, and 2-hour postprandial plasma glucose levels < 140 mg/dL.

Source: Adapted with permission from American Diabetes Association. American Diabetes Association. Clinical practice recommendations 2005: standards of medical care in diabetes. Diabetes Care. 2005;28(Suppl 1):S4–S36; and from American Diabetes Association. Preconception care of women with diabetes. Diabetes Care. 2004;27(Suppl 1):S76–S78. Copyright © 2004, 2005 American Diabetes Association.

TABLE 4.6 Lipid and Blood Pressure Goals for Adults With Diabetes

	Goal
LDL cholesterol	< 100 mg/dL
Triglycerides	< 150 mg/dL
HDL cholesterol	> 40 mg/dL*
Blood pressure	< 130/80 mm Hg

Abbreviations: HDL, high-density lipoprotein; LDL, low-density lipoprotein.

*Increasing HDL goal by 10 mg/dL has been suggested for women.

Source: Adapted with permission from American Diabetes Association. Clinical practice recommendations 2005: standards of medical care in diabetes. Diabetes Care. 2005;28(Suppl 1):S4–S36. Copyright © 2005 American Diabetes Association.

TABLE 4.7 Definitions of Abnormal Albumin Excretion*†

	Spot Collection, µg/mg creatinine	Timed Collection, µg/min	24-Hour Collection, mg/24 h
Normal	< 30	< 20	< 30
Microalbuminuria	30–299	20–199	30–299
Clinical albuminuria	≥ 300	≥ 200	≥ 300

*Because of variability in urinary albumin excretion, two of three specimens collected within a 3- to 6-month period should be abnormal before considering patients to have crossed one of these diagnostic thresholds.

†Exercise within 24 hours, infection, fever, congestive heart failure, marked hyperglycemia, and marked hypertension may elevate urinary albumin excretion over baseline values.

Source: Reprinted with permission from American Diabetes Association. Clinical practice recommendations 2004: nephropathy in diabetes. Diabetes Care. 2004;27(Suppl 1):S79–S83. Copyright © 2004 American Diabetes Association.

Comorbid Conditions

Much of the morbidity and mortality associated with diabetes is not due to the acute effects of hyperglycemia or hypoglycemia, but instead, results from the cumulative effects of an elevated blood glucose level on body tissues and comorbid conditions, such as dyslipidemia, hypertension, and renal disease (1,13,25). Clinical goals for blood pressure, lipids, and renal status are summarized in Tables 4.6 and 4.7. Chapter 13 reviews etiology of long-term complications of diabetes in greater detail, and Chapters 22 and 23 review clinical management and meal planning strategies for cardiovascular disease and renal disease.

SUMMARY

Dietetics professionals need to understand the underlying disease pathologies of diabetes and its associated comorbidities, to appropriately individualize nutrition therapy and educational interventions. Dietetics professionals who have a clear understanding of diabetes, metabolism, and current clinical recommendations for blood glucose, lipid, and blood pressure management will be prepared to serve as valuable active members of the diabetes care team.

REFERENCES

1. American Diabetes Association Web site. Basic diabetes information: facts and figures. Available at: http://www.diabetes.org/diabetes-statistics/national-diabetes-fact-sheet.jsp. Accessed January 7, 2004.

2. Boyle JP, Honeycutt AA, Narayan KMV, Hoerger TJ, Geiss LS, Chen H, Thompson TJ. Projection of diabetes burden through 2050: impact of changing demography and disease prevalence in the U.S. *Diabetes Care.* 2001;24:1936–1940.

3. Diabetes Control and Complications Trial Research Group: The effect of intensive treatment of diabetes on the development and progression of long-term complications in insulin-dependent diabetes mellitus. *N Engl J Med.* 1993;329:977–986.

4. UK Prospective Diabetes Study Group: Intensive blood-glucose control with sulphonylureas or insulin compared with conventional treatment and risk of complications in patients with type 2 diabetes (UKPDS 33). *Lancet.* 1998;352:837–853.

5. Diabetes Prevention Program Research Group. Reduction in the incidence of type 2 diabetes with lifestyle intervention or metformin. *N Engl J Med.* 2002;346:393–403.

6. American Diabetes Association. Clinical practice recommendations 2004: diagnosis and classification of diabetes mellitus. *Diabetes Care.* 2004;27(Suppl 1):S5–S10.

7. Ratner RE. Pathophysiology of the diabetes disease state. In: Franz M, ed. *A Core Curriculum for Diabetes Education: Diabetes and Complications.* Chicago, Ill: American Association of Diabetes Educators; 2003:3–18.

8. Thai A-C, Eisenbarth GS. Natural history of IDDM. *Diabetes Rev.* 1993;1:1–14.

9. Ward WK, Beard JC, Halter JB, Pfeifer MA, Porte D. Pathophysiology of insulin secretion in non-insulin-dependent diabetes mellitus. *Diabetes Care.* 1984; 7:491–502.

10. Rossetti L, Giaccari A, DeFronzo RA. Glucose toxicity. *Diabetes Care.* 1990;13:610–630.

11. LeRoith D, Zick Y. Recent advances in our understanding of insulin activation and insulin resistance. *Diabetes Care.* 2001;24:588–597.

12. American Diabetes Association and National Institute of Diabetes and Digestive and Kidney Diseases. Position statement: the prevention or delay of type 2 diabetes. *Clin Diabetes.* 2001;19:127–130.

13. American Diabetes Association. Clinical practice recommendations 2005: standards of medical care in diabetes. *Diabetes Care.* 2005;28(Suppl 1):S4–S36.

14. American College of Endocrinology (ACE) and American Association of Clinical Endocrinologists (AACE) Consensus Panel. American College of Endocrinology consensus statement on guidelines for glycemic control. *Endocrine Pract.* 2002;8(Suppl 1):5–11.

15. Expert Panel on the Detection, Evaluation and Treatment of High Blood Cholesterol in Adults. Executive summary of the Third Report of the National Cholesterol Education Program (NCEP) Expert Panel on the Detection, Evaluation, and Treatment of High Blood Cholesterol in Adults (Adult Treatment Panel III). *JAMA.* 2001;285:2486–2497.

16. Alberti KG, Zimet PZ. Definition, diagnosis, and classification of diabetes mellitus and its complications. Part 1: diagnosis and classification of diabetes mellitus provisional report of a WHO consultation. *Diabet Med.* 1998;15:539–553.

17. Ford ES, Giles WH, Dietz WH. Prevalence of the metabolic syndrome among US adults. Findings from the Third National Health and Nutrition Examination Study. *JAMA.* 2002;287:356–359.

18. Isomaa B, Almgren P, Tiinamaija T, Forsen B, Lahti K, Nissen M, Taskinen MR, Groop L. Cardiovascular morbidity and mortality associated with the metabolic syndrome. *Diabetes Care.* 2001;24:683–689.

19. Dunaif A, Thomas A. Current concepts in the polycystic ovary syndrome. *Ann Rev Med.* 2001;52: 401–419.

20. American Diabetes Association. Clinical practice recommendations 2004: gestational diabetes. *Diabetes Care* 2004;27(Suppl 1):S88–S90.

21. Biastre S. Gestational diabetes. In: Franz M, ed. *A Core Curriculum for Diabetes Education: Diabetes and Complications.* Chicago, Ill: American Association of Diabetes Educators; 2001:73–97.

22. American Diabetes Association. Clinical practice recommendations 2004: screening for type 2 diabetes. *Diabetes Care.* 2004;25(Suppl 1):S11–14.

23. American Diabetes Association. Consensus statement: postprandial blood glucose. *Diabetes Care.* 2001;24:775–778.

24. American Diabetes Association. Clinical practice recommendations 2004: preconception care of women with diabetes. *Diabetes Care.* 2004;27(suppl 1):S76–S78.

25. American Diabetes Association. Clinical practice recommendations 2004: nephropathy in diabetes. *Diabetes Care.* 2004;27(Suppl 1):S79–S83.

ADDITIONAL RESOURCES

American Diabetes Association. *Medical Management of Type 1 Diabetes.* 4th ed. Alexandria, Va: American Diabetes Association; 2003.

American Diabetes Association. *Medical Management of Type 2 Diabetes.* 5th ed. Alexandria, Va: American Diabetes Association; 2005.

5

Diabetes Prevention

Judith Wylie-Rosett, EdD, RD, and Linda M. Delahanty, MS, RD

CHAPTER OVERVIEW

- Lifestyle changes, such as increased energy intake and decreased physical activity, promote obesity, which in turn is a risk factor for type 2 diabetes. Genetic susceptibility also appears to play a strong role in the occurrence of type 2 diabetes in certain populations.
- Lifestyle modification, including nutrition therapy, is the cornerstone of type 2 diabetes prevention and treatment.
- Evidence suggests that there are clinical precursors to type 2 diabetes, that it is possible to delay and/or prevent type 2 diabetes, and that nutrition therapy has an important role in type 2 diabetes prevention.

CLINICAL PRECURSORS TO TYPE 2 DIABETES

Type 2 diabetes results from the following:

- *A deficit in early insulin secretion*—Blunted early insulin secretion leads to postprandial hyperglycemia, which may contribute to progressive beta-cell deterioration, further exacerbating early insulin secretion deficiency.
- *Insulin resistance of muscle, liver, and adipose tissue*—As a result of obesity, insulin becomes less effective. Increased demand due to insulin resistance causes insulin levels to rise. If the pancreas

cannot produce enough insulin to compensate for increased requirement, blood glucose rises.

Prediabetes

Prediabetes is defined as a blood glucose level above normal but below the level diagnostic for diabetes based on either impaired fasting glucose (IFG) or impaired glucose tolerance (IGT) (1,2) (see Table 4.3 in Chapter 4). There is growing evidence that prediabetes is associated with insulin resistance, greater risk of progression to type 2 diabetes, and an increased risk of cardiovascular disease and death (2). Intervention during the prediabetes period can prevent the development of overt type 2 diabetes (2).

The American Diabetes Association recommends screening for prediabetes (IFG or IGT) in high-risk, asymptomatic, undiagnosed adults and children within the health care setting (2). Measurement of fasting plasma glucose and the 2-hour value in an oral glucose tolerance test are safe, acceptable, predictive, and widely available tests used to detect prediabetes. Box 4.2 in Chapter 4 presents a detailed list of risk factors. In brief, screening for prediabetes should be considered for the following individuals (2):

- Individuals 45 years old or older, particularly if their body mass index (BMI) is 25 or higher.
- Overweight individuals younger than 45 years old if they have another risk factor for diabetes.

Repeat screening at 3-year intervals is suggested (2).

The National Diabetes Education Program has launched a diabetes prevention campaign, "Small Steps, Big Rewards: Prevent Type 2 Diabetes," which targets those individuals with prediabetes. Materials are available on the National Diabetes Education Program Web site (3).

Metabolic Syndrome

Impaired fasting glucose is just one component of metabolic syndrome, also referred to as insulin resistance syndrome, syndrome X, dysmetabolic syndrome, and multiple metabolic syndrome (4–6). Insulin resistance is a key characteristic of individuals with metabolic syndrome and is often accompanied by hypertension and dyslipidemia. When insulin-resistant individuals cannot maintain the high insulin levels required to overcome insulin resistance, type 2 diabetes develops.

Metabolic syndrome denotes a constellation of metabolic abnormalities in serum or plasma insulin/glucose ratios, lipids (triglycerides, low-density lipoprotein [LDL] cholesterol subtypes, and/or high-density lipoprotein [HDL] cholesterol), uric acid level, coagulation factor imbalance, and vascular physiology (6). The criteria for metabolic syndrome established by the American Association of Clinical Endocrinologists include the following:

- Major criteria
  - Insulin resistance (denoted by hyperinsulinemia relative to glucose levels) or
  - Acanthosis nigricans
  - Central obesity (waist circumference greater than 102 cm [40 inches] for men and greater than 88 cm [35 inches] for women)
  - Dyslipidemia (HDL cholesterol less than 45 mg/dL for women and less than 35 mg/dL for men, or triglycerides greater than 150 mg/dL)
  - Hypertension
  - Impaired fasting glucose or type 2 diabetes
  - Hyperuricemia
- Minor features
  - Hypercoagulability
  - Polycystic ovary syndrome
  - Vascular endothelial dysfunction
  - Microalbuminuria
  - Coronary heart disease

The National Cholesterol Education Program Adult Treatment Panel III (NCEP ATP III) defined metabolic syndrome as the presence of three or more of the following risk determinants (4):

- Increased waist circumference (> 102 cm [> 40 inches] for men; > 88 cm [> 35 inches] for women)
- Elevated triglycerides (≥ 150 mg/dL)
- Low HDL cholesterol (< 40 mg/dL in men; < 50 mg/dL in women)
- Hypertension (≥ 130 /≥ 85 mm Hg)
- Impaired fasting glucose (≥ 110 mg/dL) (subsequently defined as ≥ 100 mg/dL based on the American Diabetes Association diagnostic criteria for diabetes)

Many of these components are not routinely evaluated and, therefore, may not be helpful in categorizing individuals. Biomarkers related to these metabolic dysfunctions are useful, however, to describe the scope of the syndrome, and in research to evaluate the effects of strategies to improve metabolic function.

Therapeutic objectives include reducing the effects of underlying causes, such as overweight or obesity and physical inactivity. Emphasis on weight reduction is to enhance LDL cholesterol–lowering and to reduce metabolic syndrome risk factors. Treatment of metabolic syndrome should address associated lipid and nonlipid risk factors, such as hypertension, prothrombotic state, and atherogenic dyslipidemia.

Increased emphasis on risks associated with metabolic syndrome has affected diagnostic coding, with the Centers for Disease Control and Prevention (CDC) establishing dysmetabolic syndrome as ICD-9 code 277.7 (6). This code denotes the constellation of abnormalities noted above in relation to metabolic syndrome. The CDC does not require that a given number of components of dysmetabolic syndrome be present to use 277.7 for dysmetabolic syndrome. Rather, the code may be used based on the professional opinion of the physician that dysmetabolic syndrome is present.

EVIDENCE FOR DELAYING AND/OR PREVENTING TYPE 2 DIABETES

Recent reviews have carefully evaluated studies indicating that lifestyle intervention can alter the natural history of type 2 diabetes and delay or possibly prevent the progression from impaired glucose regulation to overt diabetes in high risk individuals (7–9). See Table 5.1 for a summary of the major diabetes prevention studies and their findings (10–18).

TABLE 5.1 Summary of Major Diabetes Prevention Trials

Study Name (Duration)	Study Population	Design and Study Interventions	Study Findings
Da Qing IGT and Diabetes Prevention Study (10) (6 y)	577 individuals identified with IGT in population screen Mean age = 44 y, mean BMI = 25.8	Quasi experimental design for study randomized by clinic (N = 33) in 4-arm trial. Control clinics: No intervention Intervention clinics: • Diet alone • Exercise alone • Diet and exercise	The cumulative incidence of diabetes at 6 years was 67.7% in the control group compared with 43.8% in the diet group, 41.1% in the exercise group, and 46.0% in the diet-plus-exercise group ($P < .05$). In a proportional hazards analysis adjusted for differences in baseline BMI and fasting glucose, the diet, exercise, and diet-plus-exercise interventions were associated with 31% ($P < .03$), 46% ($P < .001$), and 42% ($P < .005$) reductions in risk of developing diabetes, respectively.
Finnish Diabetes Prevention Study (FDPS) (11,12) (6 y; interim analysis at 3.3-y midpoint)	522 individuals with IGT Mean age = 55 y (range 40–64 y), mean fasting glucose = 110 mg/dL, mean BMI = 31	2-arm randomized trial Control arm: Brief diet and exercise counseling Intervention arm: Intensive individualized instruction on weight reduction, food intake, and increasing physical activity	58% relative risk reduction in the incidence of diabetes in intervention arm. In interim analysis, intervention group showed significantly greater improvements in each intervention goal. After 1 and 3 years, weight reductions were 4.5 and 3.5 kg in the intervention group and 1.0 kg and 0.9 kg in the control group, respectively. Measures of glycemia and lipemia improved more in the intervention group.
Diabetes Prevention Program (DPP) (13) (2.8 y)	3234 ethnically diverse individuals with IGT Mean age = 51 y (range 25–85), mean fasting glucose = 106 mg/dL (range 95–125 mg/dL), mean BMI = 34	3-arm randomized trial* Control arm: Placebo pills plus information on diet and exercise in annual 20- to 30-min individual session Intensive lifestyle arm: education to address diet, exercise, and behavior in 16-session core program during the first 24 weeks, follow-up sessions (usually monthly), and booster educational campaigns. Minimum treatment goals were 7% weight loss and 150 min/wk physical activity. Medication arm: 850 mg metformin twice daily plus information on diet and exercise in annual 20- to 30-min individual session	58% relative risk reduction (cumulative incidence 48%–66%) in the progression to diabetes with intensive lifestyle and a 31% relative risk reduction (cumulative incidence 17%–43%) with metformin. The estimated cumulative incidence of diabetes at three years was 28.9%, 21.7%, and 14.4% in the placebo, metformin, and lifestyle-intervention groups, respectively. Half of the participants in the lifestyle-intervention group achieved the 7% weight-loss goal at the end of the curriculum (at 24 weeks), and 38% had a weight loss ≥ 7% at the time of the most recent visit; the proportion of participants who met the goal of at least 150 min/wk physical activity (assessed on the basis of logs kept by the participants) was 74% at 24 weeks and 58% at the most recent visit.

(continued)

TABLE 5.1 *(Continued)*

Study Name (Duration)	Study Population	Design and Study Interventions	Study Findings
STOP-NIDDM (14) (3.3 y)	1429 individuals with IGT Mean age = 55 y, mean fasting glucose = 100–139 mg/dL, BMI > 31	Double-blind, 2-arm trial: placebo group vs acarbose group (100 mg acarbose or placebo 3 times daily)	Diabetes developed in 221 (32%) patients randomized to acarbose and 285 (42%) randomized to placebo (relative risk reduction 25%, $P = .0015$). 211 (31%) of 682 patients in the acarbose group and 130 (19%) of 686 on placebo discontinued treatment early, usually due to treatment side effects.
Troglitazone in the Prevention of Diabetes (TRIPOD) (15) (2.5 y)	266 Hispanic women with recent gestational diabetes Mean age = 35 y, mean fasting glucose = 94 mg/dL, mean BMI = 30	Double-blind 2-arm trial: placebo group vs troglitazone group	There was a 56% relative risk reduction in the progression to diabetes in the troglitazone group. After a > 8-month washout period, the preventive effects of the drug were still observed.
Fasting Hyperglycemia Study (16,17) (1 y)	227 individuals Fasting glucose = 99–137 mg/dL, mean weight = 180 lb	2-by-2 factorial design. Participants were randomized to reinforced or basic healthy living advice and to sulfonylurea treatment or control group.	Participants in the reinforced advice arm had better fitness measures ($P = .007$), but did not have better FPG, glucose tolerance, A1C, or lipid livels than the basic advice treatment arm. The sulfonylurea treatment arm had a reduction in FPG (108–100 mg/dL; $P < .001$) and A1C (5.8%–5.6%; $P < .0002$), but the placebo did not (FPG, 108–108 mg/dL; A1C, 5.7%–5.6%, NS).
Malmö Feasibility Trial (18) (5 y)	181 men with IGT in the intervention program vs 79 who would not or could not participate Mean age = 48 y	A 5-y protocol, including dietary treatment and/or increase of physical activity or training with annual check-ups.	The lifestyle intervention was associated with a 63% relative risk reduction; the accumulated incidence of diabetes was 10.6% with intervention vs 28.6% with no intervention. Glucose tolerance normalized in > 50% of intervention particpants. Blood pressure, lipid levels, and hyperinsulinaemia were reduced. Improvement in glucose tolerance was correlated to weight reduction (r = 0.19, $P < .02$) and increased fitness (r = 0.22, $P < .02$).

Abbreviations: BMI, body mass index; CI, confidence interverval; FPG, fasting plasma glucose; IGT, impaired glucose tolerance; OGTT, oral glucose tolerance test.
*The study initially had a fourth study arm (troglitazone). It was discontinued because of liver toxicity.

The Da Qing Impaired Glucose Tolerance and Diabetes Prevention Study was conducted using a quasi experimental design in which 33 clinics were randomized to four intervention conditions that included a control, dietary intervention alone, exercise alone, and combined diet and exercise intervention. At-risk individuals with impaired glucose tolerance were identified in a population screening. All the interventions resulted in a reduced incidence of diabetes (10).

The Finnish Diabetes Prevention Study was the first randomized controlled trial that provided evidence that diabetes could be prevented in individuals with impaired glucose tolerance by providing a lifestyle intervention (11,12). The Diabetes Prevention Program (DPP), which was a much larger trial, strengthened the evidence base and provided evidence that an intensive lifestyle intervention was more effective than medication in diabetes prevention (13). Both the Finnish study and DPP found a 58% relative risk reduction in the incidence of diabetes in the lifestyle intervention groups (11,13), and DPP found that the intensive lifestyle was much more effective than metformin, which achieved a 31% relative risk reduction (13).

Other randomized diabetes prevention studies include the STOP-NIDDM trial, which found that acarbose achieved a 25% relative risk reduction compared with placebo (14); the Troglitazone in the Prevention of Diabetes (TRIPOD) trial, which found a 56% relative risk reduction in developing diabetes with troglitazone compared with placebo (15); and the Fasting Hyperglycemia Study, a two-by-two factorial study, which found improvement with sulfonylurea treatment but not reinforced lifestyle advice (16,17). The Malmö Prevention Project found that individuals with impaired glucose tolerance who chose to be in diet and exercise intervention had a 12-year mortality rate that was similar to individuals with normal glucose tolerance, and less than half the rate of those who did not participate in the lifestyle intervention (18,19). Because the individuals were not randomized, it is difficult to assess how much the two groups with impaired glucose tolerance differed.

Finnish Diabetes Prevention Study

Overview

Lifestyle interventions for the Finnish Diabetes Prevention Study (11) included counseling with a nutritionist seven times during the first year and every 3 months thereafter throughout the course of the study. Goals included the following:

- Weight reduction of 5% or more
- Total fat intake less than 30% of energy consumed
- Saturated fat intake less than 10% of energy consumed
- Fiber intake of at least 15 g/1,000 kcal
- Moderate exercise of at least 30 min/day— endurance exercise with circuit-type resistance training sessions also offered

Frequent consumption of whole-meal products, vegetables, berries and fruit, low-fat milk and meat products, soft margarines, and vegetable oils rich in monounsaturated fatty acids was recommended. The average follow-up was 3.2 years.

Findings

The mean weight loss by the end of year 2 was 3.5 kg in the intervention group and 0.8 kg in the control group. The risk of developing diabetes was reduced by 58% in the intervention group; this risk reduction was directly associated with the lifestyle changes. None of the individuals who had reached all five lifestyle goals by the 1-year visit developed type 2 diabetes, whereas approximately one third of the individuals who did not reach any of the targets developed type 2 diabetes (11,12).

Diabetes Prevention Program

Overview

In the DPP (13,20), intense lifestyle intervention education was provided primarily by case managers or lifestyle coaches; the majority were registered dietitians. The lifestyle intervention included the following four components:

1. A 16-session structured "core curriculum" delivered in individual sessions during the first 24 weeks; topics of the first 16 sessions incorporate nutrition, exercise, and behavioral topics. The educational materials are available for download at the DPP Study Documents Web site (21).
2. Tailored individual intervention with contacts at least monthly (see Table 5.2 for a list of some of the individual intervention topics; materials are available for download at the DPP Study Documents Web site [21]).
3. A tool-box approach to tailor strategies to each individual's barriers to success (see Table 5.3 [22]).
4. Four- to eight-week "after core" group classes and campaigns to help sustain lifestyle goals and motivation and to offer peer support.

The following features of the lifestyle change process were designed to assist with weight loss (13,20):

- *Goal setting.* Each participant received goals for fat and energy intake (see Table 5.4 [20]), weight loss, and activity level.
- *Self-monitoring.* Participants monitored portions, calories, fat, and physical activity. Weight graphs and record-keeping booklets were used.

TABLE 5.2 Tailored Individual Intervention Topics*

Nutrition	Activity	Behavior
• Binge eating	• Staying active on vacation	• Handling holidays/vacations
• Emotional eating	• Make it fun	• Motivation
• Food cues	• Focus on flexibility	• Problem solving
• Fat in foods	• Getting moving after work	• Self-monitoring
• Meal planning/cooking	• Just do it commitment	• Self-talk

*Materials are available for download at the Diabetes Prevention Program Study Documents Web site (http://www.bsc.gwu.edu/dpp).
Source: Data are from reference 21.

TABLE 5.3 Tool-Box Strategies for Barriers to Lifestyle Change

Barriers	Tool-Box Strategies
Activity	
• Inconsistent self-monitoring	• Use problem solving
• Illness/injury	• Try new self-monitoring approach
• Aches and pains	• Identify exercise event/class
• Internal cues (stress/emotions)	• Borrow self-help materials
• Diminished motivation	• Acquire pedometer
• Time management problems	• Set up motivational strategy/ incentive/contract
• Significant life events	• Use exercise physiologist/trainer
• Access to exercise equipment	• Meet with behavioral therapist
• Weather	
Weight Loss	
• Inaccurate self-monitoring	• Use problem solving
• Poor cooking/shopping skills	• Change self-monitoring approach
• Vacation/work or family demands	• Increase contact frequency
• Internal cues (stress, binge eating, depression, emotional eating)	• Lower calorie/fat-gram goals
• Significant life events	• Obtain structured menus
• Time management problems	• Use meal replacements
• Diminished motivation	• Borrow self-help materials
• Bored with meal plan	• Use incentives/contracts

*Materials are available for download at the Diabetes Prevention Program Study Documents Web site (http://www.bsc.gwu.edu/dpp). Go to Lifestyle Balance During Core Manual, Appendix G.
Source: Data are from reference 22.

- *Frequent contact.* Each participant met with a lifestyle coach at least 16 times during the first 24 weeks of the study, followed by a minimum of monthly contact (and in some cases weekly contact) for the remainder of the study. Frequent contact assisted participants in staying focused on their goals and self-monitoring skills.
- *Problem solving.* Constant focus on the problem-solving approach to behavior change was critical to success.
- *Managing high-risk situations to help ensure long-term success.* Participants learned strategies to manage eating-out situations, the impact of stress on eating and exercise routines, slips or lapses, negative self-talk, and problem food cues.

Goals were to achieve, and to maintain throughout the trial, at least a 7% weight loss by decreasing daily energy intake by 500 to 1,000 kcal, eating less than 25% of energy from fat, and increasing physical activity to moderate activity at least 150 minutes per week. Average follow-up was 2.8 years (13).

Findings

When compared with the placebo control, intensive lifestyle intervention reduced the risk of developing type 2 diabetes by 58%, and metformin reduced the risk of developing type 2 diabetes by 31% (13). Metformin was as effective as lifestyle intervention in individuals 24 to 44 years old, or in those with a BMI of greater than 35. However, it was nearly ineffective in older adults (60 years or older) or in those with a lower BMI (< 30). Treatment effects did not differ based on sex, race, or ethnic group (13).

In the entire study, the average weight loss in the lifestyle intervention group was 5.6 kg (13). Researchers found the following:

- For every kilogram of weight lost, a 13% risk reduction for developing type 2 diabetes was noted (23).
- For every kilogram of weight lost, participants reporting the lowest percentage of calories from fat had a greater decrease in the risk for developing diabetes (23).
- Among the participants in the placebo arm, 29% developed overt diabetes during the 3 years of follow-up, compared with 22% in the metformin arm and 14% in the intensive lifestyle arm (13).

For each case of diabetes that was prevented in the DPP, the intensive lifestyle intervention cost was $15,800 and the metformin treatment cost was $31,300 (24). If similar lifestyle changes could be achieved in a group intervention with ten participants, the cost per case of diabetes prevented would decrease to $4,000. If generic metformin were used, the cost per case of diabetes prevented would decrease to $11,000. Because lifestyle intervention was considerably more effective in preventing diabetes, the cost per case of diabetes prevented was lower than for metformin-treated subjects (24).

Although longer-term follow-up is needed to determine the effects of intervention on cardiovascular risk, lifestyle intervention did reduce the magnitude of some cardiovascular disease factors (25–27).

NUTRITION THERAPY AND DIABETES PREVENTION

Type 2 Diabetes in Adults

Findings from the major diabetes prevention studies underscore the importance of education and lifestyle intervention in delaying or preventing type 2 diabetes. Use of drug therapy to prevent or delay type 2

TABLE 5.4 Diabetes Prevention Program Lifestyle Intervention: Fat, Energy, and Weight-Loss Goals

Initial Weight, lb	Fat Goal, g/d*	Energy Goal, kcal/d	Weight-Loss Goal, lb†
120–170	33	1200	8.5–12
175–215	42	1500	12–15
220–245	50	1800	15–17
250–300	55	2000	17–21

*To provide approximately 25% of energy from fat.
†Weight-loss goal equals 7% of initial weight.
Source: Data are from reference 20.

diabetes appears to be less effective and less beneficial (2). Nutrition therapy guidelines for delaying and preventing type 2 diabetes include the following:

- *Moderate, sustained weight loss of 5% to 10% of body weight* (11,23). A variety of meal-planning approaches can assist in weight loss, with intervention tailored to each individual's particular cultural beliefs, traditions, and lifestyles (20).
- *An active lifestyle including at least 30 minutes of modest physical activity daily* (11,23). Individuals should be encouraged to increase activity as they make food and behavior changes.
- *Reduced intake of fat, particularly saturated fat* (28). Current recommendations focus on controlling or reducing body weight by regular physical activity and avoidance of excessive energy intake from all sources, particularly by decreasing fat and saturated fats and by increasing consumption of fiber-rich carbohydrates, vegetables, and fruits (2,7–9).
- *Increased intake of whole grains and dietary fiber* (28). Recent studies suggest that an increased intake of whole grains and dietary fiber is associated with reduced risk for type 2 diabetes (29–32).
- *Moderate alcohol intake* (28). Light to moderate alcohol intake in nondiabetic adults has been related to improved insulin sensitivity and reduced risk for type 2 diabetes. Insufficient data exist to support specific alcohol recommendations for diabetes prevention (28).

Type 1 Diabetes

For type 1 diabetes, no nutrition recommendations can be made regarding prevention, although breastfeeding may be beneficial (28). An NIH-sponsored multicenter study, the Diabetes Prevention Trial 1 (DPT-1), was designed to determine whether low-dose insulin administered orally or by injections could delay or prevent type 1 diabetes in individuals at significant risk of developing the disease within 5 years. The DPT-1 randomly assigned 339 individuals at high risk (> 50% risk) for disease development, based on signs of autoimmune beta-cell destruction and low insulin response to an intravenous glucose challenge, to receive insulin or to serve as control subjects. The rate of development of diabetes was identical (60%) in both groups, which indicates that injection of low-dose insulin does not delay or prevent type 1 diabetes. A second arm of the DPT-1,

using oral insulin in those at moderate risk (25%-50% risk) of developing diabetes, is ongoing (33).

SUMMARY

Prediabetes and metabolic syndrome are associated with increased risk for developing type 2 diabetes. Evidence suggests that type 2 diabetes can be delayed or prevented by lifestyle intervention.

REFERENCES

1. American Diabetes Association. Position statement: diagnosis and classification of diabetes mellitus. *Diabetes Care*. 2005;28(Suppl 1):S37–S42.
2. American Diabetes Association. Position statement: standards of medical care in diabetes. *Diabetes Care*. 2005;28(Suppl 1):S4–S36.
3. National Diabetes Education Program. HHS/NDEP Diabetes Prevention Campaign. Available at: http://www.ndep.nih.gov/index.htm. Accessed January 10, 2005.
4. Expert Panel on Detection, Evaluation, and Treatment of High Blood Cholesterol in Adults. Executive summary of the Third Report of the National Cholesterol Education Program (NCEP) Expert Panel on Detection, Evaluation, and Treatment of High Blood Cholesterol in Adults (Adult Treatment Panel III). *JAMA*. 2001; 285:2486–2497.
5. ACE position statement. *Endocrine Pract*. 2003; 9;240–252.
6. New ICD-9-CM Code for Dysmetabolic Syndrome X. Available at: http://www.aace.com/members/socio/syndromex.php. Accessed January 10, 2005.
7. Tuomilehto J, Lindström J. The major diabetes prevention trials. *Curr Diab Rep*. 2003;3:115–122.
8. Steyn NP, Mann J, Bennett PH, Temple N, Zimmet P, Tuomilehto J, Lindstrom J, Louheranta A. Diet, nutrition, and the prevention of type 2 diabetes. *Pub Health Nutr*. 2004;7:147–165.
9. Davies MJ, Tringham JR, Troughton J, Khunti KK. Prevention of type 2 diabetes mellitus. A review of the evidence and its application in a UK setting. *Diab Med*. 2004;21:403–414.
10. Pan XR, Li GW, Hu YH, Wang JX, Yang WY, An ZX, Hu ZX, Lin J, Xiao JZ, Cao HB, Liu PA, Jiang XG, Jiang YY, Wang JP, Zheng H, Zhang H, Bennett PH, Howard BV. Effects of diet and exercise in preventing NIDDM in people with impaired glucose tolerance. The Da Qing IGT and Diabetes Study. *Diabetes Care*. 1997;20:537–544.
11. Tuomilehto J, Lindstrom J, Eriksson JG, Valle TT, Hamalainen H, Ilanne-Parikka P, Keinanen-Kiukaanniemi

S, Laakso M, Louheranta A, Rastas M, Salminen V, Uusitupa M; Finnish Diabetes Prevention Study. Prevention of type 2 diabetes mellitus by changes in lifestyle among subjects with impaired glucose tolerance. *N Engl J Med.* 2001;344:1343–1350.

12. Lindstrom J, Louheranta A, Mannelin M, Rastas M, Salminen V, Eriksson J, Uusitupa M, Tuomilehto J; Finnish Diabetes Prevention Study Group. The Finnish Diabetes Prevention Study (DPS): lifestyle intervention and 3-year results on diet and physical activity. *Diabetes Care.* 2003;26:3230–3236.

13. Diabetes Prevention Program Research Group. Reduction in the incidence of type 2 diabetes with lifestyle intervention or metformin. *N Engl J Med.* 2002;346:393–403.

14. Chiasson JL, Josse RG, Gomis R, Hanefeld M, Karasik A, Laakso M for the STOP-NIDDM Trial. Acarbose for prevention of type 2 diabetes mellitus: the STOP-NIDDM randomised trial. *Lancet.* 2002;359:2072–2077.

15. Azen SP, Peters RK, Berkowitz K, Knos S, Xing A, Buchanan TP, for the TRIPOD Study group. TRIPOD (TRoglitazone In the Prevention of Diabetes): a randomized, placebo controlled trial of troglitazone in women with prior gestational diabetes. *Contr Clin Trials.* 1998;19:217–231.

16. Dyson PA, Hammersley MS, Morris RJ, Holman RR, Turner RC. The Fasting Hyperglycemia Study II. Randomized controlled trial of reinforced healthy-living advice in subject in increasing but not diabetic fasting plasma glucose. *Metabolism.* 1997;46(12 suppl 1):50–55.

17. Karunakaran S, Hammersley MS, Morris RJ, Turner RC, Holman RR. The Fasting Hyperglycaemia Study: III. Randomized controlled trial of sulfonylurea therapy in subjects with increased but not diabetic fasting plasma glucose. *Metabolism.* 1997;46(12 Suppl 1):56–60.

18. Eriksson KF, Lindgarde F. Prevention of type 2 (non-insulin-dependent) diabetes mellitus by diet and physical exercise. The 6-year Malmö feasibility study. *Diabetologia.* 1991;34:891–898.

19. Erikkson KF, Lindgarde F. No excess 12-year mortality in men with impaired glucose tolerance who participated in the Malmö Prevention trial with diet and exercise. *Diabetologia.* 1998;41:1010–1016.

20. Delahanty LM, Begay SR, Coocyate N, Hoskin M, Isonaga M, Levy E, Mikami K, Ka'iulani Odom S, Szamos K. The effectiveness of lifestyle intervention in the Diabetes Prevention Program (DPP): application in diverse ethnic groups. *On the Cutting Edge.* 2002;23(6):30–36.

21. Diabetes Prevention Program Study Documents Web site. Available at: http://www.bsc.gwu.edu/dpp. Accessed January 10, 2005.

22. Wing R, Gillis B. Lifestyle Balance: The Diabetes Prevention Program's Lifestyle Change Program. 1996. Available at: http://www.bsc.gwu.edu/dpp/lifestyle/lsmop1.pdf. Accessed January 10, 2005.

23. Diabetes Prevention Program Research Group. Effects of changes in weight, diet, and physical activity on risk of diabetes with intensive lifestyle intervention in the Diabetes Prevention Program (DPP). *Diabetes.* 2002;51(Suppl 2):A28.

24. Diabetes Prevention Program Research Group. Within-trial cost-effectiveness of lifestyle intervention or metformin for the primary prevention of type 2 diabetes. *Diabetes Care.* 2003;26:2518–2523.

25. Diabetes Prevention Program Research Group. Hypertension, insulin, and proinsulin in participants with impaired glucose tolerance. *Hypertension.* 2002;40:679–686.

26. Diabetes Prevention Program Research Group. Impact of lifestyle and metformin therapy on cardiovascular (CVD) risk factors and events in the Diabetes Prevention Program. *Diabetes.* 2003;52(Suppl 1):A169.

27. Diabetes Prevention Program Research Group. The effects of intensive lifestyle intervention (ILS) and metformin (MET) on C-reactive protein (CRP), tissue plasminogen activator (TPA) and fibrinogen (FIB) in the Diabetes Prevention Program. *Diabetes.* 2003;52(Suppl 1):A18.

28. American Diabetes Association. Position statement: evidence-based nutrition principles and recommendations for the treatment and prevention of diabetes and related complications. *J Am Diet Assoc.* 2002;102;109–118.

29. Meyer KA, Kushi LH, Jacobs DR Jr, Slavin J, Sellers TA, Folsom AR. Carbohydrates, dietary fiber, and incident type 2 diabetes in older women. *Am J Clin Nutr.* 2000;71:921–930.

30. Liu S, Manson JE, Stampfer MJ, Hu FB, Giovannucci E, Colditz GA, Hennekens CH, Willett WC. A prospective study of whole-grain intake and risk of type 2 diabetes mellitus in US women. *Am J Public Health.* 2000;90:1409–1415.

31. Fung TT, Hu FB, Pereira MA, Liu S, Stampfer MJ, Colditz GA, Willett WC. Whole-grain intake and risk of type 2 diabetes: a prospective study in men. *Am J Clin Nutr.* 2002;76:535–540.

32. Pereira MA, Jacobs DR Jr, Pins JJ, Raatz SK, Gross MD, Slavin JL, Seaquist ER. Effect of whole grains on insulin sensitivity in overweight hyperinsulinemic adults. *Am J Clin Nutr.* 2002;75:848–855.

33. American Diabetes Association. Position statement: prevention of type 1 diabetes. *Diabetes Care.* 2004;27(Suppl 1):S133.

ADDITIONAL RESOURCES

American Diabetes Association. Diabetes prevention. Available at: http://www.diabetes.org/diabetes-prevention.jsp. Accessed August 25, 2004.

Barceló A, Vovides Y. The Pan American Health Organization and World Diabetes Day. *Revista Panamericana de Salud Pública/Pan Am J Public Health.* 2001;10:297–299.

Benjamin SM, Valdez R, Geiss LS, Rolka DB, Narayan KM. Estimated number of adults with prediabetes in the US in 2000: opportunities for prevention. *Diabetes Care.* 2004;26:645–649.

Diabetes Prevention Program Research Group. The Diabetes Prevention Program: a description of the lifestyle intervention. *Diabetes Care.* 2002;25:2165- 2171.

Engelgau MM, Narayan KM, Vinicor F. Identifying the target population for primary prevention: the trade-offs. *Diabetes Care.* 2003;25:2098–2099.

Expert Committee on the Diagnosis and Classification of Diabetes Mellitus. Follow-up report on the diagnosis of diabetes mellitus. *Diabetes Care.* 2003;26:3160–3167.

Ginsberg HN. Treatment for patients with the metabolic syndrome. *Am J Cardiol.* 2003;91(suppl 7A):29E-39E.

Hanley AJ, Wagenknecht LE, D'Agostino RB Jr, Zinman B, Haffner SM. Identification of subjects with insulin resistance and beta-cell dysfunction using alternative definitions of the metabolic syndrome. *Diabetes.* 2003;52: 2740–2747.

Meigs JB. Epidemiology of the insulin resistance syndrome. *Curr Diab Rep.* 2003;3:73–79.

National Center for Chronic Disease Prevention and Health Promotion. National diabetes fact sheet. Available at: http://www.cdc.gov/diabetes/pubs/general.htm. Accessed August 25, 2004.

World Health Organization. *Obesity: Preventing and Managing the Global Epidemic.* Geneva, Switzerland: World Health Organization; 2000.

World Health Organization. *Using Domestic Law in the Fight against Obesity.* Geneva, Switzerland: World Health Organization; 2003.

Wylie-Rosett J, Delahanty L. An integral role of the dietitian: implications of the Diabetes Prevention Program. *J Am Diet Assoc.* 2002;102:1065–1068.

Part 3

Diabetes Management

6

Evidence-Based Nutrition Care and Recommendations

Lea Ann Holzmeister, RD, CDE, and Patti Geil, MS, RD, FADA, CDE

CHAPTER OVERVIEW

- Evidence from randomized controlled trials, observational studies, and meta-analyses supports the clinical effectiveness of medical nutrition therapy (MNT) in diabetes (1,2).
- MNT has a significant effect on improving metabolic control in individuals with diabetes when delivered using a systematic standardized process. Nutrition practice guidelines (NPGs) for type 1, type 2, and gestational diabetes have been developed to enable the dietetics professional to provide "best practice" nutrition care for individuals with diabetes.
- Use of a standardized process does not equate to standardized care; dietetics professionals need to be familiar with evidenced-based nutrition recommendations for individuals with diabetes (3–5) and should use critical thinking and decision-making skills when providing care, so that care can be individualized (6).

EVIDENCE FOR THE EFFECTIVENESS OF MNT

Pastors et al have published a comprehensive review of the evidence for the effectiveness of MNT in diabetes

management (1). The authors cite randomized controlled trials, observational studies, and meta-analyses that demonstrated metabolic outcomes, such as improved blood glucose level and A1C when MNT was either implemented independently or was delivered as part of an overall diabetes self-management training program The randomized controlled nutrition therapy outcome studies documented the following:

- Decreases in A1C of approximately 1% in newly diagnosed type 1 diabetes, of 2% in newly diagnosed type 2 diabetes, and of 1% in type 2 diabetes with an average duration of 4 years
- Reductions in use of health services and costs, suggesting that MNT is cost effective

In addition to MNT effectiveness studies, strong evidence suggests that interventions, such as intensive lifestyle modifications based on healthy eating and physical activity, are effective in delaying or preventing the onset of type 2 diabetes by 58% to 71% (7).

The way in which MNT is delivered can influence its effectiveness. NPGs are systematically developed statements designed to assist practitioner decisions about appropriate health care for specific clinical circumstances. The American Dietetic Association (ADA) provides NPGs for type 1, type 2, and gestational diabetes

(8,9). These NPGs are evidence-based, field-tested descriptions of the "best practice" nutrition care for individuals with diabetes. Research has documented that, when registered dietitians (RDs) implemented NPGs in their practice, A1C was reduced by an average of 1% to 2% in individuals with diabetes (10,11).

GOALS OF MNT FOR INDIVIDUALS WITH DIABETES

The three main goals of MNT for individuals with diabetes are as follows (3–5):

1. *To attain and maintain optimal metabolic outcomes.* The patient's blood glucose level should be in the normal range or as close to normal as is safely possible. The lipid and lipoprotein profile should reduce the individual's risk for macrovascular disease. Blood pressure level should be in a range that reduces the risk for vascular disease.
2. *To prevent and treat the chronic complications of diabetes.* Nutrient intake and lifestyle should be modified, as appropriate, for the prevention and treatment of obesity, dyslipidemia, cardiovascular disease, hypertension, and nephropathy.
3. *To improve health through healthful food choices and physical activity.* Treatment should address individual nutrition needs, considering the patient's personal and cultural preferences, lifestyle, individual wishes, and willingness to change.

Franz and associates' 2002 technical review (4) and the American Diabetes Association's nutrition recommendations (3) and standards (5) provide principles and recommendations according to the level of evidence available. Major nutrition recommendations are listed in Tables 6.1 through 6.6 (4,5). The scientific principles have been ranked based on the American Diabetes Association grading system. The highest ranking, A, is assigned when there is supportive evidence from multiple, well-conducted studies; B is an intermediate rating indicating some evidence; C is a lower ranking indicating limited evidence; and E represents recommendations based on expert consensus or clinical experience.

For information on nutrition recommendations for special populations (eg, older adults, pregnant women, or young people with diabetes), comorbidities of diabetes (eg, hypertension, dyslipidemia, or nephropathy), and acute complications, see Chapters 12 through 17 and Chapters 21 through 23.

IMPLICATIONS

Franz et al's 2002 technical review (4) and the American Diabetes Association's recommendations (3,5) aim to translate research data and clinically applicable evidence into nutrition care. The goal of evidence-based recommendations is to improve the quality of clinical judgments and facilitate cost-effective diabetes care. However, effective MNT considers nutrition recommendations based on scientific evidence as well as on individual circumstances, preferences, cultural and ethnic backgrounds, and lifestyles. The nutrition recommendations incorporate the need for healthy food choices and an active lifestyle.

The diabetes nutrition prescription is determined by considering diabetes treatment goals, desired outcomes, and lifestyle changes that the patient is willing and able to make. Components of MNT include monitoring of metabolic parameters, such as glucose, A1C, lipids, blood pressure, body weight, and renal function, when appropriate, as well as quality of life. Monitoring of these components is essential to assess the need for changes in therapy and to ensure successful outcomes.

The American Diabetes Association's evidence-based nutrition recommendations for diabetes distinguish MNT for treating and managing diabetes from MNT for preventing or delaying the onset of diabetes. Evidence for specific lifestyle goals and strategies for the prevention of diabetes are included in the American Diabetes Association's nutrition recommendations for diabetes care (3–5). For more information on prevention of diabetes, see Chapter 5.

The American Diabetes Association's evidence-based nutrition recommendations emphasize the importance of the dietetics professional, specifically the RD's knowledge and skill in diabetes management (3,5). The dietetics professional has the greatest expertise in providing MNT. However, all health care team members involved in diabetes treatment and management should understand MNT and should support the patient's need to make lifestyle changes.

TYPE 1 AND TYPE 2 DIABETES NPGS

The ADA's Nutrition Care Process (NCP) is a "systematic problem-solving method that dietetics professionals use to critically think and make decisions to address nutrition-related problems and provide safe and effective quality nutrition care" (6). The NCP articulates the consistent and specific steps a dietetics professional would

TABLE 6.1 Carbohydrate Recommendations for Both Type 1 and Type 2 Diabetes

Recommendations	Evidence Rating*
Foods containing carbohydrate from whole grains, fruits, vegetables, and low-fat milk are important components and should be included in a healthful diet.	A
Both the amount (grams) of carbohydrate as well as the type of carbohydrate in a food influence blood glucose level. Monitoring total grams of carbohydrate, whether by use of exchanges or carbohydrate counting, remains a key strategy in achieving glycemic control. The use of the glycemic index/glycemic load can provide an additional benefit over that observed when total carbohydrate is considered alone.	B
Low-carbohydrate diets (total carbohydrate < 130 g/d) are not recommended in the management of diabetes.	E
Carbohydrate and monounsaturated fat together should provide 60%–70% of energy intake.	E
Because sucrose does not increase glycemia to a greater extent than isocaloric amounts of starch, sucrose and sucrose-containing foods do not need to be restricted by people with diabetes; however, they should be substituted for other carbohydrate sources or, if added, should be covered with insulin or other glucose-lowering medication.	A
Sucrose and sucrose-containing foods should be eaten in the context of a healthful diet.	E
Fructose reduces postprandial glycemia when it replaces sucrose or starch. However, consumption of fructose in large amounts may have adverse effects on plasma lipids.	B
The use of added fructose as a sweetening agent is not recommended.	C
There is no reason to recommend that individuals with diabetes avoid naturally occurring fructose in fruits, vegetables, and other food.	E
The use of sugar alcohols as sweetening agents appears to be safe. Sugar alcohols may cause diarrhea, especially in children.	B
It is unlikely that sugar alcohols in the amounts likely to be ingested in individual food servings or meals will contribute to a significant reduction in total energy or carbohydrate intake.	E
Resistant starches have no established benefit for people with diabetes.	C

Nonnutritive Sweeteners

Nonnutritive sweeteners are safe when consumed within the adequate daily intake levels established by the Food and Drug Administration.	A
It is unknown whether use of nonnutritive sweeteners improves long-term glycemic control or assists in weight loss.	E

*Evidence ratings follow American Diabetes Association grading system. The highest ranking, A, is assigned when there is supportive evidence from multiple, well-conducted studies; B is an intermediate rating indicating some evidence; C is a lower ranking indicating limited evidence; and E represents recommendations based on expert consensus or clinical experience.
Source: Adapted from Franz MJ, Bantle JP, Brunzell JD, Chiasson J-L, Garg A, Holzmeister LA, Hoogwerf BJ, Mayer-Davis E, Mooradian AD, Purnell JQ, Wheeler M. Evidence-based nutrition principles and recommendations for the treatment and prevention of diabetes and related complications (technical review). *Diabetes Care.* 2002;25:148–198, with permission from the American Diabetes Association. Copyright © 2002, American Diabetes Association; and from American Diabetes Association. Standards of medical care in diabetes. *Diabetes Care.* 2005;28(Suppl 1):S4–S36 with permission from the American Diabetes Association. Copyright © 2005, American Diabetes Association.

TABLE 6.2 Carbohydrate Recommendations Specific to Type 1 and Type 2 Diabetes

Recommendations	Evidence Rating*
Type 1	
Individuals receiving intensive insulin therapy should adjust their premeal insulin dosages based on the carbohydrate content of meals.	B
Individuals receiving fixed daily insulin dosages should try to be consistent in day-to-day carbohydrate intake.	C
Percentage of carbohydrate should be based on an individual nutrition assessment.	B
Dietary fiber intake is encouraged for the general public. However, there is no evidence to recommend that people with diabetes consume a greater amount of fiber.	B
Type 2	
As for the general population, consumption of fiber is to be encouraged. Although large amounts of dietary fiber (approx 50 g/d) may have beneficial effects on glycemia, insulinemia, and lipidemia, it is not known whether such high levels of fiber intake can be maintained.	B
Carbohydrate and monounsaturated fat should together provide 60%–70% of energy intake. However, the individual's metabolic profile and need for weight loss should be considered when determining the monounsaturated fat content of the diet. Increasing fat intake may result in increased energy intake.	E

*Evidence ratings follow American Diabetes Association grading system. The highest ranking, A, is assigned when there is supportive evidence from multiple, well-conducted studies; B is an intermediate rating indicating some evidence; C is a lower ranking indicating limited evidence; and E represents recommendations based on expert consensus or clinical experience.
Source: Adapted from Franz MJ, Bantle JP, Brunzell JD, Chiasson J-L, Garg A, Holzmeister LA, Hoogwerf BJ, Mayer-Davis E, Mooradian AD, Purnell JQ, Wheeler M. Evidence-based nutrition principles and recommendations for the treatment and prevention of diabetes and related complications (technical review). *Diabetes Care.* 2002;25:148–198, with permission from the American Diabetes Association. Copyright © 2002, American Diabetes Association.

TABLE 6.3 Protein Recommendations for Both Type 1 and Type 2 Diabetes

Recommendations	Evidence Rating*
In individuals with controlled type 2 diabetes, ingested protein does not increase plasma glucose concentrations, although ingested protein is just as potent a stimulant of insulin secretion as carbohydrate.	B
For persons with diabetes, there is no evidence to suggest that usual protein intake (15%–20% of total daily energy) should be modified if renal function is normal.	E
For diabetic individuals, especially those with less-than-optimal glycemic control, the protein requirement may be greater than the recommended dietary allowance but should not be greater than usual intake.	B
Contrary to advice often given to patients with diabetes, the available evidence suggests the following: • Dietary protein does not slow the absorption of carbohydrate. • Dietary protein and carbohydrate do not raise plasma glucose later than carbohydrate alone and thus do not prevent late-onset hypoglycemia.	B
It may be prudent to avoid protein intake > 20% of total daily energy.	C
The long-term effects of diets high in protein and low in carbohydrate are unknown. Although such diets may produce short-term weight loss and improved glycemia, it has not been established that weight loss is maintained. The long-term effect of such diets on plasma low-density lipoprotein cholesterol is also a concern.	E

*Evidence ratings follow American Diabetes Association grading system. The highest ranking, A, is assigned when there is supportive evidence from multiple, well-conducted studies; B is an intermediate rating indicating some evidence; C is a lower ranking indicating limited evidence; and E represents recommendations based on expert consensus or clinical experience.
Source: Adapted from Franz MJ, Bantle JP, Brunzell JD, Chiasson J-L, Garg A, Holzmeister LA, Hoogwerf BJ, Mayer-Davis E, Mooradian AD, Purnell JQ, Wheeler M. Evidence-based nutrition principles and recommendations for the treatment and prevention of diabetes and related complications (technical review). *Diabetes Care.* 2002;25:148–198, with permission from the American Diabetes Association. Copyright © 2002, American Diabetes Association.

TABLE 6.4 Fat Recommendations for Both Type 1 and Type 2 Diabetes

Recommendations	Evidence Rating*
< 10% of energy intake should be derived from saturated fats. Individuals with LDL cholesterol ≥ 100 mg/dL may benefit from lowering saturated fat intake to < 7% of energy intake.	A
Dietary cholesterol intake should be < 300 mg/d. Individuals with LDL cholesterol ≥ 100 mg/dL may benefit from lowering dietary cholesterol to < 200 mg/d.	A
Intake of *trans* fatty acids should be minimized.	B
Current fat replacers/substitutes approved by the FDA are safe for use in food.	A
To lower plasma LDL cholesterol, energy derived from saturated fat can be reduced if concurrent weight loss is desirable, or it can be replaced with carbohydrate or monounsaturated fat if weight loss is not a goal.	A
Polyunsaturated fat intake should be approximately 10% of energy intake.	C
In weight-maintaining diets, when monounsaturated fat is replaced with carbohydrate, it may beneficially affect postprandial glycemia and plasma triglycerides but not necessarily fasting plasma glucose or A1C.	B
Incorporation of two to three servings (approximately 2 g) of plant stanol or sterol food per day, substituted for similar food, will lower total and LDL cholesterol.	B
Reduced-fat diets, when maintained long-term, contribute to modest loss of weight and improvement in dyslipidemia.	B
Two or more servings of fish per week provide dietary n-3 polyunsaturated fat and can be recommended.	B
Monounsaturated fat and carbohydrate together should provide approximately 60%–70% of energy intake. However, increasing fat intake may result in increased energy intake.	E
Fat intake should be individualized and designed to fit ethnic and cultural backgrounds.	E
Use of low-fat food and fat replacers/substitutes by individuals with diabetes may reduce total fat and energy intake and thereby facilitate weight loss.	E

Abbreviations: FDA, Food and Drug Administration; LDL, low-density lipoproteins.
*Evidence ratings follow American Diabetes Association grading system. The highest ranking, A, is assigned when there is supportive evidence from multiple, well-conducted studies; B is an intermediate rating indicating some evidence; C is a lower ranking indicating limited evidence; and E represents recommendations based on expert consensus or clinical experience.
Source: Adapted from Franz MJ, Bantle JP, Brunzell JD, Chiasson J-L, Garg A, Holzmeister LA, Hoogwerf BJ, Mayer-Davis E, Mooradian AD, Purnell JQ, Wheeler M. Evidence-based nutrition principles and recommendations for the treatment and prevention of diabetes and related complications (technical review). *Diabetes Care.* 2002;25:148–198, with permission from the American Diabetes Association. Copyright © 2002, American Diabetes Association.

TABLE 6.5 Micronutrient Recommendations for Both Type 1 and Type 2 Diabetes

Recommendations	Evidence Rating*
There is no clear evidence of benefit from vitamin or mineral supplementation in individuals with diabetes who do not have underlying deficiencies. Exceptions include folate for prevention of birth defects (strong evidence) and calcium for prevention of bone disease (some evidence).	B
Although difficult to ascertain, if deficiencies of vitamins and minerals are identified, supplementation can be beneficial.	B
Routine supplementation of the diet with antioxidants is not advised, because of uncertainties related to long-term efficacy and safety.	B
Select populations, such as elderly individuals, pregnant or lactating women, strict vegetarians, and people on calorie-restricted diets, may benefit from supplementation with a multivitamin.	E
In individuals with diabetes, there is no evidence to suggest long-term benefit from herbal preparations.	E

*Evidence ratings follow American Diabetes Association grading system. The highest ranking, A, is assigned when there is supportive evidence from multiple, well-conducted studies; B is an intermediate rating indicating some evidence; C is a lower ranking indicating limited evidence; and E represents recommendations based on expert consensus or clinical experience.
Source: Adapted from Franz MJ, Bantle JP, Brunzell JD, Chiasson J-L, Garg A, Holzmeister LA, Hoogwerf BJ, Mayer-Davis E, Mooradian AD, Purnell JQ, Wheeler M. Evidence-based nutrition principles and recommendations for the treatment and prevention of diabetes and related complications (technical review). *Diabetes Care.* 2002;25:148–198, with permission from the American Diabetes Association. Copyright © 2002, American Diabetes Association.

TABLE 6.6 Alcohol Recommendations for Type 1 and Type 2 Diabetes

Recommendations	Evidence Rating*
If individuals choose to drink, daily intake should be limited to one drink for adult women and two drinks for adult men. One drink is defined as a 12-oz beer, 5-oz glass of wine, or 1.5-oz glass of distilled spirits. The type of alcoholic beverage consumed does not make a difference.	B
When moderate amounts of alcohol are consumed with food, blood glucose level is not affected. To reduce risk of hypoglycemia, alcohol should be consumed with food.	B
Ingestion of light-to-moderate amounts of alcohol does not raise blood pressure; excessive, chronic ingestion of alcohol raises blood pressure and may be a risk factor for stroke.	A
Pregnant women and people with medical problems, such as pancreatitis, advanced neuropathy, severe hypertriglyceridemia, or alcohol abuse, should be advised against ingesting alcohol.	A
There are potential benefits from the ingestion of moderate amounts of alcohol, such as decreased risk of type 2 diabetes, coronary heart disease, and stroke. (B)	B
Alcoholic beverages should be considered in addition to the regular food/meal plan for all patients with diabetes. No food should be omitted.	E

*Evidence ratings follow American Diabetes Association grading system. The highest ranking, A, is assigned when there is supportive evidence from multiple, well-conducted studies; B is an intermediate rating indicating some evidence; C is a lower ranking indicating limited evidence; and E represents recommendations based on expert consensus or clinical experience.
Source: Adapted from Franz MJ, Bantle JP, Brunzell JD, Chiasson J-L, Garg A, Holzmeister LA, Hoogwerf BJ, Mayer-Davis E, Mooradian AD, Purnell JQ, Wheeler M. Evidence-based nutrition principles and recommendations for the treatment and prevention of diabetes and related complications (technical review). *Diabetes Care.* 2002;25:148–198, with permission from the American Diabetes Association. Copyright © 2002, American Diabetes Association.

use when delivering MNT. The ADA's diabetes-specific NPGs provide a framework that enables the dietetics professional to deliver clinically effective as well as cost-effective nutrition care for individuals with diabetes. The NPGs are clinical applications of the NCP (see Chapter 1 for more on NCP).

Nutrition therapy varies for different types of diabetes. However, the underlying goal for all nutrition care for individuals with diabetes, regardless of type, is to attain and maintain optimal metabolic outcomes, including blood glucose level, lipid and lipoprotein profiles, and blood pressure level.

Type 1 Diabetes

Key Nutrition Principles

In individuals with type 1 diabetes, the insulin plan must be integrated into their lifestyle while considering food and physical activity preferences (3). For individuals receiving intensive insulin therapy, this means adjusting premeal insulin dosages based on the total carbohydrate content of each meal and snack, using an insulin-to-carbohydrate ratio. For individuals on a fixed daily dose of insulin, consistency of carbohydrate is the main recommendation. Although the carbohydrate content of the meal determines the premeal insulin dose, the protein and fat content of the diet should also be consid-

ered, to avoid weight gain and adverse effects on blood lipids. Physical activity is another key consideration in the nutrition care plan for people with type 1 diabetes. Additional carbohydrate may be needed for unplanned exercise. For planned exercise, reduction in the insulin dosage may be the best choice to prevent hypoglycemia.

Care Plan Flow

Working with an individual with diabetes to implement the key nutrition principles for type 1 diabetes is a systematic process, as outlined in the NPGs for type 1 diabetes (8). For information on the steps in the process and for a description of the steps, see Table 6.7 (8). Before the first patient encounter, the RD should collect

TABLE 6.7 Nutrition Practice Guidelines Steps for Type 1 and Type 2 Diabetes

Step	Description
Collect referral data	Necessary data include diagnosis; reason for referral/expected clinical outcome; diabetes therapy/duration/control level; medical history; medication plan; laboratory data (A1C, lipids, blood pressure, and renal function, if applicable); medical clearance for exercise, client care goals; input from health care team.
Identify assessment considerations	Considerations include the client's relevant medical history; present health status; diabetes knowledge, skill level, attitudes, and motivation; cultural influences; health beliefs/attitudes; self-efficacy; support systems; readiness to learn/change behaviors; barriers to learning; psychosocial and economic issues.
Collect assessment data	Necessary data include client goals; level of glycemic control; diabetes medication (insulin and/or oral agent) plan; usual schedule, usual food intake (meal times, composition, and macronutrient content), height and weight (BMI), physical activity level, blood glucose monitoring skills.
Perform intervention	Determine level of care: initial, continuing or ongoing, intensive. Prescribe nutrition care plan. Review MNT rationale/guidelines. Answer questions/concerns. Teach food/meal planning skills. Provide appropriate educational tools. Teach/fine-tune self-management skills. Promote problem-solving skills. Encourage physical activity. Encourage blood glucose monitoring. Provide counseling/support. Negotiate/establish short- and long-term goals (blood glucose, A1C, lipids, blood pressure, eating, exercise, weight). Develop/schedule follow-up plan.
Document care plan	Documentation should include client's short- and long-term goals, client's progress, nutrition prescription, the food/meal plan, educational topics covered, degree of patient acceptance and understanding, anticipated adherence, successful behavior changes, additional needed skills or information, additional recommendations, plans for ongoing care, and referrals to other providers, as needed.

Abbreviations: BMI, body mass index; MNT, medical nutrition therapy.
Source: Adapted from *American Dietetic Association Medical Nutrition Therapy Evidence-Based Guides for Practice: Nutrition Practice Guidelines for Type 1 and Type 2 Diabetes* [CD-ROM]. Chicago, Ill: American Dietetic Association; 2001, with permission from the American Dietetic Association.

referral data. During the first visit, time is spent assessing individual needs, collecting clinical data, developing an education and care plan, and providing an intervention. At subsequent visits, outcome data are collected and reviewed. The dietetics professional should track outcome measures, such as A1C, and should carefully document the evaluation, outcomes, and plan for ongoing care after each visit. Evaluation considerations are in Table 6.8. The level of care determines the optimal number of visits. See Figure 6.1 (12) for information from the NPGs on visits for initial, continuing, and follow-up care.

Type 2 Diabetes

Key Nutrition Principles

Lifestyle strategies centered on healthy eating and physical activity are key to nutrition therapy for type 2 diabetes (3). Individuals with type 2 diabetes are often overweight and insulin resistant, so their treatment plan emphasizes reduced energy intake and increased physical activity. Common comorbidities, such as dyslipidemia and hypertension, will also be improved with reductions in saturated fat, cholesterol, and sodium. The weight-loss programs with the most effective long-term success are structured and intensive, emphasizing lifestyle changes, education, reduced fat and energy intake, regular physical activity, and regular contact with the health care team. In type 2 diabetes, spacing of meals is determined by an individual's glucose control and medication, if any, which may affect nutrition therapy.

Care Plan Flow

The principles of delivery of the nutrition care plan are much the same as those for type 1 diabetes (see Tables 6.7 and 6.8) (8). For type 2 diabetes, the NPG outlines two levels of care: initial follow-up and ongoing care. See Figure 6.1 (12) for information on the specific number of visits recommended for people with type 2 diabetes.

TABLE 6.8 Evaluation Considerations: Type 1 and Type 2 Diabetes

Evaluate	Frequency

Self-monitoring:
• Food record
  ◦ macronutrient content of meal and snacks
  ◦ meal times
  ◦ snack frequency/content
• BG and medication record
  ◦ BG values
  ◦ Oral agent and/or insulin doses
• Activity/exercise patterns
  ◦ time and frequency
	Every visit

Specific behavior changes, per intervention plan	Every visit
Schedule changes	Every visit
Weight	Every visit
Height	Initial visit
A1C	Initially: ~ 4–6 weeks after lifestyle or medication changes; then 3–4 times a year
Lipid profile	Initially: 6 months after lifestyle or medication changes; then annually
Blood pressure	Every visit

Abbreviation: BG, blood glucose.
Source: Reprinted from American Dietetic Association Medical Nutrition Therapy Evidence-Based Guides for Practice: Nutrition Practice Guidelines for Type 1 and Type 2 Diabetes [CD-ROM]. Chicago, Ill: American Dietetic Association; 2001, with permission from the American Dietetic Association.

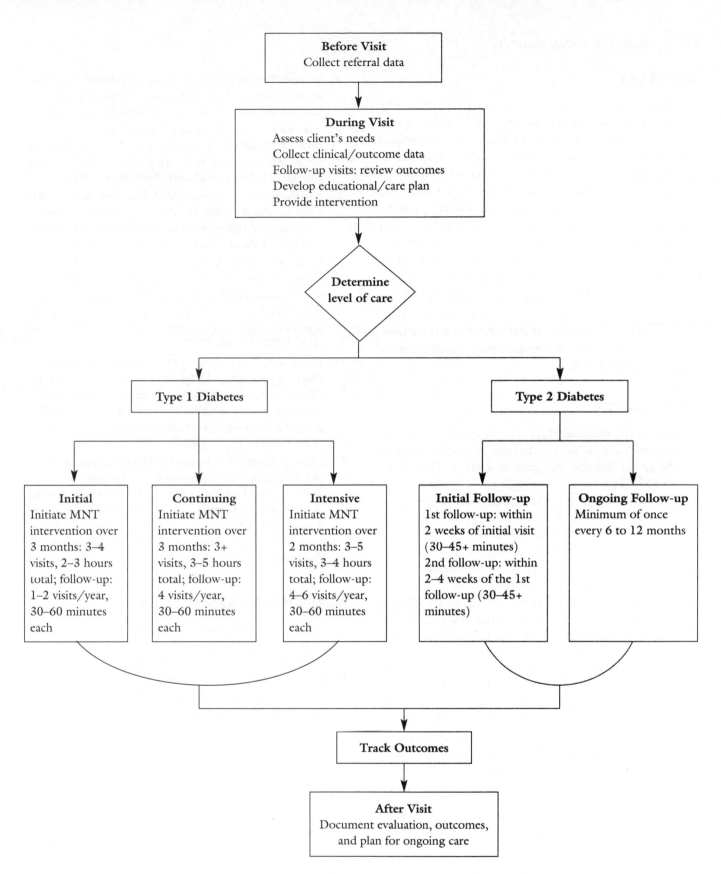

FIGURE 6.1 Diabetes nutrition practice guidelines for type 1 and type 2 diabetes. Adapted from *American Dietetic Association Medical Nutrition Therapy Evidence-Based Guides for Practice: Nutrition Practice Guidelines for Type 1 and Type 2 Diabetes* [CD-ROM]. Chicago, Ill: American Dietetic Association; 2001, with permission from the American Dietetic Association.

SUMMARY

Nutrition intervention has been noted to have the largest statistically significant effect on diabetes metabolic control (1,2,10,11). Evidence from randomized controlled trials, observational studies, and meta-analyses supports the clinical effectiveness of MNT in diabetes (1,2). NPGs have been developed and field tested with the goal of providing the dietetics professional with a road map to the "best practice" nutrition care for individuals with diabetes (10,11). Current recommendations for MNT for diabetes are based on scientific principles as well as on individual circumstances, preferences, and cultural and ethnic lifestyles (3–5). Effective MNT for diabetes combines scientific evidence with a systematic process of delivering care to ensure high-quality and cost-effective nutrition management of individuals with diabetes.

REFERENCES

1. Pastors JG, Warshaw H, Daly A, Franz M, Kulkarni K. The evidence for the effectiveness of medical nutrition therapy in diabetes management. *Diabetes Care*. 2002; 25:608–613.

2. Pastors JG, Franz MJ, Warshaw H, Daly A, Arnold M. How effective is medical nutrition therapy in diabetes care? *J Am Diet Assoc*. 2003;103:827–831.

3. American Diabetes Association. Nutrition principles and recommendations in diabetes (position statement). *Diabetes Care*. 2004;27(suppl):S36–S46.

4. Franz MJ, Bantle JP, Brunzell JD, Chiasson J-L, Garg A, Holzmeister LA, Hoogwerf BJ, Mayer-Davis E, Mooradian AD, Purnell JQ, Wheeler M. Evidence-based nutrition principles and recommendations for the treatment and prevention of diabetes and related complications (technical review). *Diabetes Care*. 2002;25:148–198.

5. American Diabetes Association. Standards of medical care in diabetes. *Diabetes Care*. 2005;28(Suppl 1):S4–S36.

6. Lacey K, Pritchett E. Nutrition care process and model: ADA adopts road map to quality care and outcomes management. *J Am Diet Assoc*. 2003;103:1061–1072.

7. Diabetes Prevention Program Research Group. Reduction in the incidence of type 2 diabetes with lifestyle intervention or metformin. *N Engl J Med*. 2002;346:393–403.

8. *American Dietetic Association Medical Nutrition Therapy Evidence-Based Guides for Practice: Nutrition Practice Guidelines for Type 1 and Type 2 Diabetes* [CD-ROM]. Chicago, Ill: American Dietetic Association; 2001.

9. *American Dietetic Association Medical Nutrition Therapy Evidence-Based Guides for Practice: Nutrition Practice Guidelines for Gestational Diabetes Mellitus* [CD-ROM]. Chicago, Ill: American Dietetic Association; 2001.

10. Franz MJ, Monk A, Barry B, McClain K, Weaver T, Cooper N, Upham P, Bergenstal R, Mazze RS. Effectiveness of medical nutrition therapy provided by dietitians in the management of non-insulin-dependent diabetes mellitus: a randomized, controlled clinical trial. *J Am Diet Assoc*. 1995;95:1009–1017.

11. Kulkarni K, Castle G, Gregory R, Holmes A, Leontos C, Power M, Snetselaar L, Splett P, Wylie-Rosett J; for the Diabetes Care and Education Dietetic Practice Group. Nutrition practice guidelines for type 1 diabetes mellitus positively affect dietitian practices and patient outcomes. *J Am Diet Assoc*. 1998;98:62–70.

12. Diabetes Care and Education Dietetic Practice Group of the American Dietetic Association. *Diabetes Nutrition Practice Guidelines Pocket Guide: A Companion Resource to the American Dietetic Association MNT Evidence-Based Guides for Practice*. Chicago, Ill: Diabetes Care and Education Dietetic Practice Group of the American Dietetic Association; 2002.

ADDITIONAL RESOURCES

Franz MJ, Reader D, Monk A. *Implementing Group and Individual Medical Nutrition Therapy for Diabetes*. Alexandria, Va: American Diabetes Association; 2002.

Leontos C, Geil P. *Individualized Approaches to Diabetes Nutrition Therapy: Case Studies*. Alexandria, Va: American Diabetes Association; 2002.

7

Physical Activity and Exercise

Charlotte Hayes, MMSc, MS, RD, CDE

CHAPTER OVERVIEW

- Physical activity and exercise play important roles in the treatment of diabetes. Regular physical activity and exercise can lead to physiologic and psychological benefits, which can improve an individual's health and quality of life (1–3).
- Physical activity is defined as "bodily movement produced by skeletal muscles that requires energy expenditure" and produces overall health benefits. Exercise, a subset of physical activity, is a "planned, structured and repetitive bodily movement done to improve or maintain one or more components of physical fitness" (4).
- Dietetics professionals who advise individuals with diabetes must understand the metabolic effects, risks, and benefits of physical activity and exercise for these individuals before making specific recommendations.

METABOLIC EFFECTS OF PHYSICAL ACTIVITY AND EXERCISE

The usual metabolic response to exercise involves a precisely regulated shift in fuel flux, which allows increasing energy demands of working muscle to be met while glucose homeostasis is maintained (3,5,6). At rest, the primary fuel source for muscle is free fatty acids (FFAs). At the onset of exercise, muscle glycogen and triglyceride stores become primary fuel sources. As exercise continues, circulating glucose, supplied first by liver glycogenolysis and then predominantly by gluconeogenesis and FFAs mobilized from adipose stores, becomes the chief fuel source (3,5,6). This metabolic response is influenced by a number of variables. Additional diabetes-specific variables can influence the response in individuals with diabetes (Box 7.1) (3).

Multiple alterations in hormonal output that occur during and after exercise ultimately govern fuel mobilization and utilization with activity (Table 7.1) (3,5). The physiologic purpose of these alterations is to maintain fuel homeostasis during and after exercise, when the demand for fuels is heightened. The magnitude of these metabolic adaptations is influenced by the energy demands of an exercise session. High-intensity, long-duration exercise demands greater metabolic adaptations than moderate physical activity requires, both during exercise and during recovery (6).

Type 1 Diabetes

For individuals with type 1 diabetes, the usual hormonal response to exercise is lacking, and this can lead to disturbances in fuel metabolism and failure to maintain fuel homeostasis (3,7). The circulating insulin level is a key determinant of blood glucose response to exercise.

BOX 7.1

Variables That Influence Metabolic Effects of Exercise

General Variables

- Level of training and fitness
- Exercise intensity, duration, type
- Age
- General health
- Nutritional state
  - Temporal relationship of exercise to food intake: fasting vs fed state
  - Caloric value and macronutrient make-up of preexercise meal or snack
- Environmental factors

Diabetes-Specific Variables

- Type 1 or insulin-treated type 2: timing of exercise in relation to timing of insulin, insulin dosages and type(s), mode of delivery
- Type 2: timing of exercise in relation to oral hypoglycemic agents and medication dosages
- Overall metabolic control
- Complications of diabetes

Source: Adapted with permission from Wasserman DH, Davis SN, Zinman B. Fuel metabolism during exercise in health and diabetes. In: Ruderman N, Devlin JT, Schneider SH, Kriska A, eds. *Handbook of Exercise in Diabetes.* Alexandria, Va: American Diabetes Association; 2002:63–99. Copyright © 2002, American Diabetes Association.

TABLE 7.1 Hormonal Adjustments to Maintain Fuel Homeostasis

Hormone	Response to Exercise	Metabolic Effects
Insulin	Decreases	Restricts use of glucose by nonexercising skeletal muscle; increases liver glycogenolysis; stimulates lipolysis
Glucagon	Increases	Stimulates hepatic glycogenolysis and gluconeogenesis
Epinephrine	Increases	Increases glucose production during latter stages of prolonged exercise; increases muscle glycogenolysis; increases adipose tissue lipolysis
Norepinephrine	Increases	Increases glycogenolysis and lipolysis
Cortisol	Increases	Promotes fatty acid (with heavy exercise) utilization; supports protein catabolism; increases hepatic glucose production

Source: Data are from references 3 and 5.

If preexercise insulin delivery does not match insulin needs during activity, risk of either hypoglycemia or of worsening hyperglycemia and ketosis can result (see Table 7.2) (3,8).

To prevent a significant "mismatch" and excessive excursions in the blood glucose level, the individual with type 1 diabetes must learn self-management skills for exercise. Self-management skills include the following:

- Monitoring blood glucose before and after exercise, to gain understanding of glycemic response. Individuals who are starting an exercise program or increasing their duration of exercise may also want to monitor blood glucose level during exercise—at least initially.
- Making appropriate decisions about how to adjust diabetes food and/or medications to accommodate future periods of increased activity.

- Evaluating the effectiveness of these decisions, and modifying strategies as needed.

Type 2 Diabetes

For individuals with type 2 diabetes, physical activity/exercise should be a primary treatment modality, because it reduces insulin resistance, a fundamental metabolic abnormality of type 2 diabetes, and it improves glucose tolerance. Specifically, physical activity/exercise increases insulin sensitivity, increases muscle uptake and utilization of glucose and FFAs, reduces liver glucose production, and reduces circulating insulin levels (2,3,8). When physical activity/exercise is performed consistently, it supports optimal improvements in glycemic control and reductions in or maintenance of body weight.

Meal planning plus physical activity/exercise should be considered complementary therapies that together

TABLE 7.2 Metabolic Response to Exercise Based on Insulin Status

Insulin Level	Liver Glucose Output	Muscle Glucose Uptake	Metabolic Effects
Low	Large increase	Moderate increase	Moderate increase in blood glucose (hyperglycemia), lipolysis, and ketones
Desirable	Large increase	Large increase	Stable blood glucose
High	Moderate increase	Large increase	Decrease in blood glucose (hypoglycemia); decreased mobilization of free fatty acids

Source: Data are from references 3 and 8.

promote optimal glycemic control. Risk of hypoglycemia is variable and depends on diabetes medication management. For individuals treated with meal planning plus physical activity alone, hypoglycemia risk is not increased—additional food intake to support euglycemia with physical activity/exercise is not necessary (5,6). For individuals on oral diabetes medications that do not contribute to hypoglycemia (see Chapter 8 on oral diabetes medications), additional food intake for exercise is generally unnecessary (6,9). For individuals treated with insulin secretagogues or insulin, hypoglycemia risk is elevated, and principles of exercise management that guide individuals with type 1 diabetes should be applied to type 2 diabetes management (9).

BENEFITS OF PHYSICAL ACTIVITY AND EXERCISE

For most people with diabetes, the benefits of physical activity far exceed the risks. Physical activity and exercise provide the following benefits:

- They have a positive impact on the metabolic abnormalities that characterize type 2 diabetes (2,3,8).
- They improve success with weight management (3,8).
- They prevent or delay the onset of type 2 diabetes for individuals with prediabetes or those at high risk for developing the condition (10,11).
- They play a central role in improving cardiovascular risk factors (ie, lipids, blood pressure, fibrinolysis); this is especially important to the long-term health of all individuals with diabetes (12–14). Physical inactivity and diabetes are both independ-

ent risk factors for development of cardiovascular disease (CVD) (13,14).
- They improve coping and stress management and reduce feelings of depression.
- They improve physical fitness and functional capacity.
- They enhance quality of life (1,2).

Exercise has not consistently been shown to improve glycemic control, as measured by A1C, for individuals with type 1 diabetes (1,3). However, individuals with type 1 diabetes who learn to precisely self-adjust their management to accommodate exercise can achieve near-normal A1C values and can certainly experience many other health benefits (eg, improved body composition, improved cardiovascular risk factors, reduced stress level, and improved well-being) by participating in regular exercise.

EXERCISE RISKS

In addition to exercise benefits, the potential risks of exercise must be considered when advising people with diabetes about physical activity and exercise. Both the acute complications, hyper- and hypoglycemia, and long-term microvascular and macrovascular complications can lead to increased exercise risk for individuals with diabetes (see Table 7.3) (6,15).

To minimize the risks and maximize the benefits of physical activity, the individual with diabetes should achieve reasonable and stable glycemic control before beginning an exercise routine; should have a thorough medical history and physical exam completed to screen for presence of microvascular, macrovascular, or neurologic complications that could be worsened by exercise (1,2,16); and should consider whether a graded exercise

TABLE 7.3 Exercise Risks Associated With Diabetes Complications

Complications	Exercise Risks
Acute	
Hypoglycemia	Can occur during or after exercise for those taking insulin or insulin secretagogues; postexercise, late-onset hypoglycemia can be severe and can occur 24–48 h after exercise
Hyperglycemia	Worsening of hyperglycemia and ketosis can occur in those with previously poor glycemic control (a fasting blood glucose level ≥ 250–300 mg/dL) and relative or absolute insulin deficiency
Chronic/preexisting	
Proliferative retinopathy	Retinal detachment, vitreous or retinal hemorrhage; elevated blood pressure
Peripheral neuropathy	Loss of protective sensation, foot ulcers, soft-tissue injury, injury to bones and joints, infection, amputation
Autonomic neuropathy	Impaired counterregulatory response to exercise, reduced heart rate and blood pressure responses to exercise, orthostatic hypotension, impaired body temperature regulation, dehydration, hypoglycemia unawareness, reduced exercise tolerance
Nephropathy	Exercise-induced proteinurea or albuminurea, elevated blood pressure
Coronary artery disease	Myocardial infarction or arrhythmia
Peripheral vascular disease	Claudication pain

Source: Data are from references 6 and 15.

test with electrocardiographic monitoring is appropriate before initiating a new exercise program (Box 7.2) (1,16,17). Individuals with diabetes are at increased risk for underlying cardiovascular disease. Findings of this screening should be used to establish an individualized physical activity program that minimizes exercise risk and maximizes gains in health and physical fitness.

EXERCISE RECOMMENDATIONS

In recent years, there has been a shift in the focus of exercise recommendations away from those that solely stress the importance of participation in traditional, structured aerobic exercise toward a broader construct that emphasizes the value of moderate, unstructured lifestyle activity (ie, physical activity) as well (18,19). The value of this broadened approach is that it allows options for physical activity participation suitable and palatable to even the most deconditioned nonexerciser.

Previously sedentary individuals can attain significant health benefits by taking steps to incorporate more lifestyle activities into their daily routines (see Table 7.4) (16,18–20). By accumulating at least 30 minutes per day of moderate activities like brisk walking, gardening, and yard work or household chores, individuals who have been inactive can make initial progress toward improving cardiorespiratory fitness, reducing cardiovascular risk factors, reducing blood pressure, and improving body composition (1,18,21).

An exercise dose-response relationship cannot be overlooked. Individuals who work to achieve and maintain higher levels of activity by participating in planned exercise can achieve even greater improvements in maximum oxygen uptake, physical fitness, and cardiovascular risk factors (Table 7.4) (16,18–20,22). However, when exercise is performed at a very strenuous, high-intensity level, it fails to offer substantially greater health benefits and increases cardiovascular risk, risk of musculoskeletal

<table>
<tr><td colspan="2">

BOX 7.2

Indications for Preexercise Graded Exercise Testing

- Known or suspected coronary artery disease (CAD), cerebrovascular disease, or peripheral vascular disease
- Autonomic neuropathy
- Age > 35 years
- Age > 25 years and
  - Type 2 diabetes of > 10 years duration OR
  - Type 1 diabetes of > 15 years duration
- Presence of additional risk factors for CAD (family history of premature CAD, tobacco use, hypertension, dyslipidemia including hypercholesterolemia, reduced high-density lipoprotein cholesterol, and/or hypertriglyceridemia, sedentary lifestyle, obesity, impaired fasting glucose)
- Microvascular disease: proliferative retinopathy or nephropathy including microalbuminurea

Source: Data are from references 1, 16, and 17.

</td></tr>
</table>

injury, and risk of aggravating existing diabetes complications (16,18).

Individualizing Physical Activity Recommendations

Physical activity and exercise recommendations should focus on the general health benefits of an active lifestyle, the specific reasons that exercise is being prescribed for an individual, and unique goals and outcomes that the individual with diabetes desires to achieve. The following are guidelines to consider when advising individuals with diabetes about physical activity and exercise goals:

- Establish an individualized program that includes physical activity, exercise, or a combination of the two (Table 7.4) (16,18–20).
- Consider individual interests, needs, and previous exercise history, as well as health status, in determining types of activities that are most suitable for an individual.
- Establish exercise recommendations that gradually and successfully lead the individual toward achieving his or her desired exercise outcomes (Table 7.5) (16,20,21).

TABLE 7.4 Lifestyle Activity for Health and Structured Exercise Goals for Improved Physical Fitness

	Lifestyle Activity for Health Goal	*Structured Exercise for Fitness Goal*
Frequency	Short, frequent intervals throughout each day; gradually work up to 10–30 min/session to total ≥ 30 min/day	3–5 day/wk
Intensity	Moderate effort	Moderate to vigorous; measure using target heart rate of 55%–79% of age-predicted maximal heart rate*
Duration	≥ 30–60 min/day	20–60 min of continuous or intermittent exercise
Type	Moderate lifestyle activity	Aerobic exercise (eg, brisk walking or biking) plus muscle strengthening and stretching
Energy expenditure	200 kcal/day or approximately 1000 kcal/wk	700–2000 kcal/wk

*Exercise intensities between 55% and 65% of maximum heart rate are most appropriate for individuals who are unfit.
Source: Data are from references 16, 18–20.

TABLE 7.5 Desired Diabetes and Exercise Outcomes and Exercise Strategies for Achievement of Outcomes

Desired Outcomes of Exercise	Strategies for Achieving Outcomes
Improved glycemic control	Type 1 diabetes: individuals with flexible insulin regimens should be able to exercise whenever they desire with appropriate adjustments in carbohydrate and insulin. Type 2 diabetes: exercise at least 3–5 days/wk on nonconsecutive days
Weight loss and maintenance	Emphasis on low-intensity, long-duration exercise ($\geq$ 60 min/day); focus on total level of energy expenditure (2000–2800 kcal/wk)
Reduced cardiovascular risk factors	Exercise intensity within established target heart rate range (55%–79% maximum heart rate); 20–60 min/session; 3–5 times/wk; focus on weekly energy expenditure (700–2000 kcal/wk)
Improved psychologic well-being	Focus on activities that are easy and comfortable for the individual to perform; consider unique capabilities and interests; assure ease of access; activities of choice should be sustainable and enjoyable.
Improved physical fitness and functional ability	Target heart rate $\geq$ 55%-65% of maximum heart rate; focus on balance of structured aerobic exercise, resistance training, and flexibility work

Source: Data are from references 16, 20, and 21.

- Recommend medically supervised exercise for some individuals, such as persons with severe diabetes complications like autonomic neuropathy. If cardiovascular status is uncertain or a stress test has not been completed, activity should be limited to a light to moderate level until further evaluation is completed.

Options for Individuals With Diabetes Complications

Safe exercise options are essential for individuals who have diabetes complications.

Proliferative Retinopathy

For individuals with proliferative retinopathy, low-impact activities, such as walking, swimming, low-impact aerobics, and stationary cycling, should be encouraged. Individuals should avoid pounding, jarring, or "head-low" activities, or those that involve heavy lifting, straining, and breath holding.

Nephropathy

For individuals with nephropathy, light- to moderate-intensity physical activity should be encouraged. These individuals should avoid intense or extreme forms of exercise and should limit elevations in blood pressure.

Peripheral Neuropathy

For individuals with peripheral neuropathy, non-weight-bearing activities, like swimming, cycling, yoga or tai chi, light chair and arm exercises, stretching, or light weight lifting, should be encouraged. These individuals should avoid repetitive weight-bearing or high-impact activities.

Peripheral Vascular Disease or Claudication

For individuals with peripheral vascular disease or claudication, intermittent (to the point of maximum tolerable pain, then rest), low-impact, weight-bearing activities, like walking, should be encouraged. These individuals should also be encouraged to engage in non–weight-bearing activities, such as swimming, cycling, stretching, and light weight lifting. Individuals with peripheral vascular disease should avoid high-impact activities.

EXERCISE SAFETY GUIDELINES AND RECOMMENDATIONS

Nutrition care for individuals with diabetes is integral to successful exercise performance and should complement other strategies that are used to optimize glycemic control. The following are important guidelines for maintaining a desirable blood glucose level with exercise.

Glucose Level

Blood glucose level must be monitored before and after exercise, or periodically during prolonged or unusually intense exercise. Frequent monitoring enables the individual with diabetes to anticipate the onset of hypo- or hyperglycemia and to take early corrective actions. Careful record keeping of blood glucose level, food, activity, and oral diabetes medications or insulin can enhance understanding of how exercise affects blood glucose level and how an individual's diabetes management plan can be altered to maintain euglycemia during and after a period of activity.

Insulin Dosages

Dosages of insulin or insulin secretagogues that can potentiate hypoglycemia (see Chapters 8 and 9) should be adjusted as needed for exercise (9). A 30% to 50% reduction in the dosage of insulin acting during the time of exercise is a generally accepted safe starting guideline (9,23,24). Greater reductions (75% to 80%) may be needed for prolonged, vigorous activity, such as hiking, cross-country skiing, or distance running (Table 7.6) (9,24). Dose reductions of insulin secretagogues may be necessary to prevent hypoglycemia during occasional periods of prolonged physical activity (9) or if a pattern of hypoglycemia emerges as a person becomes more physically fit and insulin sensitive, as a result of routine exercise training.

TABLE 7.6 Sample Guidelines for Reducing Premeal Rapid-Acting Insulin for Exercise

Level of Exercise*	% Dose Reduction	
	30 Min of Exercise	60 Min of Exercise
Very light	25	50
Moderate	50	75
Vigorous	75	—

*Very light = 25% VO$_2$, ~ 30% maximum heart rate; moderate = 50% VO$_2$, ~ 60% maximum heart rate; vigorous = 75% VO$_2$, ~ 80% maximum heart rate.
Source: Adapted from Rabasa-Lhoret R, Bourque J, Ducros F, Chiasson J. Guidelines for premeal insulin dose reduction for postprandial exercise of different intensities and durations in type 1 diabetic subjects treated intensively with a basal-bolus insulin regimen (ultralente-lispro). Diabetes Care. 2001;24:625–630, with permission from the American Diabetes Association. Copyright © 2001, American Diabetes Association.

Timing of Exercise

Individuals with diabetes should consider timing of exercise in relation to peak action times of insulin or oral diabetes medications. It is safest to exercise at times when glucose-lowering medications are not "peaking" (9). Individuals should also consider timing of exercise in relation to planned meals and snacks. Exercise that is performed 1 to 2 hours postprandially generally reduces risk of hypoglycemia and may blunt the postmeal blood glucose rise. This generality may not hold true for individuals who use one of the short-acting insulin analogs that peak 30 to 60 minutes after injection (9).

Food Intake

Decisions regarding intake of additional food before, during, or after exercise should be individualized based on the following factors:

- Preexercise blood glucose level
- Use of insulin or oral diabetes medication
- Time of last meal in relation to exercise
- Macronutrient composition of preexercise meals and snacks
- Time of day that exercise is performed
- Exercise intensity
- Exercise duration
- Level of training and fitness
- Previously measured metabolic response to exercise

Carbohydrate Intake

Individuals with diabetes should adjust carbohydrate intake before, during, and after exercise, as necessary to maintain adequate glycemic control and to optimize exercise performance. Additional carbohydrate foods can be consumed:

- As a preexercise meal or snack 1 to 3 hours before the start of exercise. An intake of 1 to 4.5 g carbohydrate per kg body weight will optimize muscle and liver glycogen stores (25).
- During prolonged (> 45–60 minutes) or intense exercise (≥ 80% maximal heart rate). Intake of 15 g of carbohydrate every 30 to 60 minutes of activity is generally a safe starting guideline (25,26).
- Postexercise, as part of planned meals and snacks, or as additional, supplemental feedings (25,26). Intake of 1.5 g carbohydrate per kg body weight within 30 minutes of an extended exercise session

(lasting > 90 minutes) and intake of an additional 1.5 g carbohydrate per kg 2 hours later will support glycogen repletion (25) and will reduce risk of postexercise hypoglycemia (26).

Individuals should consume only enough extra carbohydrate to maintain blood glucose level in the desired target range. Excess carbohydrate and calorie intake can easily counter the energy deficit created by exercise and can result in elevated postexercise blood glucose readings. It can also prevent weight loss or promote weight gain.

Fluid Intake

Individuals should drink fluids before, during, and after exercise. Two cups of fluid should be consumed within 2 hours of starting exercise. During exercise, 1 cup of water should be consumed for every 30 to 60 minutes of activity. Beverages that contain at least 8% carbohydrate, such as sports drinks or diluted fruit juices (50% dilution), can be useful because they supply fluid as well as fuel for prolonged activity (≥ 60 minutes). Individuals should continue to consume additional fluids after exercise (25). If rehydration is the sole reason for consuming fluids after exercise, then water or another calorie-free beverage will be adequate. If glycogen repletion and maintenance of euglycemia postexercise is a consideration, then carbohydrate-containing beverages are appropriate options.

Other Recommendations

Individuals with diabetes should be cognizant of additional safety recommendations during periods of physical activity. Preexercise insulin should be injected at a site away from muscles that will be contracting and actively doing work if an insulin dose is taken within 30 minutes of the onset of activity (3,9). (Individuals using rapid-acting insulin do not need to consider injection site.)

Individuals should exercise only with caution during periods of poor glycemic control. If the fasting blood glucose level is higher than 250 mg/dL, urine ketones should always be tested. Insulinopenia and poor metabolic control are indicated by (a) the combination of a fasting blood glucose value of 250 mg/dL and positive ketones or (b) a fasting blood glucose value higher than 300 mg/dL with or without ketones. Exercise should be delayed until better metabolic control is achieved (1,3).

If hypoglycemia is suspected, exercise should be delayed until the blood glucose value is verified by self-monitoring of blood glucose. A blood glucose value less than 70 mg/dL must be treated appropriately. A source of carbohydrate should be readily available for treatment of hypoglycemia (see Chapter 12 on hypoglycemia). Ideally, the blood glucose level will be 90 to 130 mg/dL before exercise is resumed (4,27).

Proper foot care is essential. Footwear should fit well and be appropriate for the activity the individual plans to do. Foot inspections for signs of irritation should be done both before and after exercise.

The individual should always wear medical identification. Extremely hot, humid, or cold environments should be avoided, and exercise clothing should be appropriate for the exercise climate.

EXERCISE COUNSELING AND MOTIVATIONAL TECHNIQUES

Mounting evidence indicates that physical activity and exercise play central roles in the treatment of diabetes. For the general population, a dose-response relationship between volume of physical activity (or level of physical fitness) and all-cause mortality is recognized (28). Individuals who are most fit tend to have the lowest rates of cardiovascular and all-cause mortality. Those who achieve a moderate level of fitness by performing 30 minutes of daily activity and accruing an energy expenditure of approximately 1,000 kcal/week, the amount encouraged by the US Surgeon General (18), reduce their all-cause mortality by 20% to 30% (28). This inverse dose-response relationship between physical fitness and mortality appears to be the same for people with diabetes. Higher levels of physical fitness independent of BMI have been shown to reduce all-cause mortality in males with diabetes (27). Even individuals who are significantly overweight or obese can reduce mortality risk by achieving a moderate level of physical fitness (29).

However, many individuals with diabetes have difficulty achieving a level of activity that supports improved health. Persons who counsel individuals with diabetes play a vital role in establishing effective physical activity and exercise interventions that will enhance exercise adoption and long-term maintenance. Theoretical, behavioral models, as well as practical considerations, provide helpful guidance to those who counsel and support individuals as they attempt to integrate physical activity or exercise into their lifestyle.

To be most effective, physical activity and exercise messages and interventions should be responsive to an individual's current readiness and willingness to change, level of self-confidence in ability to perform exercise, and outcome expectations (2) (see Chapter 3 for more information on counseling). Beyond behavioral models, application of key, practical considerations can increase likelihood of success with physical activity and exercise adoption and adherence. For example, individuals should gain heightened awareness of the amount of time they spend sitting and, in other ways, being sedentary and take steps to reduce "inactive time."

Dietetics professionals should consider ease of access when recommending physical activity and exercise options and should determine whether potential obstacles to access could become barriers. Examples of possible barriers include needs for special equipment, training, or instruction; travel to a distant facility; dependence on an exercise partner; and seasonal activity limitations (2).

Counselors should evaluate ease of performance and should determine whether an activity is suitable for an individual with unique physical attributes or limitations or specific lifestyle issues (2). The importance of maintaining a comfortable level of exercise effort should be stressed. Rating of Perceived Exertion is an easy-to-use tool that can guide individuals toward an appropriate level of exercise effort. The individual should gradually move toward a higher level of activity by increasing exercise duration and frequency before focusing on intensity (2). The counselor should ensure correct performance of an activity, to prevent discomfort or injuries that could cause setbacks. Supervised exercise may be appropriate for individuals who have physical limitations or who lack confidence in their ability to exercise. The eventual transition to home-based exercise may lead to better adherence long-term.

PRACTICAL TOOLS

Practical tools that are inexpensive, easy-to-access, and easy-to-use can help motivate individuals to exercise and to achieve physical activity goals. Pedometers, resistance bands, small hand-held or leg weights, stability balls, and fitness videos are examples of simple fitness tools that people can use in their homes or at work during short activity breaks. Although these tools can add variety, novelty, and interest to an activity routine and prevent boredom and dropping out, they can potentially contribute to injury if not used correctly. Indications for correct use, as well as precautions, should be addressed when advising people about use of any new exercise equipment or exercise options.

SUMMARY

Physical activity and exercise play integral roles in the treatment of diabetes. Programs should be carefully developed so that potential exercise risks are minimized and benefits are maximized. Recommendations should be guided by findings of a preexercise medical history and assessment and should lead to desired metabolic and psychosocial outcomes.

REFERENCES

1. American Diabetes Association. Position statement: physical activity/exercise and diabetes. *Diabetes Care.* 2004; 27(Suppl 1):S58–S62.

2. Albright A, Franz M, Hornsby G, Kriska A, Marrero D, Ullrich I, Verity LS. American College of Sports Medicine position stand: exercise and type 2 diabetes. *Med Sci Sports Exerc.* 2000;32:1345–1355.

3. Wasserman DH, Davis SN, Zinman B. Fuel metabolism during exercise in health and diabetes. In: Ruderman N, Devlin JT, Schneider SH, Kriska A, eds. *Handbook of Exercise in Diabetes.* Alexandria, Va: American Diabetes Association; 2002:63–99.

4. Physical activity and cardiovascular health. *NIH Consens Statement.* 1995;13(3):1–33.

5. McArdle WD, Katch FI, Katch VL. The endocrine system and exercise. *Exercise Physiology: Energy, Nutrition, and Human Performance.* 4th ed. Baltimore, Md: Williams & Wilkins; 1996:356–388.

6. Mullooly CA, Hanson Chalmers K. Physical activity/exercise. In: Franz MJ, ed. *A Core Curriculum for Diabetes Educators.* 5th ed. Chicago, Ill: American Association of Diabetes Educators; 2003:61–92.

7. Raguso CA, Coggan AR, Gastadelli A, Sidossis LS, Bastyer EJ III, Wolfe RR. Lipid and carbohydrate metabolism in IDDM during moderate and intense exercise. *Diabetes.* 1995;44:1066–1074.

8. Young JC. Exercise prescription in individuals with metabolic disorders, practical consideration. *Sports Med.* 1995; 19:43–45.

9. Berger M. Adjustment of insulin and oral agent therapy. In: Ruderman N, Devlin JT, Schneider SH, Kriska A, eds. *Handbook of Exercise in Diabetes.* Alexandria, Va: American Diabetes Association; 2002:365–376.

10. Knowler WC, Barrett-Connor E, Fowler SE, Hamman RT, Lachin JM, Walker EA, Nathan DM. Reduction in the incidence of type 2 diabetes with lifestyle intervention or metformin. *N Engl J Med.* 2002;346:393–403.

11. Tuomilhehto J, Lindstrom J, Eriksson JG, Walle TT, Hanalainen H, Ilanne-Parikka P, Keinanen-Kiukaanniema S, Laakso M, Louheranta A, Rastas M, Salminen V, Uusitupa M. Prevention of type 2 diabetes mellitus by changes in lifestyle among subjects with impaired glucose tolerance. *N Engl J Med.* 2001;344:1343–1350.

12. Fletcher GF, Balady G, Blair SN, Blumenthal J, Caspersen C, Chaitman B, Epstein S, Sivarajan Froelicher ES, Froelicher VF, Pina IL, Pollock ML. Statement on exercise:

benefits and recommendations for physical activity programs for all Americans. *Circulation.* 1996;94:857–862.

13. Grundy SM, Garber A, Goldberg R, Havas S, Holman R, Lamendola C, Howard WJ, Savage P, Sowers J, Vega GL. Prevention Conference VI: diabetes and cardiovascular disease, writing group IV: lifestyle and medical management of risk factors. *Circulation.* 2002;105:153–158.

14. Stewart KJ. Exercise training and cardiovascular consequences of type 2 diabetes and hypertension: plausible mechanisms for improving cardiovascular health. *JAMA.* 2002;288:1622–1631.

15. Marrero DG. Initiation and maintenance of exercise in patients with diabetes. In: Ruderman N, Devlin JT, Schneider SH, Kriska A, eds. *Handbook of Exercise in Diabetes.* Alexandria, Va: American Diabetes Association; 2002:289–309.

16. Gordon NF. The exercise prescription. In: Ruderman N, Devlin JT, Schneider SH, Kriska A, eds. *Handbook of Exercise in Diabetes.* Alexandria, Va: American Diabetes Association; 2002:269–288.

17. American College of Sports Medicine. *ACSM's Guidelines for Exercise Testing and Prescription.* 6th ed. Philadelphia, Pa: Lippincott, Williams & Wilkins; 2000.

18. US Department of Health and Human Services. *Physical Activity and Health: A Report of the Surgeon General.* Atlanta, Ga: US Dept of Health and Human Services, Centers for Disease Control and Prevention, National Center for Chronic Disease Prevention and Health Promotion; 1996.

19. Physical activity. In: *Dietary Reference Intakes for Energy, Carbohydrates, Fiber, Fat, and Protein (Macronutrients).* Available at: http://www.nap.edu. Accessed November 19, 2002.

20. Wing RR. Exercise and weight control. In: Ruderman N, Devlin JT, Schneider SH, Kriska A, eds. *Handbook of Exercise in Diabetes.* Alexandria, Va: American Diabetes Association; 2002;355–363.

21. Pratt M. Benefits of lifestyle activity vs structured exercise. *JAMA.* 1999;281:375–376.

22. Dunn AL, Marcus BH, Kampert JB, Garcia ME, Kohl HW III, Blair SN. Comparison of lifestyle and structured interventions to increase physical activity and cardiorespiratory fitness. *JAMA.* 1999;281:327–334.

23. Schiffrin A, Parikh S. Accommodating planned exercise in type 1 diabetic patients on intensive treatment. *Diabetes Care.* 1985;8:337–342.

24. Rabasa-Lhoret R, Bourque J, Ducros F, Chiasson J. Guidelines for premeal insulin dose reduction for postprandial exercise of different intensities and durations in type 1 diabetic subjects treated intensively with a basal-bolus insulin regimen (ultralente-lispro). *Diabetes Care.* 2001;24:625–630.

25. Coleman E. Carbohydrate and exercise. In: Rosenbloom C, ed. *Sports Nutrition: A Guide for the Professional Working With Active People.* Chicago, Ill: American Dietetic Association; 2000:13–31.

26. Franz MJ. Nutrition, physical activity and diabetes. In: Ruderman N, Devlin JT, Schneider SH, Kriska A, eds. *Handbook of Exercise in Diabetes.* Alexandria, Va: American Diabetes Association; 2002:321–337.

27. American Diabetes Association. Standards of medical care in diabetes. *Diabetes Care.* 2004;27(Suppl 1):S15–S35.

28. Lee I-M, Skerrett P. Physical activity and all-cause mortality: what is the dose-response relation? *Med Sci Sports Exerc.* 2001;33(suppl):S459–S471.

29. Church T, Cheng Y, Earnest C, Barlow C, Gibbons L, Priest E, Blair S. Exercise capacity and body composition as predictors of mortality among men with diabetes. *Diabetes Care.* 2004;27:83–88.

ADDITIONAL RESOURCES

Publications

ACSM Fitness Book. 3rd ed. Champaign, Ill: Human Kinetics Publishers; 2003.

Colberg S. *The Diabetic Athlete.* Alexandria, Va: American Diabetes Association; 2000.

Hayes C. *The I Hate to Exercise Book for People with Diabetes.* Alexandria, Va: American Diabetes Association; 2000.

Videos

Armchair Fitness: An Aerobic Workout for People of All Ages. Available from: CC-M Productions, 7755 16th St, NW, Washington, DC 20012; 800/453-6280 or 202/453-6280.

Fitness Forever: The Exercise Program for Healthy Aging. Available from: Fitness Forever, 13820 Donner Pass Rd, Truckee, CA 96161; 800/985-5185 or 530/550-9866.

Web Sites

American Heart Association. Choose to Move. Available at: http://www.justmove.org. Accessed December 20, 2004.

America on the Move. Available at: http://www.americaonthemove.org. Accessed December 20, 2004.

Diabetes Exercise and Sports Association. Available at: http://www.diabetes-exercise.org. Accessed December 20, 2004.

Health Partners 10,000 Steps Program. Available at: http://www.10k-steps.com. Accessed December 20, 2004.

National Institute of Diabetes and Digestive and Kidney Diseases. Active at Any Size. Available at: http://win.niddk.nih.gov/publications/active.htm. Accessed December 20, 2004.

Shape Up America. Available at: http://www.shapeup.org/fitness.html. Accessed December 20, 2004.

8

Oral Diabetes Medications

Janine Freeman, RD, CDE

CHAPTER OVERVIEW

- Use of oral glucose-lowering medications is indicated for individuals with type 2 diabetes who are unable to achieve glycemic control through medical nutrition therapy (MNT) and regular physical activity.
- Five classes of oral glucose-lowering medications, each of which works through a different mechanism of action, are currently available to improve glycemic control in individuals with type 2 diabetes (Table 8.1) (1–8).
- With few exceptions, oral glucose-lowering medications lower glycosylated hemoglobin (A1C) by approximately 1% to 2% (2).

ORAL DIABETES MEDICATIONS AND GLYCEMIC CONTROL

As type 2 diabetes progresses, hepatic glucose production increases and endogenous insulin production decreases, which results in the need for medication to adequately control glycemia in most people. Oral glucose-lowering medications address two primary defects in insulin secretion and insulin action in type 2 diabetes (Figure 8.1): (*a*) insulin resistance (characterized by increased production and impaired suppression of hepatic glucose and decreased glucose uptake by muscle) and (*b*) impaired insulin secretion (ie, insulin deficiency) by the pancreas.

The expected improvement in glycemic control varies with the individual and is dependent on the following factors (9):

- Baseline glycemic control
- Stage of progression of type 2 diabetes
- Concurrent lifestyle changes
- Adherence to lifestyle modification and medication therapy
- Additive effects of other oral glucose-lowering medications
- Other factors independently affecting blood glucose (such as stress, illness, or steroid drugs)

CLASSES OF ORAL DIABETES MEDICATIONS

There are five classes of oral diabetes medications: sulfonylureas, meglitinides, biguanides, thiazolidinediones (TZDs), and alpha-glucosidase inhibitors. Each type has nutrition implications, outlined in Table 8.2 (2,10,11).

Sulfonylureas

The primary mechanism of action of sulfonylureas, referred to as insulin secretagogues, is to enhance insulin secretion from the pancreas. Sulfonylureas, therefore, are ineffective when there is little or no pancreatic beta cell

TABLE 8.1 Characteristics of Oral Diabetes Medications*

Medication	Brand Name	Recommended Dosage	Primary Action	Potential for Weight Gain	Potential for Hypoglycemia	Appropriate for Use in Renal Insufficiency	Appropriate for Use in Hepatic Insufficiency
Sulfonylureas (2nd generation)							
Glyburide	Diabeta, Micronase	1.25–10 mg/day single or divided dose	Increases pancreatic secretion of insulin	Yes	Yes	Yes	No
	Glynase Prestabs	0.75–12 mg/day					
Glipizide	Glucotrol	2.5–20 mg/day single or divided dose		Yes	Yes	Yes	No
Glipizide GITS	Glucotrol XL	5–20 mg once a day		Yes	Yes	Yes	No
Glimepiride	Amaryl	1–4 mg once a day		Yes	Yes	Yes	No
Meglitinides							
Nateglinide	Starlix	120 mg before meals	Increases pancreatic production of insulin (short-acting)	Yes	Yes	Yes	Yes
Repaglinide	Prandin	0.5–4.0 mg before meals		Yes	Yes	Yes	Use with caution
Biguanides							
Metformin	Glucophage	500–2000 mg/day in divided dosage with meals	Suppresses hepatic glucose output	No	No	No	No
Metformin extended-release	Glucophage XR	500–2000 mg once a day with evening meal		No	No	No	No
Thiazolidinediones							
Rosiglitazone	Avandia	2–8 mg once a day	Increases insulin sensitivity in muscle and adipose tissue	Yes	No	Yes	No
Pioglitazone	Actos	15–45 mg once a day		Yes	No	Yes	No
Alpha-Glucosidase Inhibitors							
Acarbose	Precose	25–100 mg before meals	Delays carbohydrate absorption	Yes	No	No	Contraindicated in patients with cirrhosis
Miglitol	Glyset	25–100 mg before meals		Yes	No	No	Contraindicated in patients with cirrhosis

(continued)

TABLE 8.1 (*Continued*)

Medication	Brand Name	Recommended Dosage	Primary Action	Potential for Weight Gain	Potential for Hypoglycemia	Appropriate for Use in Renal Insufficiency	Appropriate for Use in Hepatic Insufficiency
Combination Therapies							
Metformin + rosiglitazone	Avandamet	1–4 mg rosiglitazone/ 500 mg metformin twice daily	Suppresses hepatic glucose output and increases insulin sensitivity	Yes	No	No	No
Metformin + glipizide	Metaglip	2.5–5 mg glipizide/ 250–500 mg metformin twice daily	Suppresses hepatic glucose output and increases pancreatic production of insulin	Yes	Yes	No	No
Metformin + glyburide	Glucovance	1.25–5 mg glyburide/ 250–500 mg metformin twice daily	Suppresses hepatic glucose output and increases pancreatic production of insulin	Yes	Yes	No	No

*When used as monotherapy.
Source: Data are from references 2–8.

function. Second-generation sulfonylureas (see Table 8.1) have all but replaced the first-generation sulfonylureas (chlorpropamide, tolbutamide, and tolazamide), because the second-generation medications have increased potency, a decreased likelihood of side effects, and less-frequent interactions with other agents. Treatment of type 2 diabetes inadequately controlled with lifestyle modification may include the use of sulfonylureas alone. They may be more effective in people who have had type 2 diabetes for less than 5 years, developed diabetes after age 40 years, have a fasting blood glucose level below 200 mg/dL, do not have dyslipidemia, and are not overweight. These agents are not necessarily ineffective in overweight individuals, but there is less likelihood

that the agent will provide an initial blood glucose–lowering effect in individuals who are overweight (12–14).

Common adverse effects of sulfonylurea therapy include weight gain (typically 2 to 5 kg) (3) and hypoglycemia. Weight gain is likely secondary to the increased insulin secretion (2), but it can also be associated with overtreatment and/or frequent treatment of hypoglycemia. Hypoglycemia risk is greater in older adults and in people with impaired liver and kidney function (2). This higher risk is due to the individual's decreased ability to metabolize and excrete the sulfonylureas, leading to increased action and levels of these drugs. Hypoglycemia risk also increases with physical activity and when carbohydrate intake is inconsistent.

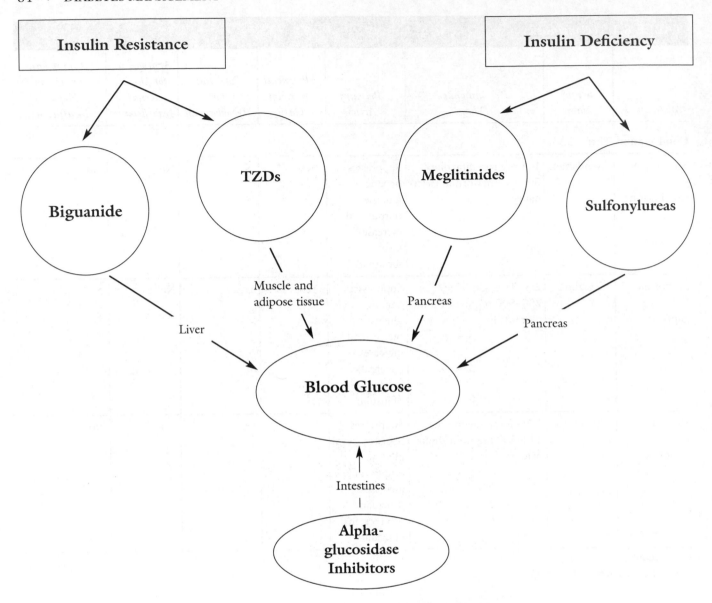

FIGURE 8.1 Type 2 diabetes oral medication sites of action. TZD = thiazolidinediones.

Meglitinides

Repaglinide and nateglinide are the two short-acting insulin secretagogues available in the United States. They exert their primary effect on postprandial blood glucose levels by rapidly stimulating insulin release from the pancreas after administration with meals (2). The effect is glucose dependent. Like sulfonylureas, meglitinides are ineffective when there is little or no pancreatic beta cell function.

Advantages of the meglitinides include greater flexibility in the timing of meals with less late postprandial hypoglycemia, because of the short duration of action

(3). Primary side effects include hypoglycemia and weight gain, which may be less pronounced than weight gain caused by sulfonylureas (4). Unlike the sulfonylureas, both nateglinide and repaglinide may be used even if renal disease is present. Repaglinide, however, should be used with caution in malnourished, elderly, or debilitated individuals, and in individuals with pituitary, adrenal, or hepatic insufficiency because those individuals are particularly susceptible to repaglinide's hypoglycemic effects (10). Both of these agents should be taken about 15 minutes before a meal. If the meal is skipped or contains less than 240 kcal, the medication should be omitted.

TABLE 8.2 Nutrition Implications of Oral Diabetes Medications

Medication Class	Potential for Hypoglycemia in Monotherapy	Hypoglycemia Treatment	Weight Effects	Meal Planning Considerations
Sulfonylureas (2nd generation)	Yes	Carbohydrate source	Potential for increase in weight	• Carbohydrate consistency is important. • Fixed schedule is necessary. • Energy restriction, reduced fat intake, regular physical activity beneficial in preventing or limiting weight gain. • Potential alcohol intolerance. • Glipizide most effective when taken on empty stomach.
Meglitinides	Yes, but less potential than with sulfonylureas	Carbohydrate source	Potential for increase in weight	• Carbohydrate consistency is important. • Taken with meals—in most cases, if meal is omitted, the corresponding dose should be omitted to prevent hypoglycemia. • Energy restriction, reduced fat intake, regular physical activity beneficial in preventing/limiting weight gain.
Biguanides	No	Not indicated	No effect to potential for slight decrease in weight	• Taken with food to reduce gastrointestinal upset. • Potential to decrease vitamin B-12 and folate absorption.
Thiazolidinediones	No	Not indicated	Potential for increase in weight	• Energy restriction, reduced fat intake, regular physical activity beneficial in preventing/limiting weight gain.
Alpha glucosidase inhibitors	No	Glucose tablets or gel, or milk, if hypoglycemia occurs in combination therapy	No effect on weight	• Taken with first bite of the meal.

Source: Data are from references 2, 10, and 11.

Biguanides

Metformin is the only biguanide available in the United States. Metformin's primary mechanism of action is to decrease hepatic glucose production by reducing gluconeogenesis (formation of glucose from noncarbohydrate sources) and by decreasing glycogenolysis (breakdown of glycogen to glucose) (2). A secondary effect is to enhance insulin sensitivity in the muscle through its impact on glucose toxicity (2).

Metformin does not stimulate the pancreas to secrete insulin and may lead to modest weight loss (4 to 6 lb during the first 6 months of treatment) (1), decreased risk of hypoglycemia (generally no risk in monotherapy), and reduced triglyceride and low-density lipoprotein (LDL) cholesterol levels (2). Persons who may benefit most from initial metformin therapy include individuals with type 2 diabetes who are overweight, have elevated cholesterol levels, and have elevated fasting blood glucose levels.

Recent studies have shown metformin to improve ovulatory function in women with polycystic ovary syndrome (PCOS) (15). Metformin has also been shown to reduce the incidence of gestational diabetes in women with PCOS and to decrease the prevalence of type 2 diabetes in individuals with impaired glucose tolerance (3). The Diabetes Prevention Program, a major clinical trial that compared the effects of diet and exercise to treatment with metformin 850 mg twice a day, showed that in overweight individuals with impaired glucose tolerance, treatment with metformin reduced type 2 diabetes risk by 31% (16).

Primary side effects with initial treatment include abdominal discomfort, diarrhea, and nausea and/or vomiting, which can be minimized by taking the medication with food, starting at a low dosage, and increasing the dosage slowly (17). Due to an increased risk of developing lactic acidosis, a rare but fatal condition, metformin is contraindicated if individuals present with any of the following (7,18):

- Binge drinking
- Heart failure that is being treated with furosemide and digoxin
- Decreased kidney function (serum creatinine > 1.5 mg/dL in males, > 1.4 mg/dL in females)
- Decreased liver function

Individuals undergoing major surgery or procedures using radiocontrast dye should discontinue metformin before the procedure and have their kidney function reassessed 48 hours after the procedure, to assure adequate kidney function before restarting metformin (9).

Thiazolidinediones

Rosiglitazone and pioglitazone are the two TZDs, referred to as insulin sensitizers, available in the United States. The primary action of TZDs is to reduce insulin resistance by increasing glucose uptake by skeletal muscle cells (3). Therefore, TZD use may be effective in overweight individuals with type 2 diabetes, because they have an increased likelihood of insulin resistance. TZDs appear to be more effective when used in earlier stages of diabetes, with greater insulin resistance and more beta cell function (19). TZDs frequently take several weeks to months to exert their full glycemic effect (3). They do not cause hypoglycemia when used as monotherapy.

An advantage of TZD use is a possible beneficial effect on lipid levels. An increase in high-density lipoprotein cholesterol concentration and a decrease in triglycerides are frequently seen. The effects on LDL cholesterol are more variable. Increases in LDL cholesterol levels appear to be due to a shift from small dense particles to the less atherogenic large and buoyant LDL particles (2).

The primary side effects of the TZDs are edema and weight gain. Weight gain tends to be more prevalent when these agents are used in combination with insulin. Dose-related weight gain is seen in monotherapy and in combination therapy. The mechanism of weight gain is unclear but probably involves a combination of fluid retention and fat accumulation (20,21). Weight should be measured when therapy is initiated and monitored in follow-up. Energy restriction, reduced fat intake, and regular exercise can be beneficial in preventing or limiting weight gain. Also, in premenopausal, anovulatory women with insulin resistance, treatment with a TZD may cause ovulation resumption and subsequent risk of pregnancy.

TZDs should not be used in individuals with hepatic dysfunction or advanced forms of congestive heart failure. Liver function testing should be done before a TZD is started, every 2 months for the first year and then periodically thereafter (20,21). TZDs are the most expensive oral glucose-lowering medications.

Alpha-Glucosidase Inhibitors

Acarbose and miglitol are the two alpha-glucosidase inhibitors (AGIs) available in the United States for treatment of type 2 diabetes. The primary effect of the AGIs, which are taken with meals, is to lower the postprandial blood glucose rise by reducing the rate of digestion of starches and disaccharides and the subsequent absorption of glucose. The efficacy of AGIs is considerably less than other oral glucose-lowering medications (2).

AGIs have no effect on weight and do not cause hypoglycemia when used as monotherapy. When used in combination with sulfonylureas or insulin, hypoglycemia may result. Hypoglycemia should be treated with glucose tablets or milk, because AGIs blunt the digestion of complex carbohydrates and delay the absorption of nonglucose carbohydrates, such as sucrose.

Primary side effects include abdominal bloating, diarrhea, and flatulence that may be self-limiting and transient when the dosage is slowly increased. AGIs should not be used in individuals with cirrhosis, elevated serum creatinine levels (> 2.0 mg/dL), or any conditions made worse by increased gas formation (2).

USE OF ORAL GLUCOSE-LOWERING MEDICATIONS

The choice of oral glucose-lowering medications is based on a number of factors that involve the individual with diabetes and medication characteristics, including the following:

- Predisposition to adverse effects
- Degree of hyperglycemia
- Mechanism of action of medication
- Medication cost

Oral glucose-lowering medications have not been approved by the Food and Drug Administration (FDA) for use in pregnancy and are generally not indicated during breastfeeding. Concerns with the use of oral glucose-lowering medications during pregnancy include the risk of fetal malformations, in which studies have yielded conflicting data, and neonatal hypoglycemia (22). These medications, however, have been studied in pregnant women, in particular sulfonylureas in gestational diabetes and metformin in pregnant women with polycystic ovarian syndrome and gestational diabetes, with positive outcomes (15).

Metformin is the only oral glucose-lowering medication currently approved by the FDA for use in children aged 10 years and older. The extended-release formulation is approved for use in individuals aged 18 years or older (18).

COMBINATION THERAPY WITH ORAL GLUCOSE-LOWERING MEDICATIONS

Because type 2 diabetes involves multiple pathophysiological factors and is progressive in nature, combination therapy using different classes of oral glucose-lowering medications is often necessary to achieve glycemic control. Combination therapy is frequently selected over monotherapy as the initial medication treatment. The United Kingdom Prospective Diabetes Study showed that after 3 years in the study, 50% of subjects were able to adequately control glycemia on a single drug. After 9 years, 75% of subjects using oral agents required combination therapy to achieve control (23).

The addition of an oral glucose-lowering medication to one of another class results in additive A1C reduction. In most cases, the additional A1C reduction is similar to the effect from using the added drug as monotherapy (3). Three types of fixed combination oral glucose-lowering medications have been approved for use in the

United States (see Table 8.1). If glycemic control cannot be attained with oral glucose-lowering medication, insulin should be used.

MANAGING HYPOGLYCEMIA RISK

Diabetes educators should assess the incidence of hypoglycemic episodes related to glucose-lowering medications. If frequent hypoglycemic episodes occur in individuals using insulin secretagogues (sulfonylureas, repaglinide, nateglinide or combinations using these medications) despite reasonable food distribution, a dosage adjustment or change in the type of medication may be needed. Care should be taken to ensure that unnecessary snacks are not being recommended by the health care team to avoid hypoglycemic episodes, thus increasing the risk of weight gain. Individuals using insulin secretagogues should be advised to consider the time action of the oral glucose-lowering medication when exercising, to avoid hypoglycemia (see Chapter 12).

WEIGHT GAIN WITH ORAL GLUCOSE-LOWERING MEDICATIONS

Weight gain is a frequent side effect when sulfonylureas are used to treat type 2 diabetes and may occur when TZDs are used, especially in combination with insulin. Metformin and AGIs can be used if weight gain is a primary issue. Emphasis on meal planning with close monitoring of portion sizes, regular physical activity, and avoidance of frequent hypoglycemia may help to prevent weight gain in these individuals. Therapy should take weight gain into consideration, but optimal blood glucose control, without adverse effects, should determine which therapy is used.

SUMMARY

Because of a better understanding of the pathophysiology of type 2 diabetes than in the past, medication therapy is now initiated earlier in the course of the disease, with either monotherapy or combination therapy. Knowledge of the actions, side effects, and contraindications of oral diabetes medications can help the dietetics professional coordinate appropriate MNT and physical activity, to assist the individual with diabetes to achieve optimal glycemic control without unwanted effects. Frequent reassessment and adjustment of therapy is necessary to maintain glycemic control, because of the progressive nature of type 2 diabetes.

REFERENCES

1. DeFronzo RA. Pharmacologic therapy for type 2 diabetes mellitus. *Ann Intern Med.* 1999;131:281–303.

2. Franz MJ. *A Core Curriculum for Diabetes Education: Diabetes Management Therapies.* Chicago, Ill: American Association of Diabetes Educators; 2003:95–154.

3. Inzucchi SE. Oral antihyperglycemic therapy for type 2 diabetes: scientific review. *JAMA.* 2002;287:360–372.

4. Marbury T, Huang WC, Strange P, Lebovitz H. Repaglinide versus glyburide: a one-year comparison trial. *Diabetes Res Clin Pract.* 1999;43:155–156.

5. Ahmann AJ, Riddle MC. Current oral agents in type 2 diabetes. *Postgrad Med.* 2002;111:32–42.

6. Metaglip [prescribing information]. Princeton, NJ: Bristol-Myers Squibb; 2002.

7. Glucovance [prescribing information]. Princeton, NJ: Bristol-Myers Squibb; 2002.

8. Avandamet [prescribing information]. GlaxoSmithKline; 2002.

9. Campbell RK, White JR. *Medications for the Treatment of Diabetes.* Alexandria, Va: American Diabetes Association; 2000.

10. Prandin [product insert]. Princeton, NJ: Novo Nordisk Pharmaceuticals, Inc; 2002.

11. Starlix [product insert]. East Hanover, NJ: Novartis Pharmaceuticals Corp; 2002.

12. Raskin P, ed. *Medical Management of Non-Insulin Dependent (Type 2) Diabetes.* 3rd ed. Alexandria, Va: American Diabetes Association; 1994.

13. Davis SN, Granner DK. Insulin, oral hypoglycemic agents, and the pharmacology of the endocrine pancreas. In: Hardman JG, Limbird LE, Molinoff PB, eds. *Goodman & Gilman's the Pharmacologic Basics of Therapeutics.* 9th ed. New York, NY: McGraw-Hill; 1996:1486–1517.

14. White JR Jr. The pharmacologic management of patients with type II diabetes mellitus in the era of new oral agents and insulin analogues. *Diabetes Spectrum.* 1996;9:227–234.

15. Glueck CJ, Wang P, Goldenberg N, Sieve-Smith L. Pregnancy outcomes among women with polycystic ovary syndrome treated with metformin. *Hum Reprod.* 2002; 17:2858–2864.

16. The Diabetes Prevention Program Research Group. Reduction in the evidence of type 2 diabetes with lifestyle intervention or metformin. *N Engl J Med.* 2002;346:393–403.

17. White JR. The pharmacological reduction of blood glucose in patients with type 2 diabetes mellitus. *Clin Diabetes.* 1998;16:58–67.

18. Glucophage [prescribing information]. Princeton, NJ: Bristol-Myers Squibb; 2002.

19. Aronoff S, Rosenblatt S, Braithwaite S, Egan JW, Mathisen AL, Schneider RL. Pioglitazone hydrochloride monotherapy improves glycemic control in the treatment of patients with type 2 diabetes: a 6-month randomized placebo-controlled dose-response study: the Pioglitazone 001 Study Group. *Diabetes Care.* 2000;23:1605–1611.

20. Actos [product insert]. Osaka, Japan: Takeda Pharmaceuticals America, Inc; 2002.

21. Avandia [product insert]. GlaxoSmithKline Group; 2002.

22. Merlob P, Levitt O, Stahl B. Oral antihyperglycemic agents during pregnancy and lactation. *Pediatr Drugs.* 2002; 4:755–760.

23. Turner RC, Cull CA, Frighi V, Holman RR, and the UKPDS Group. Glycemic control with diet, sulfonylurea, metformin, or insulin in patients with type 2 diabetes mellitus. *JAMA.* 1000;281:2005–2012.

9

Insulin Therapy

Jan Kincaid Rystrom, MEd, RD, CDE

CHAPTER OVERVIEW

- Insulin is a vital diabetes management tool when used in conjunction with medical nutrition therapy, physical activity, and, when appropriate, oral diabetes medications. A clear understanding of the pharmacokinetics of insulin, as well as the ability to recognize trends in blood glucose data, is essential to recommend changes in meal plans and insulin plans and to determine appropriate insulin-to-carbohydrate ratios.
- Insulin is classified based on the expected onset, peak, and duration of action.
- Algorithms can be used to introduce and adjust insulin levels.
- Syringes and pens are the two most common methods of insulin administration, whereas insulin pumps offer variable and adjustable insulin dosing to meet individual needs. Noninvasive methods of insulin delivery are in development.
- Common side effects from insulin use are hypoglycemia and weight gain.

INSULIN FUNCTION

Endogenous insulin is a hormone secreted by the beta cells of the pancreas in response to changes in blood levels of glucose and other nutrients. When the pancreas is stimulated, proinsulin is cleaved into insulin and c-peptide.

Insulin and c-peptide are secreted into the bloodstream in equal amounts. Normal daily insulin secretion of a healthy, nonpregnant, nonobese adult is 0.5 to 0.7 units per kg of body weight. Measurement of direct insulin levels is difficult, because insulin is rapidly removed from the blood as it is used. Measurement of c-peptide can be used as a clinical indicator of endogenous insulin production and to determine type of diabetes.

Insulin is responsible for the following:

- Facilitating glucose transport from the circulation into muscle and adipose cells
- Suppressing glucose production in the liver
- Regulating cellular glucose, lipid, and protein metabolism
- Promoting growth in specific cell types

Diabetes is most commonly categorized as either type 1 diabetes (an absolute deficiency of insulin secretion due to destruction of the beta cells) or as type 2 diabetes (a relative deficiency of insulin secretion in combination with insulin resistance). The goal of insulin replacement is to mimic endogenous insulin.

The discovery and development of insulin revolutionized the treatment of diabetes. Insulin provided the first pharmacological treatment for people who otherwise would have been prescribed starvation diets and comfort care until their inevitable demise. Since the introduction

TABLE 9.1 Types of Insulin*

Insulin Type	Brand Name (Manufacturer†)	Onset Action, h	Peak Action, h	Duration, h	Notes
Rapid-acting					
Aspart	Novolog (Novo Nordisk)	0.25–0.5	1–3	3–5	Approved for pump use
Lispro	Humalog (Eli Lilly & Co)	0.25–0.5	0.5–2.5	< 5	Approved for pump use
Short-acting					
Regular	Humulin R (Eli Lilly & Co)	0.5–1	2–4	5–8	
	Novolin R (Novo Nordisk)	0.5	2.5–5	8	
Intermediate-acting					
NPH	Novolin N (Novo Nordisk)	1–2	4–12	18–26	Usually dosed twice daily
	Humulin N (Eli Lilly & Co)	2–4	4–10	14–18	Usually dosed twice daily
Lente	Humulin L (Eli Lilly & Co)	1–3	6–15	18–26	
	Novolin L (Novo Nordisk)	2.5	7–15	22	
Long-acting (basal)					
Ultralente	Humulin U (Eli Lilly & Co)	4–6	8–30	24–36	
Insulin glargine	Lantus (Aventis)	2	No pronounced peak	> 24	Cannot be mixed with other insulins. A clear, long-acting insulin (others are cloudy). Low pH can produce irritations at the injection site.
Combinations (mixed)					
70/30	Humulin 70/30 (Eli Lilly & Co)	0.5–1	Dual	10–16	70% NPH, 30% Regular
	Novolin 70/30 (Novo Nordisk)	0.5	Dual	24	70% NPH, 30% Regular
70/30	Novolog Mix 70/30 (Novo Nordisk)	0.25–0.5	Dual	10–16	70% aspart protamine suspension, 30% aspart
50/50	Humulin 50/50 (Eli Lilly & Co)	0.5–1	Dual	10–16	50% NPH, 50% Regular
75/25	Humalog Mix 75/25 (Eli Lilly & Co)	0.25–0.5	Dual	10–16	75% lispro protamine suspension, 25% lispro

*Insulin action is dependent on many different factors, including the insulin dose.

†Manufacturers: Avenits, Bridgewater, NJ 08807-2854; Eli Lilly and Company, Indianapolis, IN 46285; Novo Nordisk, Princeton, NJ 08540.

of the first animal-derived insulin in 1922, insulin and insulin delivery systems have been steadily improved and refined.

TYPES OF INSULIN

Virtually all insulin prescribed in North America today is purified human recombinant DNA. These very pure insulins are extremely well tolerated, resulting in fewer antibody and allergy issues than those associated with animal-derived insulins of the past.

Insulin is classified based on the expected onset, peak, and duration of action (1). The dietetics professional must have an understanding of these factors before developing a care plan and meal plan. Table 9.1 summarizes the onset action, peak action, and duration on insulin types available.

A major advancement in insulin production in the past 10 years has been the development of insulin analogs lispro, aspart, glulisine (approved by the Food and Drug Administration but not yet available for consumers) glargine, and detemir (not yet on the market). Insulin analogs are produced from human insulin, with a structural change in the amino acid order of the insulin that affects the rates of absorption. Lispro, aspart, and glulisine have much faster rates of absorption than regular insulin; glargine and detemir insulins are long-acting insulins, with no peak action time.

The standard packaging of insulin in the United States is 10-mL glass vials containing 100 units per mL (U-100), or 1,000 units per vial. Regular insulin is available by prescription in U-500 concentration (500 units per mL or 5,000 units per vial). The more-concentrated insulin is useful to persons with pronounced insulin resistance, who would otherwise require large-volume doses.

INSULIN PLANS

Several algorithms based on body weight are used for the introduction and adjustment of insulin. See Table 9.2 (2–5) for a comparison of these algorithms. Many of these algorithms are based on conventional wisdom and should be used as general starting guidelines. People with type 1 diabetes, or those with type 2 diabetes who require insulin, typically receive one half to two thirds of their insulin dose as intermediate- or long-acting insulin, to cover basal insulin requirements. The remaining one third to one half of the daily insulin dose is given as rapid- or short-acting insulin before meals, to control postprandial glycemia.

Insulin plans are as varied as the practitioners prescribing the insulin. The best plan is one that can be maintained and that produces blood glucose control within target range (6). Insulins are often combined into plans according to the time activity of the insulin. When evaluating an individual's insulin plan, the dietetics professional should consider the time activity of each type of insulin used and the impact that time activity will have on the individual's eating schedule.

Fixed and Flexible Insulin Plans

There are two main categories of insulin plans—fixed and flexible. See Table 9.3 for a description of each plan and its advantages and disadvantages. Fixed-dose plans may include one, two, three, or more daily doses of insulin; the number or amount of insulin doses does not vary, unless as directed by the health care provider. The fixed-dose plan is often used by, but not typically recommended for, free-living persons (7).

Flexible plans allow fine-tuning of the insulin dose according to many factors, including the following:

- Current blood glucose level
- Planned carbohydrate intake
- Planned activity level

The dietetics professional must be able to work with the individual on a flexible plan, to identify blood glucose trends (see Chapter 11), to support the method of carbohydrate identification best suited to that person (see Chapter 18), and to understand the kinetics of insulin, in order to suggest dose changes.

Sliding Scale Insulin

The sliding scale is an algorithm used to determine a premeal insulin dose based on the blood glucose at that moment. There is no adjustment for amount of food to be eaten or prediction of postmeal activity. As a result, sliding scale insulin can (and often does) result in acute complications from hypo- and hyperglycemia (8). Sliding scale insulin is not designed to provide mealtime or basal coverage, but frequently it is misused in the inpatient setting to do so. Sliding scales are sometimes used to treat hyperglycemia in individuals managed by nutrition therapy or oral diabetes medications. It is inappropriate to use only a sliding scale with an individual requiring insulin therapy. Sliding scales are still commonly used in acute-care or long-term-care facilities,

TABLE 9.2　Insulin Algorithms

Type of Diabetes	Total Daily Insulin Dose	Details
Type 1 diabetes	0.6 U/kg body weight	½–⅔ basal insulin (glargine, ultralente, or NPH); ⅓–½ rapid- or short-acting insulin given before meals (2) **Basal insulin:** • *Glargine*: 0.3 U glargine/kg body weight. • *NPH*: 0.2 U NPH × weight in kg before breakfast + 0.1 U NPH × weight in kg at bedtime *or* 0.1 U NPH × weight in kg 3 times/day given every 8 hours. • *Ultralente*: 0.1 U ultralente × weight in kg before breakfast + 0.2 U ultralente × weight in kg before dinner. **Bolus insulin:** • 1 U rapid- or short-acting insulin for every 10 to 15 g carbohydrate eaten. • Adjust bolus doses as needed to correct postprandial glucose levels (2).
Type 1 diabetes with trace to small ketones or Type 2 diabetes with BMI ≤ 27	0.3–0.5 U/kg body weight	**Flexible plan:** • For individuals with an unpredictable schedule, willing to take 3 to 4 injections per day, desiring optimal control and convenience. • ½ *bolus insulin* (aspart, lispro, glulisine) equally distributed for meals or given according to insulin:carbohydrate ratio. • ½ *basal insulin* (glargine once daily; or ultralente before breakfast and ultralente before dinner or bedtime; or ultralente before breakfast and NPH at bedtime for cases of dawn phenomenon*) (3). **Fixed plan:** • For individuals with consistent food intake who want simplified plan of 2 to 3 injections per day. • ⅔ daily dose at breakfast, ⅓ daily dose at evening meal; at breakfast give 1:2 bolus/basal insulin, at dinner give 1:1 bolus/basal insulin. • Bolus insulin is lispro, aspart, glulisine, or regular; basal insulin is NPH; 70/30 or 75/25 may be used (3).
Type 1 diabetes with moderate to large ketones or type 2 diabetes with BMI ≥ 27	0.5–0.7 U/kg body weight	**Flexible plan:** • For individuals with an unpredictable schedule, willing to take 3 to 4 injections per day, desiring optimal control and convenience. • ½ *bolus insulin* (aspart, lispro, glulisine) equally distributed for meals or given according to insulin:carbohydrate ratio. • ½ *basal insulin* (glargine once daily; or ultralente before breakfast and ultralente before dinner or bedtime; or ultralente before breakfast and NPH at bedtime for cases of dawn phenomenon) (3). **Fixed plan:** • For people with consistent food intake who want simplified plan of 2 to 3 injections per day. • ⅔ daily dose at breakfast, ⅓ daily dose at evening meal. • At breakfast give 1:2 bolus/basal insulin.

(*continued*)

TABLE 9.2 *(Continued)*

Type of Diabetes	Total Daily Insulin Dose	Details
		• At dinner give 1:1 bolus/basal insulin. • Bolus insulin is lispro, aspart, glulisine, or regular; basal insulin is NPH; 70/30 or 75/25 may be used (3).
Type 2 diabetes on no oral diabetes medications		• For cases of predominantly daytime hyperglycemia: 10 U intermediate-acting insulin in the morning. • For cases of marked fasting hyperglycemia: 10 U intermediate-acting insulin at bedtime (4).
Type 2 diabetes with suboptimal glycemic control on oral diabetes medications		• 10–15 U intermediate-acting insulin twice daily with discontinuation of oral medications; or 10–15 U intermediate- or long-acting insulin at bedtime; or 10–15 U 70/30 before dinner with continuation of oral medications. • Increase insulin dose by 5–10 U increments weekly until fasting glucose level is less than 120 (5).
Type 2 diabetes on oral diabetes medications	0.1–0.2 U/kg ideal body weight	• Intermediate-acting insulin at bedtime, or long-acting insulin at bedtime, or 75/25 or 70/30 insulin before evening meal. • Continue oral medications; adjust insulin dose until glucose goals met. • If glucose goals not met consider changing to multidose therapy (5).

Abbreviation: BMI, body mass index.
* Dawn phenomenon is an increase in blood glucose in diabetes in the early morning (4–8 am), most likely due to increased glucose production in the liver after an overnight fast.
Source: Adapted with permission from *Insulin BASICS Clinical Guidelines* (3). © 2002 International Diabetes Center, Minneapolis, USA. Data are from references 2–5.

because the physician can write a simple order for a scaled insulin dose based on blood glucose results; the order can be easily interpreted and implemented by the nursing staff (9).

INSULIN ADMINISTRATION

The two most common methods of insulin administration are via syringes and pens. It is important to select the administration method most appropriate for each individual (see Table 9.4).

Syringes

Injection by syringe was the original method of insulin administration. Early glass syringes required careful handling and cleaning; the needles were large, crude, and required regular sharpening. Disposable syringes were introduced in the mid-1960s. Today's disposable syringes have fine, beveled needles that are shorter in length and

lubricated for ease of injection and minimal tissue damage. New short-needle syringes may be less distressing in appearance, especially to people who are not enthusiastic about injecting. Short-needle syringes have also been helpful for very lean individuals and for children, to prevent intramuscular injection, which can result in an unpredictable onset of insulin action (10). Short needles are typically recommended for use in people with normal or near-normal body mass index.

Standard syringes in the United States are designed for U-100 insulin. U-500 insulin must be used with syringes specifically designed for U-500 insulin. Some syringes are clearly marked to accommodate increments of one-half units. See Table 9.5 (11) for a comparison of insulin syringes.

Pens

A pen device, popular in Europe for a decade but only recently debuting in the North American market, is

TABLE 9.3 Insulin Plans

Insulin Plan Type	Description	Example of Use	Advantages	Disadvantages	Patient Selection/Indications for Use
Fixed	Constant dose of basal insulin, may be combined with standard mealtime dose of rapid- or short-acting insulin. Premixed insulins may be used.	• 30 U of 70/30 insulin taken before breakfast and dinner. • 15 U lispro plus 25 U NPH taken before breakfast and 10 U lispro and 20 U NPH taken before dinner.	• Simple, easy to understand • Few daily injections	• Less flexible dosing • Dose cannot be adjusted to treat hyperglycemia, for variable carbohydrate intake, or for change in usual activity level	• Type 2 diabetes and new to insulin • Type 2 diabetes with consistent schedules and eating patterns • Individuals unable or unwilling to calculate mealtime insulin dose based on carbohydrate intake • Individuals with physical disabilities • Individuals with limited motivation for diabetes management • Individuals living in controlled settings where meals, medications, and activities are consistent and predictable
Flexible*	Basal insulin (intermediate-acting or long-acting) given once or twice daily in addition to bolus insulin (short- or rapid-acting insulin).	• Lispro dose before all meals taken according to planned carbohydrate intake plus correction dose to treat hyperglycemia and dose of glargine taken at bedtime.	• Allows adjustment of insulin dose to treat hyperglycemia, variable carbohydrate intake, or alteration in usual activity level	• Three or more daily injections • More complicated • Requires extra training to understand insulin plan and become competent in making insulin dosing decisions	• Type 1 diabetes • Individuals requiring flexible insulin plan due to schedule or personal preference • Individuals desiring to vary carbohydrate intake • Individuals motivated to check blood glucose 3 to 4 times daily and learn carbohydrate counting

*Also known as multiple daily injections (MDI) or intensive insulin therapy.

about the size of large marking pen. Pens are either reusable (with a prefilled glass cartridge) or disposable. Disposable pens contain either 150 units or 300 units of insulin. Insulin cartridges and prefilled pens are available for rapid-acting, regular, NPH, and some premixed insulins. The pens allow a single-use needle to be screwed onto the end for injection. The dose is "dialed up," and a button is pressed to inject the insulin. The needle is discarded and replaced for each injection. As with all devices, optimal absorption requires correct loading, dosing, and injecting techniques (see Box 9.1).

Adaptive Devices

Injection using a vial and syringe has serious drawbacks for individuals with visual impairments and manual dexterity difficulties. Vision impairments can make drawing up the correct dosage difficult. Adaptive devices are available to hold the vial and syringe, to magnify the cartridge, and to provide tactile and audio confirmation of the doses. Table 9.6 (11) identifies insulin delivery aids for individuals with visual or physical impairments. Individuals with limited dexterity may have difficulty manip-

TABLE 9.4 Insulin Administration

Administration Method	Advantages	Disadvantages	Patient Selection
Syringe and vial	• Least expensive administration method	• Requires manual dexterity, and good vision	• Individuals who mix two types of insulin and prefer a minimal number of injections per day
Insulin pen	• Convenient, portable, inconspicuous • Uses shortest needles available (⁵⁄₁₆ in)	• More expensive • May require additional injections if multiple types of insulin are used • Glargine currently not available in disposable pen	• Individuals with manual dexterity problems and low levels of vision • Individuals who frequently take injections away from home

TABLE 9.5 Insulin Syringes (for use with U-100 insulin)

Syringe Type, cc (U)	Appropriate Administration, units of insulin	Needle Gauge	Needle Size, in
1 (100)	50–100	28	½ and ⁵⁄₁₆
		29	½
		30	½ and ⁵⁄₁₆
		31*	⁵⁄₁₆
½ (50)	30–50	28	½
		29	½
		30	⁵⁄₁₆, ⅜, and ½
		31*	⁵⁄₁₆
³⁄₁₀ (30)	< 30	28	½
		29	½
		30†	⁵⁄₁₆, ⅜, and ½
		31*†‡	⁵⁄₁₆

*Smallest gauge needle available.
†Available in ½-unit scale.
‡Useful for children and thin people.
Source: Data are from reference 11.

BOX 9.1

Insulin Pen: General Instructions for Use*

1. Gently turn the insulin pen up and down 10 times to be sure the insulin is evenly mixed. Avoid shaking the pen to mix the insulin because this could create air bubbles.
2. Use an alcohol swab to wipe the rubber seal on the end of the pen.
3. Attach and uncap a pen needle.
4. Prime the pen (also called giving an air shot) by turning the dial to 2 units and press the injection button all the way down until a drop or stream of insulin is seen (do not inject this insulin). Prime every time to make sure insulin is flowing and to remove air bubbles. If there's no insulin flow, then replace the needle.
5. Dial the pen to the number of units to be injected. If a full dose cannot be dialed, the pen does not contain enough insulin to administer that dose. The partial dose can be administered with the remaining dose administered from a new pen/cartridge. Alternately, use a new pen/cartridge for the entire dose.
6. Select an injection site. Insert the needle into the skin and press the injection button down completely. Keep the needle in the skin with the button pushed all the way down for five to six seconds to ensure the full dose has been delivered.
7. Pull the needle out of the skin.
8. Remove the needle from the pen and dispose of the needle in a sharps container. Always remove used needles after every injection, to prevent insulin from leaking, to prevent bubbles from forming in the cartridge, and to ensure sterility.
9. Place the cap back on the pen for storage.

*It is recommended that each manufacturer's specific directions be followed.

TABLE 9.6 Insulin Delivery Aids for Individuals With Visual or Physical Impairments*

Delivery Aid	Product Name (Manufacturer†)	Description
Syringe magnifiers	BD Magni-Guide (BD) Insul-eze (Palco Labs) Syringe Magnifier (Apothecary Products) Tru-Hand (Whittier Medical)	Devices designed to magnify syringe calibrations on syringes of various sizes.
Nonvisual insulin measurement	Count-a-Dose (Medicool, Inc)	Syringe-filling device, which uses a click wheel to fill syringe; click is heard and felt as wheel is rotated.
	Load-Matic (Palco Labs)	Allows individual to load syringes by touch alone. Aligns needle with bottle top; fills syringe by 10-U or single-unit increments.
Needle guides and vial stabilizers	Inject Assist (Apothecary Products) Injection Safety Guard (Apothecary Products) Insul-Cap (Palco Labs)	Guides needle into insulin vial. Provides stability to insulin bottle as syringe is filled.
	NeedleAid (NeedleAid, Ltd)	Stabilizing guide for injection using a syringe or insulin pen.
Vial syringe guides	Vial Syringe Guide (Apothecary Products)	Connects insulin syringe to insulin bottle.

*Listing is not intended to be all-inclusive.
†Manufacturers: Apothecary Products, Burnsville, MN 55337-1295; BD, Franklin Lakes, NJ 07417-1883; Medicool, Inc, Torrance, CA, 90501; NeedleAid, Ltd, Dartmouth, NS Canada B2X 3P3; Palco Labs, Santa Cruz, CA 95062; Whittier Medical, North Andover, MA 01845.
Source: Adapted with permission from American Diabetes Association. Diabetes Forecast: Resource Guide 2004 (11). Copyright © 2004, American Diabetes Association.

ulating the syringe and the vial, especially when mixing insulins. Mixing insulin is also a complex, multistep process, which may be too difficult for some individuals. Including an occupational therapist and physical therapist in the assessment and treatment of patients with visual or physical impairments can be useful.

Other Injection Devices

The effects of arthritis, vision changes, and self-care attitudes can make insulin use challenging for even the most motivated person. Other injection devices are now available, in response to the growing use of insulin by older persons. For a description of alternate injection devices, see Table 9.7 (11). One such device has a prefilled insulin cartridge and a dial similar to an egg timer, which is used to select the dose. A large button allows for ease of insulin delivery. Another of the prefilled insulin car-

tridge devices combines a blood glucose meter with an injection device. Insulin users can carry their insulin and meter in one compact unit.

Needle-free injection devices, or jet injectors, are useful for individuals with extreme needle phobia. The device uses pressure to create a thin stream of insulin that penetrates the skin and is deposited into the subcutaneous tissue in a fraction of a second. Once large and cumbersome, these injectors are now smaller in size. The initial hardware and ongoing supply costs can still be a deterrent to use.

Insulin Injection Training

Specific training for the injection of insulin is vital for people with diabetes. Figure 9.1 (12) provides step-by-step instructions for the administration of insulin using a vial and syringe. Dietetics professionals should check

TABLE 9.7 Injection Devices

Device (Manufacturer*)	Description	Indications for Use/Comments	Limitations
InnoLet injection device (Novo Nordisk)	Prefilled injection device. Dial used to select insulin dose is similar to egg timer with easy-to-read numbers. Button used to inject insulin is large.	Easy to use. Appropriate for individuals with dexterity problems, visual impairments.	Available only with regular, NPH, and 70/30 insulins. Does not allow mixing of insulins.
In Duo (Novo Nordisk)	Prefilled insulin cartridge combined with blood glucose meter.	Convenient to carry insulin and meter in a single unit. Appropriate for individuals who take aspart insulin before each meal or use 70/30 insulin.	Available only with 70/30 and aspart insulins.
Jet injectors: Advanta Jet (Activa Brand Products, Inc); Advanta Jet ES (Activa Brand Products, Inc); Gentle Jet (Activa Brand Products, Inc); Injex 30 (Equidyne Systems, Inc); Medi-Jector Vision (Antares Pharma, Inc); Vitajet 3 (Bioject, Inc)	Needleless devices that release a tiny jet stream of insulin, which is forced through the skin with pressure.	Appropriate for individuals with fear of needles. Some devices are designed for use with visual impairments.	May cause bruising. Initial expense and ongoing supply costs may be a deterrent to use.

*Manufacturers: Activa Brand Products, Inc, Charlottetown, PEI, Canada, CIE 2B3; Antares Pharma, Inc., Minneapolis, MN 55441; Bioject, Inc., Portland, OR 97224; Equidyne Systems, Inc., San Diego, CA 92128; Novo Nordisk Pharmaceuticals, Inc., Princeton, NJ 08540.

Source: Data are from reference 11.

state regulations to determine whether the scope of practice allows piercing the skin such as during instruction on insulin administration. If piercing the skin is not permitted, the dietetics professional may consider becoming a certified medical assistant or having the individual requiring instruction practice on a model and then inject him- or herself.

Injection Sites

It is important for people with diabetes on insulin to rotate injection sites, to prevent local irritation. Areas for injections must be selected individually and are determined by presence of scar tissue, amount of subcutaneous body fat, and the individual's preferences. Insulin absorption is most rapid in the abdomen, followed by the arms, thighs, and buttocks (13). Exercise or massage at the injection site may cause more rapid insulin absorption. It can be useful to teach individuals to rotate within one area

of the body rather than rotating to a different part of the body, in order to decrease the variability in absorption from day to day.

Insulin Pumps

Insulin pumps are pager-sized, battery-driven devices, used to deliver insulin. Each pump holds a single cartridge containing either regular or rapid-acting (aspart, lispro) insulin. The insulin is delivered through flexible tubing that attaches the pump to the person by way of an infusion set. Continuous subcutaneous insulin infusion (CSII), also known as "pump therapy," allows the individual with diabetes and the health care team to create variable and adjustable insulin dosing, to meet the insulin needs of the individual. For this reason, CSII is popular with those who desire the opportunity to fine-tune their insulin doses, as well as with children, adolescents, athletes, and others with very active and unpredictable

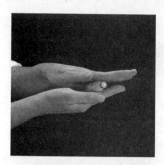

1. First wash your hands.

Then gently mix the insulin by:
- rolling the vial between the palms of your hands
- or, turning the vial over from end to end a few times

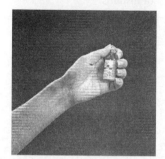

2. If this is a new vial, remove the flat, colored cap, but not the rubber stopper or the metal band under the cap.

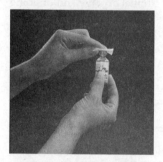

3. Clean the rubber stopper with an alcohol swab.

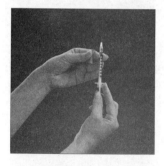

4. Remove the cover from the needle.

Pull the plunger back to pull air into the syringe.

Pull back until the tip of the plunger is at the line for the number of units required.

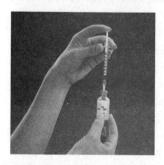

5. Push the needle through the rubber stopper.

Make sure the tip of the needle is not in the insulin.

Press the plunger to push air into the vial of insulin.

FIGURE 9.1 Insulin administration using a vial and syringe. Reprinted with permission from *Managing Your Diabetes: Comprehensive Patient Education Program*. Indianapolis, Ind.: Eli Lilly and Company. Copyright © 2001, Eli Lilly and Company. (12).

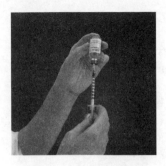

6. Turn the vial and syringe upside down. Now the tip of the needle should be in the insulin.

Holding the vial with one hand, use the other to pull back on the plunger, which will pull insulin into the syringe. Stop when the plunger is at the line for your dose.

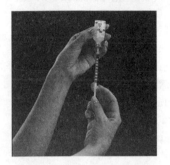

7. Look at the insulin in the syringe. If you see any air bubbles:

- use the plunger to push the insulin back into the vial. Then slowly pull the plunger back to the line for your dose of insulin.
- repeat this until there are no large air bubbles in the syringe.

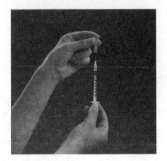

8. Make sure the tip of the plunger is at the line showing your dose of insulin.

Double-check your dose. Magnifiers are available if needed to help you see more clearly.

Pull the needle out of the rubber stopper.

If you need to lay the needle down before taking your shot, put the cover back on the tip to protect it.

FIGURE 9.1 (*Continued*)

lifestyles (14). Women planning pregnancies, or those managing diabetes while pregnant, benefit from being able to match rapidly changing insulin needs and achieve tight glycemic goals (15).

Pumps deliver insulin in two ways:

1. Basal insulin is preprogrammed to replace the intermediate or long-acting insulin of an intensified insulin plan. The pump can be programmed with different basal rates at different times of day, in order to meet the individual's insulin needs.
2. Bolus insulin doses are administered to cover food intake and to correct hyperglycemia.

Advantages

Pump therapy offers many advantages, including a reduced fear of nocturnal hypoglycemia (6) and immediate improvement in blood glucose control (6). Insulin can be delivered in basal rate increments of 0.05 units.

Differences in insulin absorption from various body sites are reduced. Dawn phenomenon effects can be managed by adjusting basal rates, to meet increased insulin needs during early-morning hours. (Dawn phenomenon refers to an increase in blood glucose in the early morning, most likely due to increased glucose production in the liver after an overnight fast.)

Pump therapy also provides for more normal and flexible lifestyles (16). The insulin bolus is matched to actual carbohydrate intake, which allows variable carbohydrate intake according to appetite and preferences. Basal rates can be temporarily decreased during periods of exercise or increased activity, or temporarily increased during times of decreased activity.

"Extended" or "time-release" bolus may be programmed to allow the bolus dose to be delivered over a set time period. For example, an individual eating a high-fat meal (pizza or prime rib) might decide to bolus

10 units over 2 hours, in order to match insulin release with prandial blood glucose rise (17).

Disadvantages

Pump therapy has its limitations. The pump user must have support systems in place, and along with family, friends, and health care team, must understand pump therapy. The pump user must be proficient in carbohydrate counting and able to calculate meal and correction bolus insulin doses (17). The pump user also must understand the effect of large amounts of protein and fat on meal absorption. See Appendix D for problem-solving tips.

Additional limitations include the following:

- Risk of skin irritation and infection at the infusion sites (16).
- Risk of technical failure of the pump.
- Potential increase in the incidence of hospital admissions for diabetic ketoacidosis, because only short-acting or rapid-acting insulin is used. If the pump fails to deliver for any reason, the result is a rapid rise in blood glucose (16).
- Increased expense of pump and supplies when compared to traditional syringe injections.

Candidates for Pump Therapy

Appropriate pump candidates have the following characteristics:

- Motivation to learn a new therapy, equipment, and problem-solving skills
- Emotional maturity to accept disease and be physically connected to pump
- Ability and willingness to test blood glucose and maintain records
- Ability to count carbohydrates and calculate carbohydrate and correction boluses
- Adequate financial resources

STORAGE OF INSULIN AND INSULIN ADMINISTRATION DEVICES

Appropriate storage of insulin is essential to ensure that the insulin does not lose potency. Dietetics professionals should advise individuals of the following storage guidelines (11,13,18). Individuals with diabetes should also read the manufacturer's insert for information specific to the product they are using.

Storage Temperature Guidelines

- Individuals with diabetes should store the insulin they are using, including pens in use, at room temperature.
- Most vials of insulin can be stored at room temperature for up to 1 month (ie, 28 days).
- Most prefilled insulin pens can be stored at room temperature for 10 to 14 days.
- Vials of insulin not in use should be stored in the refrigerator.
- Insulin vials and pens that are refrigerated should be stored between 36°F and 46°F.
- Extreme temperatures (eg, storing in a freezer or a car glove compartment) should be avoided. Insulin loses its potency if frozen.
- Use room-temperature insulin for injections; injecting cold insulin may make the injection painful or cause local irritation (13).
- Opened or unopened bottles of insulin should be discarded after staying at room temperature for 1 month (13).

Expiration Date Guidelines

Individuals with diabetes must check expiration dates before using insulin. Insulin should not be used beyond the expiration date.

Product Clarity Guidelines

- Insulin should be examined before use to make sure it looks normal (eg, no particles or discoloration). Cloudiness or discoloration of clear insulins, or clumping or frostiness of insulin suspensions, indicates that the insulin may have lost potency and that it should not be used.
- Individuals using regular insulin, aspart, lispro, or glargine should know that the insulin is supposed to be clear, and that if it is not (ie, they see particles or discoloration), they should not use it.
- Individuals using NPH, ultralente, or lente, should know that the insulin is supposed to be cloudy, and that if they see crystals in the insulin or on the inside of the bottle or small particles or clumps in the insulin, they should not use it.

INSULIN SIDE EFFECTS

To help individuals on insulin therapy understand the causes of actual, and sometimes perceived, adverse effects, dietetics professionals should be aware of adverse effects from insulin.

Hypoglycemia

The most common side effect of insulin therapy is hypoglycemia, defined as a blood glucose level less than 70 mg/dL. Most all people using insulin will experience hypoglycemia at some point. Therefore, it is vital that individuals taking insulin receive education on the signs, symptoms, and treatment guidelines for hypoglycemia (see Chapter 12).

Weight Gain

Many people new to insulin therapy attribute associated weight gain to the insulin, when in fact the weight gain actually results from improvement in glycemic control. With improved glycemic control, the body captures and uses (or stores) glucose instead of losing it through the urine. A single injection of glargine or NPH insulin is not associated with significant weight gain (2). The combination that best minimizes weight gain in type 2 diabetes is metformin plus glargine or NPH insulin given at bedtime (2).

Troubleshooting

Dietetics professionals can aid individuals on insulin therapy by understanding problems that may arise with insulin therapy (see Table 9.8) (6).

OVERCOMING RESISTANCE TO USING INSULIN

Dietetics professionals can play a key role in educating individuals with diabetes on the importance of adequate glycemic control and can help gain acceptance to insulin therapy. The following strategies can be useful:

- Discuss that despite the individual's best efforts at following an appropriate diabetes management plan, adequate glycemic control has not been achieved, hence the need for insulin.

TABLE 9.8 Complications of Insulin Therapy

Complication	Description	Comments/Recommendations
Atrophy	Concaving or pitting of fatty tissue; an immune response related to the species/source of insulin and purity of insulin	• Use of human or highly purified pork insulins reduces incidence of atrophy. • Inject in areas of body without atrophy or around the periphery of atrophied areas.
Hypertrophy	Fatty thickening of lipid tissue	• Rotation of injection sites prevents hypertrophy. • Avoid injecting in areas with hypertrophy or inject around the periphery of hypertrophied areas.
Local allergic reaction	Most often a rash	• Allergies are rare. • Local reactions are much less common with purified human insulins.
Systemic allergic reaction	Anaphylaxis, serum sickness	• Appear to be immunologically mediated. • Zinc or protamine in the insulin, preservatives, rubber or latex stoppers have all been implicated in allergic reactions. • Desensitization to insulin is necessary. (The insulin manufacturer would need to be contacted for the desensitization kit and the procedure to follow.)

Source: Reprinted with permission from White JR, Campbell RK. Pharmacologic therapies for glucose management. In: *A Core Curriculum for Diabetes Education.* 5th ed. American Association of Diabetes Educators; Chicago, Ill: 2003:95–154.

- Reinforce the short-term benefits of improved glycemia, including improved energy levels and decreased nocturia.
- Review importance of glycemic control to prevent long-term complications.
- Review new devices available for insulin therapy, including small-gauge, short needles; insulin pens; and assistive devices for vision and physical impairments.

COMBINATION THERAPY

Type 2 diabetes has long been recognized as a progressive disease. Diminished insulin production, along with worsening insulin resistance, leads to deteriorating blood glucose control (19). Because glycemic control can help prevent progressive macro- and microvascular complications, treatment plans for individuals with type 2 diabetes have expanded beyond oral therapy, to include insulin alone or in combination with oral diabetes medications (20,21). Insulin is required when a combination of oral diabetes medications is unable to maintain the A1C at less than 7% (21). (See Chapter 8 for information on the oral diabetes medications.) The dietetics professional must understand the unique action of these drugs, especially when insulin is added, when developing a nutrition therapy plan of care.

IMPLICATIONS FOR NUTRITION THERAPY

An important component of diabetes self-management is mastering skills to support insulin therapy, including identifying and quantifying carbohydrate foods and calculating correction doses. The dietetics professional must be able to assess each individual's learning style, ability and motivation to learn, and lifestyle, to determine which meal-planning method to use. (See Chapter 18 for the variety of meal-planning options.)

Carbohydrate Counting

Carbohydrate counting takes practice, record keeping, and patience. Primary goals of carbohydrate counting are (a) to help keep food intake consistent at each meal/snack, or (b) to establish an insulin-to-carbohydrate ratio for use in determining how much preprandial short- or rapid-acting insulin is needed to "cover" the foods to be eaten.

A typical starting ratio is 1 unit of rapid- or short-acting insulin per 15 g of carbohydrate to be consumed.

This ratio is highly individualized and variable, based on factors such as body weight, insulin resistance, hormones, and activity level. The dietetics professional can help use food records, insulin dose data, and blood glucose results to identify appropriate insulin-to-carbohydrate ratios. (See Chapter 18 for more information on carbohydrate counting and on calculating insulin-to-carbohydrate ratios). Most individuals find that blood glucose control improves with carbohydrate counting. Additionally, carbohydrate counting can aid in weight control, as awareness of food intake and portion increase.

Insulin Adjustment

Dietetics professionals can make important contributions to improving the glycemic control through the following actions:

- Reviewing blood glucose records from log books or downloaded blood glucose monitor data, to identify times of day with suboptimal glycemic control (see Chapter 10 for more information).
- Reviewing premeal insulin dose timing, to identify possible causes for suboptimal postprandial blood glucose control. Rapid-acting insulins should be administered immediately before eating, and short-acting insulins should be administered 30 to 45 minutes before eating, so that the insulin peaks at the same time the food is digested and absorbed.
- Comparing carbohydrate intake at each meal to corresponding rapid- or short-acting insulin dose taken at each meal, to identify inconsistent carbohydrate intake when using a fixed insulin plan or inaccuracy in calculating insulin dose based on carbohydrate intake when using flexible insulin plans.
- Counseling caretakers of children with unpredictable food intake to try injecting insulin immediately after eating, when actual carbohydrate intake can be quantified.
- Counseling individuals with gastroparesis or nausea (due to conditions such as gastrointestinal illness, chemotherapy, or pregnancy) who may vomit the meal before the calories are absorbed, to take insulin after the meal to prevent postprandial hypoglycemia.
- Recommending changes in the meal plan based on blood glucose response in coordination with the health care team member who is adjusting diabetes medication(s).

- Communicating with the provider prescribing insulin when, upon review of glucose records and current eating habits, it is clear that further changes in the meal plan or timing adjustments in the insulin doses will not improve or correct the postprandial blood glucose results (e-mail from IB Hirsch, November 17, 2002).

FINANCIAL ASSISTANCE FOR INDIVIDUALS USING INSULIN

There are many resources that can help individuals who need financial assistance to acquire insulin, including the following:

- *Lilly Cares.* Approval for up to 4 months of free insulin is possible. Required form must be completed by individual with diabetes and returned to Lilly with a prescription from the physician. The prescription must have specific dosing (eg, patient using 20 units basal, 20 units bolus daily). The individual is mailed a letter of approval and must take the approval letter, along with another prescription, to the pharmacy, to receive the 4-month supply. Proof of income is not required. Program information is available at 800/545-6962.
- *Lilly Answers.* This program requires tax forms and income information. The individual with diabetes completes the form. Upon approval, the total cost of a 30-day supply of Humalog is $12. Ask the physician writing the prescription to take into consideration extra insulin, such as that needed to prime an insulin pump. For further information, call 877/RXLILLY, or go to the program's Web site (http://www.lillyanswers.com; accessed January 23, 2005).
- *Lilly sales representatives.* Representatives may make coupons available to individuals with diabetes for two free bottles of insulin in a 12-month period.
- *Novo Nordisk A/S: Patient Assistance Program.* This program provides a one-time-only 3-month supply of insulin. Obtain application form from Novo Pharmaceutical sales representative and a prescription signed by the physician.
- *Diabetes Trust Foundation.* This foundation provides supplemental support for families who have insurance but need assistance with the copayments for diabetes supplies and pumps. Additional information is available from the foundation Web site (http://diabetestrustfoundation.org; accessed January 23, 2005) or by calling 800/577-1383.
- *Insulin pump companies.* Insulin pump companies may offer scholarship programs, to help individuals make insulin pump therapy affordable. Contact specific insulin pump companies for more information (Web sites are listed in "Additional Resources" at the end of this chapter).

TREATMENTS ON THE HORIZON

Until a cure for diabetes is developed, many individuals with diabetes look toward noninvasive methods of insulin delivery.

Inhaled Insulin

Inhaled intrapulmonary delivery of insulin is one alternative to injections that is being researched (22). Inhaled insulin doses are taken immediately before meals, with reported postprandial glucose control. The insulin is delivered to the lungs, using a handheld inhalation system that contains either dry powder or liquid insulin. Initial human trials have demonstrated the effectiveness of this insulin delivery system; however, further research is needed on the long-term pulmonary safety of inhaled insulin (23). With additional study and development, inhaled insulin could become a viable alternative to injection insulin therapy for some individuals with diabetes.

Implantable Insulin Pumps

"Closed loop" or "artificial pancreas" systems combine an implantable insulin pump with a continuous glucose sensor device to create nearly physiologic blood glucose regulation. The technology has shown promising results in animal testing, and human trials are now under way. Continual progress is being made to refine the durability and size of the implantable devices, to extend battery life, and to develop the surgeries required for implantation.

Human Amylin

Recent attention has been given to the glucose regulation role of amylin, a polypeptide neuroendocrine hormone that is secreted with insulin by the beta cells in response to nutrients. Three key actions of amylin are as follows:

1. It suppresses postprandial glucagon secretion and subsequent hepatic glucose production.
2. It modulates nutrient delivery from the stomach to the small intestine, which reduces postprandial glucose concentrations.
3. It reduces food intake by influencing satiety (24).

Research shows promising results in blood glucose control when administering synthetic amylin in combination with insulin therapy for both type 1 and type 2 diabetes. The dosing and delivery methods, however, still must be studied and approved for human use.

Glucagon-like Peptide-1

Glucagon-like peptide-1 (GLP-1) is a hormone produced in cells lining the intestine in response to a meal. Many of the actions of GLP-1 are similar to human amylin. The functions of GLP-1 include the following:

- Stimulation of insulin production and secretion
- Simultaneous reduction of glucagon response
- Reduction in the rate of food passing from the stomach into the intestine
- Increased number of insulin-producing beta cells

The body destroys GLP-1 within a few minutes, and because GLP-1 is a protein, it cannot be given orally. Research is under way with injections of synthetic GLP-1, which is not rapidly destroyed by the body. Recent study results involving type 2 diabetes indicate improvements in fasting glucose levels, reduction in A1C levels, weight loss, and reduction in appetite (25). Studies have also demonstrated that subcutaneous GLP-1 can improve glycemic control in type 1 diabetes (26).

Another strategy is to produce a drug to inhibit the body's enzyme that destroys GLP-1. Studies providing an orally active inhibitor to people with type 2 diabetes have demonstrated reductions in fasting glucose levels, prandial glucose excursions, and mean glucose levels (27).

SUMMARY

There are different types of insulin with varying rates of absorption and activity. These insulins can be combined into insulin plans that are individualized on the basis of lifestyle, schedule, eating preferences, and need for flexibility.

Insulin can be delivered using syringes, pens, or pumps. Adaptive aids are available for individuals with visual and physical impairments. Insulin pump therapy has been proven to be safe and effective and to improve the lifestyles of people with diabetes. Development of insulin administration therapies that may eliminate the need for injections continues.

Dietetics professionals can contribute to the diabetes management team by helping individuals with diabetes understand insulin therapy and by prescribing an appropriate meal plan to match the insulin plan that best meets each individual's needs.

REFERENCES

1. American Diabetes Association. *The Diabetes Ready-Reference Guide for Health Care Professionals.* Alexandria, Va: American Diabetes Association; 2000.
2. American Diabetes Association. *Practical Insulin: A Handbook for Prescribers.* Alexandria, Va: American Diabetes Association, 2002.
3. International Diabetes Center, Park Nicollet Institute. *Insulin Basics: Clinical Guidelines.* Minneapolis, Minn: International Diabetes Center; 2002.
4. Starting insulin therapy. In: Kelley DB, ed. *Medical Management of Type 2 Diabetes.* Alexandria, Va: American Diabetes Association, 1998:66–71.
5. Abrahamson M, Beaser R, Blair E, Ganda O, Rosenzweig J. Joslin Diabetes Center & Joslin Clinic Clinical Guideline for Pharmacological Management of Type 2 Diabetes. Available at: http://diabetesmanagement.joslin.org/Guidelines/Pharm_ClinGuide.pdf. Accessed January 23, 2005.
6. White JR, Campbell RK. Pharmacologic therapies for glucose management. In: *A Core Curriculum for Diabetes Education.* 5th ed. American Association of Diabetes Educators; Chicago, Ill: 2003:95–154.
7. Lorber DL. Sliding scale insulin [letter]. *Diabetes Care.* 2001;24:2011.
8. Hirsch IB, Farkas-Hirsch R. Sliding scale or sliding scare: it's all sliding nonsense. *Diabetes Spectrum.* 2001;14:79–81.
9. Gaster B, Hirsch IR. Sliding scale insulin use and rates of hyperglycemia. *Arch Intern Med.* 1998;158:95.
10. Tubiana-Rufi N, Belarbi N, Du Pasquier-Fediaevsky L, Polak M, Kakou B, Leridon L, Hassan M, Czernichow P. Short needles (8mm) reduce the risk of intramuscular injections in children with type 1 diabetes. *Diabetes Care.* 1999;22:1621–1625.
11. American Diabetes Association. Special resource guide 2004. *Diabetes Forecast.* 2004;57:RG14-RG37.
12. Eli Lilly and Company. *Managing Your Diabetes: Comprehensive Patient Education Program.* Indianapolis, Ind: Eli Lilly and Company; 2001.

13. American Diabetes Association. Insulin administration (position statement). *Diabetes Care.* 2004;27(suppl): S106–S107.

14. Walsh J, Roberts R. Pumping Insulin: Everything You Need for Success With an Insulin Pump. 3rd ed. San Diego, Calif: Torrey Pines Press; 2000.

15. Pickup J, Keen H. Continuous subcutaneous insulin infusion at 25 years: evidence base for the expanding use of insulin pump therapy in type 1 diabetes. *Diabetes Care.* 2002;25:593–598.

16. Lenhard MJ, Reeves GD. Continuous subcutaneous insulin infusion: a comprehensive review of insulin pump therapy. *Arch Intern Med.* 2001;161:2293.

17. Bolderman KM. *Putting Your Patients on the Pump.* Alexandria, Va: American Diabetes Association; 2002.

18. 2004 reference guide. *Diabetes Interview.* 2004;138(13): 23–35.

19. UK Prospective Diabetes Study (UKPDS) Group. Intensive blood-glucose control with sulphonylureas or insulin compared with conventional treatment and risk of complications in patients with type 2 diabetes (UKPDS 33). *Lancet.* 1998;352:837–852.

20. Inzucchi SE. Oral antihyperglycemic therapy for type 2 diabetes: scientific review. *JAMA.* 2002;287:360–372.

21. Ahmann AJ, Riddle MC. Current oral agents for type 2 diabetes; many options, but which to choose when? *Postgrad Med.* 2002;111:32.

22. Skyler JS, Cefalu WT, Kourides IA, Landschulz WH, Balagtas CC, Cheng SL, Gelfand RA. Efficacy of inhaled human insulin in type 1 diabetes mellitus: a randomized proof-of-concept study. *Lancet.* 2001;357:331–335.

23. Royle P, Waugh N, McAuley L, McIntyre L, Thomas S. Inhaled insulin in diabetes mellitus. *Cochrane Database Syst Rev.* 2003. Available at: http://www.update-software.com/abstracts/ab003890.htm. Accessed January 23, 2005.

24. Amylin: a brief review of physiological functions. Carmel, Ind: Amylin Pharmaceuticals; 2001.

25. Item #3 revisited from July 17, 2001, issue 61. Diabetes in Control Web site. Issue 97, item 3 (2002). Available at: http://www.diabetesincontrol.com/issue97/item3.shtml. Accessed Jan. 23, 2005.

26. Behme MT, Dupre J, McDonald TJ. Glucagon-like peptide 1 improved glycemic control in type 1 diabetes. *BMC Endocr Disord.* 2003;3:3. Available at: http://www.biomedcentral.com/1472–6823/3/3. Accessed January 23, 2005.

27. Ahren B, Simonsson E, Larsson H, Landin-Olsson M, Torgeirsson H, Jansson PA, Sandqvist M, Bavenholm P, Efendic S, Eriksson JW, Dickinson S, Holmes D. Inhibition of dipeptidyl peptidase IV improves metabolic control over a 4-week study period in type 2 diabetes. *Diabetes Care.* 2002;25:869–875.

ADDITIONAL RESOURCES

General Diabetes and Insulin Information

Children With Diabetes. Available at: http://www.childrenwithdiabetes.com. Accessed January 23, 2005.

Diabetes Mall (books, food scales, resources). Available at: http://www.diabetesnet.com. Accessed January 23, 2005.

Lilly Diabetes.com. Available at: http://www.lillydiabetes.com/index.jsp. Accessed December 20, 2004.

Novo Nordisk. Available at: http://www.novonordisk.com. Accessed December 20, 2004.

Insulin Pumps

Insulin Pumpers (includes chat rooms, articles, links to other sites). Available at: http://www.insulin-pumpers.org. Accessed December 20, 2004.

Animas. Available at: http://www.animascorp.com. Accessed December 20, 2004.

Deltec Cozmo. Available at: http://www.delteccozmo.com. Accessed December 20, 2004.

Disetronic. Available at: http://www.disetronic.com. Accessed December 20, 2004.

Medtronic Minimed. Available at: http://www.minimed.com. Accessed December 20, 2004.

Insulin Pumps for Children

Grandmasandy.com (downloadable book for kids on pumps; games for kids with diabetes). Available at: http://www.grandmasandy.com. Accessed December 20, 2004.

Kids Pumping. Available at: http://www.kidspumping.com. Accessed December 20, 2004.

Pumpwear Inc. Available at: http://www.pumpwearinc.com. Accessed December 20, 2004.

10

Monitoring

Amy Fischl, MS, RD, BC-ADM, CDE

CHAPTER OVERVIEW

- To maintain metabolic control and to prevent complications (see Chapters 12 and 13 for further information), the following parameters should be monitored in individuals with diabetes: blood glucose; glycosylated hemoglobin (A1C); glycosylated serum albumin (fructosamine); ketones, urine and blood; lipids; microalbumin; and blood pressure.
- Methods for monitoring blood glucose include laboratory tests and self-monitoring of blood glucose (SMBG), via fingertips and alternate sites.
- Inadequate blood samples and uncalibrated monitors are some common user errors with blood glucose monitors.
- The process of tracking diabetes care has been simplified by computerized data management systems.
- Continuous glucose monitoring systems provide information on blood glucose fluctuations; the effect of physical activity on blood glucose; the duration of basal insulin; and insulin-to-carbohydrate ratios and the effect on postprandial blood glucose.

GLUCOSE MONITORING

Glucose monitoring is essential for establishing optimal treatment of diabetes and for making proactive management decisions to help prevent hypoglycemia and hyper-

glycemia. Blood glucose can be monitored using the following methods:

- Self-monitoring of capillary blood glucose using a blood glucose monitor (also known as a blood glucose meter)
- Laboratory glucose
- A1C
- Glycosylated serum albumin (fructosamine)
- Other blood glucose monitoring devices

As mentioned above, the parameters that should be monitored include blood glucose; A1C; glycosylated serum albumin (fructosamine); ketones, urine and blood; lipids; microalbumin; and blood pressure. See Table 10.1 (1,2) for monitoring frequency and goals for each of these parameters for people with diabetes aged 18 years or older (see Chapter 15 for information on children from birth through adolescence and Chapter 17 on diabetes in pregnancy and lactation).

SELF-MONITORING OF BLOOD GLUCOSE

Blood glucose monitors became available to the public in the early 1980s. Around the same time, recruitment for the Diabetes Control and Complications Trial (DCCT)

TABLE 10.1 Monitoring Frequency and Goals for Individuals With Diabetes 18 Years or Older*

Parameter	Recommended Monitoring Frequency	Goal
Plasma blood glucose, mg/dL	• Determined by individual needs and goals.	Preprandial: 90–130 Postprandial[†]: < 180
A1C	• At initial assessment, to document glycemic control. • Then at least 2 times per year in individuals with stable glycemic control who are meeting treatment goals; or • Quarterly in individuals not meeting treatment goals or whose therapy has changed.	< 7.0% (American Diabetes Association) ≤ 6.5% (American College of Endocrinology)
Fructosamine	• At 2- to 3-week intervals in short-term follow-up.	Varies depending on measurement method
Ketones (blood and urine)	• Routinely during illness in all individuals with diabetes. • In individuals with type 1 diabetes when blood glucose is consistently > 300 mg/dL. • Regularly monitor urine ketones in individuals trying to lose weight via energy restriction.	Negative
Total cholesterol, mg/dL	• Annually or more frequently, as needed, to achieve goals. In adults with low-risk values, rescreen every 2 years.	< 200
LDL cholesterol, mg/dL	• Annually or more frequently, as needed, to achieve goals. In adults with low-risk values, rescreen every 2 years.	< 100
HDL cholesterol, mg/dL	• Annually or more frequently, as needed, to achieve goals. In adults with low-risk values, rescreen every 2 years.	Men: > 40 Women: > 50
Triglycerides	• Annually or more frequently, as needed, to achieve goals. In adults with low-risk values, rescreen every 2 years.	< 150
Urinary microalbumin	• Type 1: annually in individuals with ≥ 5-y history of diabetes. • Type 2: annually beginning at diagnosis, and during pregnancy.	< 30 mg/24-h urine collection, or < 30 mg/g creatinine in spot urine collection
Blood pressure, mm Hg	• Check at every routine visit.	< 130/80

Abbreviations: HDL, high-density lipoprotein; LDL, low-density lipoprotein.
*See Chapter 17 for glycemic goals during pregnancy.
[†]1–2 hours after start of meal.
Source: Data are from references 1 and 2.

was initiated (3). One arm of the study used SMBG with blood glucose monitors, which increased the validity of blood glucose monitors. Before the advent of SMBG, individuals with diabetes often had their blood glucose measured only once or twice a year, with urine glucose testing serving in between as a crude estimate of blood glucose. The accuracy and quantitative results offered by blood glucose monitors was a significant achievement (4).

Uses

SMBG allows individuals with diabetes to assess their responses to therapy and to determine whether glycemic goals are being met. SMBG results can be useful in the following ways (1):

- To provide immediate feedback on blood glucose control
- To prevent hypoglycemia
- To adjust diabetes medications
- To adjust diabetes medical nutrition therapy
- To adjust physical activity

Timing and Frequency

The timing and frequency of SMBG should be determined by the needs and goals of each individual with diabetes (1). Times to monitor blood glucose include before meals, 1 to 2 hours after meals, and at bedtime; in the middle of the night (3 am); before, during, and after exercise or physical activity; and before driving.

In general, monitoring more frequently is important when determining the effect of a certain type or amount of food, when adjusting diabetes medication, when determining the effect of weight loss and/or exercise or activity (5–10), or when altering exercise or physical activity. The frequency of monitoring is also important when schedule changes, stress, or illness occur, when a new nondiabetes medication is initiated that affects either blood glucose (eg, steroids) or the ability to recognize low blood glucose (eg, some blood pressure medications), or when the patient is pregnant.

Tracking blood glucose, medication dosages, food and beverage intake, physical activity, and other factors affecting blood glucose (such as stress or illness) in a log is key to identifying patterns and aiding in individualizing the treatment plan (11). SMBG can enhance individual participation in diabetes management and can lead to a greater understanding of the therapy.

Type 1 Diabetes

Most individuals with type 1 diabetes should monitor three or more times each day (1). Individuals using insulin pump therapy require frequent testing at initiation of pump therapy to fine-tune the basal rate.

Type 2 Diabetes

The timing and frequency of SMBG for individuals with type 2 diabetes should be adequate to assist in reaching glucose goals. If type 2 diabetes is managed with medical nutrition therapy and exercise, initially SMBG is recommended once or twice daily at alternating times throughout the day (eg, Monday—before breakfast and lunch; Tuesday—before dinner and bedtime). Alternating test times can help contain costs of testing supplies while still providing an overall picture of blood glucose control. Once an understanding of premeal blood glucose control is established, and premeal blood glucoses are within target, the effect of meals can be further assessed by also monitoring after meals. To limit SMBG to twice a day, evaluate one meal each day (eg, Wednesday—before and after breakfast; Thursday—before and after dinner). In addition, keeping a food diary for the meal(s) corresponding to the results assists in determining the amount of carbohydrate tolerated per meal.

If type 2 diabetes is managed with the addition of oral glucose-lowering medication, once to twice daily testing, rotating test times each day is suggested. With good control, monitoring should be continued at least several times per week at various times throughout the day, particularly focusing on postmeal results, to assess lifestyle effects (such as nutrition and physical activity). Testing at various times is important to determine a 24-hour profile of blood glucose levels, but testing at consistent times is important to determine a pattern in blood glucose levels. If type 2 diabetes is managed with the addition of insulin, more frequent monitoring (such as three or more times a day) may be suggested.

Pregnancy

While optimal blood glucose targets and testing plans for gestational diabetes have not been established, many centers recommend 4 tests per day (fasting and 1 to 2 hours after all meals). Pregnant women taking insulin should monitor three or more times daily (1); premeal and bedtime monitoring may also be required. There is no consensus or national standard regarding ketone testing in pregnancy. Some clinics ask women to test the first urine specimen of the day for ketones. Other centers suggest ketone testing only when there is concern that the woman's energy or carbohydrate intake in insufficient. The goal is a negative result (see Chapter 17).

BLOOD GLUCOSE MONITORS

Technology is constantly evolving, providing a greater variety of blood glucose monitors for individuals to choose from. Combination blood glucose meters that also monitor other parameters (total cholesterol, high-density lipoproteins [HDL], triglycerides, and ketones) are now available. See Table 10.2 for a listing of monitors and the manufacturers' contact information.

Blood glucose monitors vary slightly in size, design, capabilities, and cost. They all run on batteries, are

TABLE 10.2 Selected Blood Glucose Monitors and Manufacturers

Manufacturer	Contact Information	Monitors
Abbot Laboratories, MediSense Products	http://www.MediSense.com 800/527-3339	ExacTech ExacTech RSG Precision Xtra Precision QID Precision Sof-Tact
Bayer Diagnostics, Ascensia Products	http://www.bayercarediabetes.com 800/348-8100	Ascensia Dex 2 Ascensia Elite Ascensia Elite XL Ascensia Breeze
BD	http://www.BDdiabetes.com	BD Latitude BD Logic
Home Diagnostics	http://www.prestigesmartsystem.com 800/342-7226	Prestige IQ Prestige LX True Track Smart System
Hypoguard USA	http://www.hypoguard.com 952/646-3200	Assure Assure II Assure 3 Hypoguard Advance QuickTek Supreme II Select GT
LifeScan	http://www.lifescan.com 800/227-8862	One Touch Basic One Touch In Duo One Touch Profile One Touch Sure Step One Touch Ultra One Touch UltraSmart
QuestStar Medical	http://www.queststarmedical.com 800/525-6718	Focus
Roche Diagnostics	http://www.accu-chek.com 800/855-8072	Accu-Chek Active Accu-Chek Advantage Accu-Chek Compact Accu-Chek Complete
TheraSense	http://www.TheraSense.com 888/522-5226	FreeStyle FreeStyle Tracker

portable, and fit in the palm of the hand, with some as small as a pager. Monitors have a small opening where a test strip is either inserted or ejected for contact with a blood sample, and they have a display screen where the blood glucose result is visible (audio monitors are available for those with severe visual impairment). Some monitors require simple cleaning. Whereas monitors measure capillary whole blood glucose, most new monitors and test strips are calibrated to yield a plasma glucose value that correlates with the laboratory blood glucose value. Plasma glucose values are approximately 15% higher than whole blood glucose values. Check the box of test strips to see if they yield a plasma or whole blood reading. Due to Food and Drug Administration standards, brand name blood glucose monitors have a fairly high degree of accuracy, if used appropriately. See Box 10.1 for a list of factors to consider when selecting a blood glucose monitor.

BOX 10.1

Factors to Consider When Selecting a Blood Glucose Monitor

- Cost of monitor and supplies
- Rebates and trade-ins
- Insurance coverage for monitor
- Insurance coverage for test strips, and if so, the number allowed per month
- Monitor size
- Display screen size
- Strip size
- Ease of opening strip package
- Required blood sample size
- Test time
- Blood glucose range
- Temperature range the monitor can be used in
- Altitude limit
- Cleaning and maintenance
- Memory, and if so, ease in accessing it
- Data management capabilities and options
- Special features
- Test site
- Ease of performing a blood glucose check
- Ease of performing a control test
- Ease of calibrating
- Technical support

PERFORMING A BLOOD GLUCOSE TEST

Before teaching SMBG, dietetics professionals should confirm that piercing the skin is within their scope of practice in the state in which they practice. If it is not, another qualified health care professional, or the patient, must perform the actual stick. Dietetics professionals should also remember that the Joint Commission for the Accreditation of Healthcare Organizations and the Centers for Medicare and Medicaid Services require hospitals and other facilities to have bedside blood glucose monitoring quality assurance programs, and the Clinical Laboratory Improvement Act of 1988 places restrictions on blood glucose monitoring performed outside the hospital setting.

Following are the steps in performing a blood glucose test:

1. Ensure the monitor is correctly calibrated for the test strips.
2. Insert or eject test strip, as appropriate.
3. Select site to provide blood sample—fingertips or alternate site as appropriate (see below for more information on alternate-site testing).
4. Clean site with warm, soapy water or alcohol, and dry well.
5. Puncture skin using a lancing device, and secure an adequate drop of blood. Lancing devices are typically provided as part of the blood glucose monitoring kit. Most allow the user to select a penetration setting. Individuals typically prefer a more shallow penetration; however, those with tough skin or poor circulation may require a deeper penetration setting. Special lancing devices or end caps are available for use at alternate sites.
6. Apply blood to designated area on test strip, or allow strips that work by capillary action to "sip" an adequate blood sample.
7. Wait for test results.

For those individuals who have difficulty securing an adequate drop of blood with finger sticks, the following strategies may help:

- Vigorously wash hands with warm water to increase circulation to the fingertips.
- Hang hand at the side for 30 seconds, to allow blood to pool in hand.
- Shake blood down into hand.
- Use a lancing device or end cap that allows a deeper puncture.

- Once the fingertip is punctured, gently "milk" blood from the bottom of the finger to the tip until an adequate size blood drop is formed.

Alternate-Site Testing

The driving force behind alternate-site testing was sore fingers. Sites alternate to the fingertips include the hand, upper arm, thigh, calf, and, most commonly, the forearm. It is important to remember that there is a lag time in blood glucose results from the fingertip to the forearm. The rate of blood flow to the finger is three to five times faster than to the arm. For alternate-site testing, warming the site by massaging the skin for about 15 seconds, or until warm, can help with blood flow.

The anastomosing network of arteries is less concentrated in the forearm, and the dermis is not as vascular as in the fingertip (12). Therefore, when glucose is changing rapidly, a difference may be noted between the glucose reading in the arm and in the finger. For many people, vigorously rubbing the arm eliminates the glucose difference between the arm and the finger, but in isolated cases it does not. If an individual tests for hypoglycemia, tests after a meal, or suffers from hypoglycemia unawareness, it is recommended that he or she test on the finger rather than at an alternate site (13).

Common User Errors

If the blood glucose test produces errors, the blood sample should be checked for adequacy. Some monitors will still register a reading even when the blood sample is inadequate; the reading, however, will be inaccurate. Monitors should be checked to make sure they are properly calibrated and not soiled. Monitor calibration may occur automatically, or it may require setting a code or inserting a strip or chip into the monitor.

Sources of test errors also include defective strips. Strips should be stored according to manufacturers' guidelines, expired strips should not be used, and control solutions should be used to verify that the meter and strips are working together properly. Monitor accuracy should be checked at least once a month (or according to manufacturer's instructions) or any time a problem is suspected. Individuals using a monitor should be encouraged to demonstrate their technique and should allow the educator an opportunity to provide feedback on technique and cleaning.

Other Factors Affecting SMBG Results

Other factors that affect SMBG results include the following:

- Hematocrit variations
- Environmental temperature and humidity
- Altitude
- Hypotension
- Hypoxia
- Triglyceride levels

COMPUTERIZED DATA MANAGEMENT

Data management systems simplify the process of tracking diabetes care. Some data management systems are part of the blood glucose monitor; others must be connected to the monitor. Data management systems automatically record blood glucose, date, and time, with each blood glucose check. Some also store other information, such as insulin type and dose, exercise, and meals. Most blood glucose monitors have the capability to download the memory to a personal computer, where the data can be plotted on a graph or chart to show blood glucose patterns. Computer programs are available for use by educators, the individual with diabetes, or both, to gain a better understanding of patterns. Meter modules are also available to attach to a personal digital assistant (PDA), which allows blood glucose values to be stored in the PDA. The program with the PDA can then generate charts, graphs, and averages from the information. In addition, other health data can be entered into the PDA, such as blood pressure, A1C results, ketones, insulin dosages, and carbohydrate intake. Overall, the more information entered, the greater the success in identifying trends and making changes in diabetes care (14,15).

OTHER BLOOD GLUCOSE MONITORING DEVICES

The ability to monitor blood glucose continuously and to observe glycemic excursions and their relationship to insulin, nutrient intake, and physical activity can help achieve better glycemic control. Currently, there are two methods for continuous glucose monitoring: (*a*) continuous glucose monitoring system (CGMS) via insertion of a small electrode into subcutaneous tissue; and (*b*) extraction of interstitial fluid via a sensor attached to a watch-like device.

Continuous Glucose Monitoring System

CGMS consists of a sterile, disposable, subcutaneous glucose sensor with an external connector, a cable that connects the sensor to the monitor, a pager-size electronic monitor that records data from the sensor, and a communication station that enables data stored in the monitor to be downloaded to a computer. See Figure 10.1 for an example.

The CGMS sensor can collect data for up to 72 hours and allows the entry of event markers (eg, for food intake, insulin, physical activity, and symptomatic hypoglycemia). It does not provide glucose results in real time, so it is best used by health care providers to note trending (16). CGMS provides valuable information on blood glucose fluctuations, the effect of physical activity on blood glucose, the duration of basal insulin, and insulin-to-carbohydrate ratios and the effect on postprandial blood glucose.

CGMS helps in meal insulin delivery, by determining the most effective way to use the dual wave bolus feature on insulin pumps. Reviewing CGMS data with the individual can demonstrate effective ways of treating hypoglycemia. By evaluating glucose trends, insulin adjustments can decrease fear of nighttime hypoglycemia and increase comfort with intensive plans. CGMS also

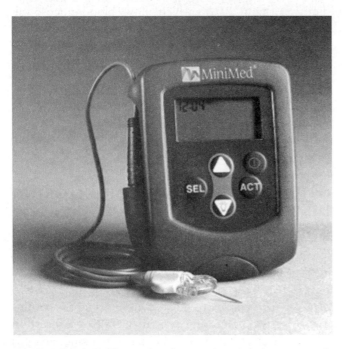

FIGURE 10.1 Example of a continuous glucose monitoring system: CGMS® System Gold™. Reprinted with permission from Medtronic, Inc.

provides insight when food digests and affects blood glucose in individuals with gastroparesis.

Many practices successfully obtain reimbursement for these services, when a reimbursement strategy is in place before the sensor is used.

Glucose Watch

There is a noninvasive watch-type device that uses interstitial fluid absorbed through a small sensor in a disposable pad on the underside of the watch, to estimate blood glucose. The watch is calibrated daily by finger stick blood glucose values, so it does not replace SMBG (17). It provides readings every 10 minutes for up to 13 hours. The readings are time-averaged glucose values and are most useful for noting blood glucose trends (17). The lag time is particularly important when glucose levels are rapidly falling (18). The watch is especially helpful for individuals experiencing hypoglycemia unawareness, nocturnal hypoglycemia, fasting hyperglycemia, and postprandial hyperglycemia, because it sounds an alarm for high or low values.

PARAMETERS REQUIRING MONITORING

Laboratory Glucose

An isolated laboratory glucose value can be useful in diagnosing diabetes (see Chapter 4) or in assessing blood glucose at a specific point in time. However, one laboratory glucose value is not helpful in evaluating overall control or blood glucose patterns.

Glycosylated Hemoglobin (A1C)

A1C is an accurate reflection of overall blood glucose control during the preceding 2 to 3 months. As a result, an A1C value should be measured approximately every 3 months, to evaluate metabolic control and to determine whether the target range is maintained. See Table 10.1 for monitoring frequency and goals of the American College of Endocrinology (19) and American Diabetes Association (1). This test can be accomplished via a blood draw, a finger stick with an at-home test kit or single-use device, or via a finger stick in the physician's office using an electronic machine. A normal A1C is 4.0% to 6.0% (range may vary slightly depending on the laboratory) (Table 10.3). A1C results can be affected by sickle cell hemoglobin and by some other blood diseases, depending on the method. A1C is not currently approved for diagnostic purposes.

TABLE 10.3 Conversion of A1C to Plasma Blood Glucose	
A1C, %	Mean Plasma Blood Glucose Level, mg/dL
6	135
7	170
8	205
9	240
10	275
11	310
12	345
13	380

Glycosylated Serum Albumin (Fructosamine)

This glycated serum protein test measures blood glucose control during the previous 2 to 3 weeks. The normal range varies depending on the method used. Fructosamine can be useful in the following circumstances:

- During pregnancy, to assess control
- In cases where a rapid assessment of overall glycemic control is needed
- During short-term follow-up of recent glycemic-lowering interventions (3)
- When there is a discrepancy between an individual's reported blood glucose values and the A1C

Ketones

Three ketone bodies (acetoacetate, 3-beta-hydroxybutyrate, and acetone) are formed as byproducts of fat metabolism in the liver. Individuals with type 1 diabetes are ketosis prone, whereas those with type 2 diabetes are generally ketosis resistant but can exhibit ketones when severely stressed by trauma or infection (2). Ketone monitoring should be performed in the following classes of individuals, because of increased risk of ketone production (1,9):

- All individuals with diabetes during illness or acute stress, especially when exhibiting symptoms of ketoacidosis (nausea, vomiting, abdominal pain). Testing should be done routinely when individuals are unwell or stressed.
- Individuals with type 1 diabetes when their blood glucose is consistently higher than 300 mg/dL.

- Pregnant women with diabetes or gestational diabetes may need to check for ketones to help identify whether food intake is adequate and to provide warning of impending metabolic decompensation (7,20) (see Chapter 17). As stated earlier in the chapter, frequency of ketone testing in pregnancy varies.
- Individuals trying to lose weight by energy restriction. If ketones are present but blood glucose is in range, ketones indicate weight loss, not impending ketoacidosis.

The desired result is negative ketones. Ketones can be measured in the blood and urine. Blood ketones may be measured by the laboratory or by a special meter for home use. Urinary ketones can be measured by the laboratory or by using a dipstick and by matching the color to a color chart. The dipstick measures acetoacetate. Urine dipstick ketone results can actually become more positive after initiation of insulin therapy, because the concentration of acetoacetate increases while 3-beta-hydroxybutyrate decreases. In this case, the more positive results are generally not cause for concern, as long as blood glucose is improving. Blood glucose monitors that also measure ketones measure 3-beta-hydroxybutyrate, and have been found to be a more accurate and current assessment of ketones than urine ketone tests (11,21). See Chapters 12 and 17 for more information on managing ketones and nutrition implications.

Lipids

Lipids should be monitored annually or more frequently, as needed, to achieve goals (see Table 10.1). In adults with low-risk values, rescreening is recommended every 2 years. Children older than 2 years should be screened when blood glucose control has been established after diagnosis with diabetes. If there is no family history and the values are low risk, then the child should be rescreened every 5 years (1). Lipids are monitored most frequently by a fasting laboratory test; however, a blood glucose monitor that measures total cholesterol, triglycerides, and HDL can be a valuable tool for home use. For more information on lipids and nutrition implications, see Chapters 13 and 22.

Microalbumin

Normal levels of albumin in the urine should be less than 30 mg per gram of creatinine in a spot urine collection or less than 30 mg per 24-hour urine collection.

The persistent presence of urinary albumin in the range of 30 to 299 mg per 24 hours (microalbuminuria) is an indicator of early-phase nephropathy in type 1 diabetes and a marker for development of nephropathy in type 2 diabetes (1). Monitoring urine for the presence of microalbuminuria is valuable for prompt diagnosis and intervention. An annual test to screen for the presence of microalbuminuria should be performed in type 1 individuals with a 5-year or greater duration of diabetes and in type 2 individuals beginning at diagnosis (1). Screening for microalbuminuria can be performed by three methods:

1. Measurement of the albumin-to-creatinine ratio in a random spot urine collection (For spot collection, the first urine void of the morning may be less variable and therefore a better indicator of kidney function.)
2. Timed collection (ie, 4 hours or overnight)
3. 24-hour urine collection with creatinine, allowing for concurrent measurement of creatinine clearance

Urinary albumin excretion is variable and can be affected by a number of factors, including exercise (within 24 hours), acute illness or fever, or infection (ie, urinary tract infection, hematuria). Urinary albumin excretion can also be affected by marked hyperglycemia or hypertension, menses, and congestive heart failure. As a result, two of three urine specimens collected within a 6-month period should be abnormal before considering an individual to have microalbuminuria (1). See Chapter 23 for further information on nephropathy and nutrition implications.

Although microalbumin is typically screened through the health care professional's office, home-test kits are available. After a urine sample is applied to the special test kit, the kit is returned to the company for interpretation.

Blood Pressure

Blood pressure should be measured at each routine visit with the goal of blood pressure under 130/80 mm Hg. If systolic blood pressure is 130 mm Hg or higher, or diastolic is 80 mm Hg or higher, then blood pressure should be rechecked on a separate day to confirm those values (1). See Table 10.1 for blood pressure monitoring frequency and goals. See Chapter 22 for further information on blood pressure.

SUMMARY

Monitoring is an essential component of routine diabetes care to maintain metabolic control and to aid in prevention of complications. The use of SMBG results is extremely important when making suggestions for meal planning, medication, and exercise adjustments. Technology is constantly evolving, particularly in relation to self-monitoring of blood glucose. New and exciting options are on the horizon.

REFERENCES

1. American Diabetes Association. Standards of medical care in diabetes (position statement). *Diabetes Care*. 2005; 28(Suppl 1):S4–S36.
2. Diabetes management therapies. In: Franz MJ, ed. *A Core Curriculum for Diabetes Education*. 5th edition. Chicago, Ill: American Association of Diabetes Educators; 2003: 187–212.
3. Diabetes Control and Complications Trial Research Group. The effect of intensive treatment of diabetes on the development and progression of long-term complications in insulin-dependent diabetes mellitus. *N Engl J Med*. 1993;329:977–986.
4. Skyler JS, Lasky IA, Skyler DL, Robertson EG, Mintz DH. Home blood glucose monitoring as an aid in diabetes management. *Diabetes Care*. 1978;1:150–157.
5. American Diabetes Association. *Medical Management of Type 1 Diabetes*. 3rd ed. Alexandria, Va: American Diabetes Association; 1998.
6. American Diabetes Association. *Medical Management of Type 2 Diabetes*. 4th ed. Alexandria, Va: American Diabetes Association; 1998.
7. American Diabetes Association. *Medical Management of Pregnancy-Complicated Diabetes*. 3rd ed. Alexandria, Va: American Diabetes Association; 2000.
8. *Therapy of Diabetes Mellitus and Related Disorders*. 3rd ed. Alexandria, Va: American Diabetes Association; 1998.
9. American Diabetes Association. *Intensive Diabetes Management*. 3rd ed. Alexandria, Va: American Diabetes Association; 2003.
10. American Diabetes Association. *Medications for the Treatment of Diabetes*. Alexandria, Va: American Diabetes Association; 2000.
11. American Diabetes Association consensus statement: self-monitoring of blood glucose. *Diabetes Care*. 1994; 17:81–86.
12. Sparks HV. *Skin and muscle*. In: Johnson PL, ed. *Peripheral Circulation*. New York, NY: Wiley; 1978:198.

13. McGarraough G, Price D, Schwartz S, Weinstein R. Physiological differences in off-finger glucose testing. *Diabetes Technol Therap.* 2001;3:367–376.

14. FreeStyle Tracker Diabetes Management System. Available at: http://www.therasense.com. Accessed September 20, 2004.

15. Accu-Check. Available at: http://www.accu-chek.com. Accessed September 20, 2004.

16. Mastrototaro JJ. The MiniMed Continuous Glucose Monitoring System. *Diabetes Technol Therap.* 2000; 2(Suppl 1):S13–S18.

17. GlucoWatch. Available at: http://www.glucowatch.com. Accessed September 20, 2004.

18. Tierney MJ, Tamada JA, Potts RO, Eastman RC, Pitzer K, Ackerman NR, Fermi SJ. The GlucoWatch biographer: a frequent, automatic and noninvasive glucose monitor. *Ann Med.* 2000;32:632–641.

19. American College of Endocrinology. Consensus statement on guidelines for glycemic control (based on Consensus Development Conference, Washington, DC, August 20 and 21, 2001). *Endocrine Pract.* 2002;8(Suppl 1):S5–S11.

20. American Diabetes Association. Gestational diabetes mellitus (position statement). *Diabetes Care.* 2003;26(Suppl 1):S103–105.

21. American Diabetes Association. Tests of glycemia in diabetes (position statement). *Diabetes Care.* 2003;26(Suppl 1):S106–108.

ADDITIONAL RESOURCES

American Diabetes Association. Management of dyslipidemia in adults with diabetes. *Diabetes Care.* 2003;26(suppl 1): S83–S86.

American Diabetes Association. Resource guide 2005. *Diabetes Forecast.* 2005;58:RG36-RG57, RG59-RG63.

American Diabetes Association. Tests of glycemia in diabetes (technical review). *Diabetes Care.* 1995;18:896–909.

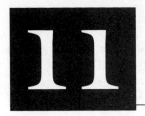

Pattern Management

Karmeen Kulkarni, MS, RD, BC-ADM, CDE

CHAPTER OVERVIEW

- Pattern management allows individuals with diabetes to self-adjust their food intake, physical activity, and/or diabetes medication, to aid in achieving "tighter" blood glucose control.
- One of the roles of registered dietitians (RDs) in pattern management is to educate individuals with diabetes on how food, physical activity, and diabetes medications affect blood glucose control.
- Because pattern management is possible only with adequate data, it is vital for individuals with diabetes to record their blood glucose, food/carbohydrate intake, physical activity, diabetes medication, and schedule.

DEFINITION OF PATTERN MANAGEMENT

Pattern management is a systematic approach to help individuals with diabetes identify patterns in their blood glucose readings to determine whether changes are needed to optimize their glucose control (1). For many years, adjustments in therapy were primarily made by the health care team during office visits, which resulted in delayed improvements in glycemic control and little input from the person with diabetes. Pattern management allows individuals with diabetes to self-adjust their food intake, physical activity, and/or diabetes medication, based on daily monitoring records. This results in more immediate improvement in glycemic control and increases self-confidence in the decision-making role.

In the past, pattern management was associated more with intensive insulin therapy to achieve optimal glycemic control and avoid or delay the onset of chronic complications (2–4). Pattern management is now routinely used for people with type 2 diabetes, to improve glycemia by making lifestyle changes and/or changes in oral diabetes medication or insulin. A review of pattern management should be a routine part of every office visit.

The Role of the Dietitian in Pattern Management

Nutrition therapy is one of the key components of glycemic control. The RD plays an important role in pattern management by educating individuals with diabetes about the effect of food, physical activity, and diabetes medications on blood glucose control, as well as by identifying individual glycemic responses to foods.

Assessment of food records helps to evaluate consistency in food/carbohydrate intake and its impact on blood glucose levels. The RD can assist in evaluating records, to determine which factors are responsible for out-of-range blood glucose patterns. Although the tendency of many health care practitioners is to focus primarily on medication adjustments, one of the RD's roles

116

is to communicate with other members of the health care team on a regular basis regarding the need for adjustments in the timing or amount of food or physical activity in lieu of medication adjustment.

Elements of Successful Pattern Management

Successful diabetes management depends on the individual's commitment to learn the required skills, to provide the essential data, and to accept responsibility for self-management decisions with support and guidance from the diabetes care team. Pattern management helps build self-management skills, which will ultimately improve glycemic control. Successful pattern management requires the following (5):

- Willingness by the person with diabetes to self-adjust their food intake, physical activity, and diabetes medication
- Frequent self-monitoring of blood glucose
- Written records of blood glucose data, diabetes medication, food intake, and physical activity
- Food/meal plan with consistency in carbohydrate intake
- Self-management training
- Frequent interaction with the diabetes care team

SELF-MONITORING OF BLOOD GLUCOSE

Regular self-monitoring of blood glucose (SMBG) and record keeping are necessary to provide the data needed for pattern management. The frequency and timing is dependent on the type of therapy and the treatment goals. For example, intensive management with basal insulin and premeal rapid-acting insulin require SMBG premeal, 2 hours postprandial, at bedtime, and occasionally at 2 or 3 am. Individuals with type 2 diabetes, managed with nutrition therapy, physical activity, and with or without oral diabetes medications, may benefit from alternating SMBG premeal, 2 hours postprandial, and at bedtime. For individuals taking insulin, fasting and premeal blood glucose results are useful to monitor the dose of basal (or background) insulin, such as NPH, glargine, or ultralente.

To adjust the mealtime rapid-acting insulins lispro and aspart, 2-hour postprandial blood glucose readings are required. The target for 2 hours postmeal is a blood glucose excursion of only 20 to 40 mg/dL (1). Two-hour postprandial blood glucose readings are also helpful to determine the glycemic response to a meal and the

effect of some oral diabetes medications. If there are any changes in therapy (ie, changes in medication, physical activity, or energy intake) or if the individual is pregnant, more frequent SMBG is required.

Barriers to SMBG

The value of SMBG has been well documented despite the resistance to monitoring demonstrated by some individuals. Blonde and colleagues (6) reviewed more than 3,000 clinical visits of 228 patients with type 2 diabetes who were seen by 65 different health care providers during a 3-year period. The patients were categorized into three groups based on the documentation of SMBG frequency. Of the patients who performed regular SMBG, 70% had A1C levels of less than 8%, compared with 22% of patients who did not perform SMBG. Thirty percent of patients who monitored regularly had A1C values greater than 8%, compared with 78% of patients who did not monitor regularly.

Before learning and using the system of pattern management, individuals with diabetes should overcome any barriers to SMBG and record keeping. The RD can assist individuals in overcoming these barriers in a positive manner by offering possible solutions (see Table 11.1) (7). For example, to reduce time involved in SMBG, a newer model meter which provides results within 5 seconds could be suggested in place of an older model that takes 40 to 45 seconds. A solution to painful fingertips might be a smaller gauge lancet or an adjustable-depth lancing device, or use of an alternate testing site, such as the forearm.

TABLE 11.1 Self-Monitoring of Blood Glucose Barriers and Possible Solutions

Barrier	Possible Solutions
Psychosocial issues	Positive reinforcement
Pain	Smaller sample size, smaller gauge lancet or adjustable-depth lancing device, alternate site testing
Convenience	All supplies self-contained
Time	Meters with faster results
Cognition	Use of results (pattern management)
Recording	Memory/data manager feature in meter

Source: Data are from reference 7.

When referring to blood glucose levels, the health practitioner should use terms such as "in range" or "out of range" rather than value-judgment terms like "good" and "bad" (1). Positive reinforcement should be provided whenever possible. For example, the RD could say, "It's great that you have been doing SMBG on a regular basis." As individuals become more comfortable with SMBG, they are able to focus on demonstrated patterns, which eventually allow them to make therapy adjustments.

Recording Data

Study results have shown the most improvement in glycemic control when individuals keep blood glucose records, review the records, and self-adjust based on principles including pattern management (1). Although most blood glucose meters today have a memory feature, that feature alone does not provide the necessary data needed for pattern management. Optimally, blood glucose values are recorded in columnar format, so that blood glucose patterns over several days can be identified at a glance, with timing, medication, physical activity, and food/carbohydrate intake also recorded. See Figure 11.1 for a sample blood glucose log.

Convincing the person with diabetes to spend the time and effort to record the data necessary for successful pattern management is initially challenging. Time, effort, and inconvenience are identified barriers to record keeping for some individuals. Frequent follow-up and encouragement by the health care team can be very helpful in maintaining motivation. Some individuals may prefer a more sophisticated data management system, which allows input of medication, grams of carbohydrate, and physical activity, in addition to blood glucose data. The system can then provide a printout of data in a format that more easily allows identification of blood

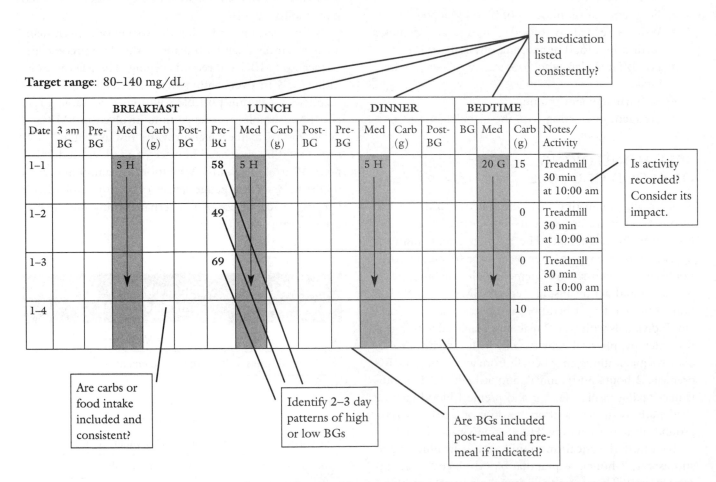

Target range: 80–140 mg/dL

Is medication listed consistently?

Date	3 am BG	BREAKFAST				LUNCH				DINNER				BEDTIME			
		Pre-BG	Med	Carb (g)	Post-BG	Pre-BG	Med	Carb (g)	Post-BG	Pre-BG	Med	Carb (g)	Post-BG	BG	Med	Carb (g)	Notes/Activity
1–1			5 H			58	5 H				5 H				20 G	15	Treadmill 30 min at 10:00 am
1–2						49										0	Treadmill 30 min at 10:00 am
1–3						69										0	Treadmill 30 min at 10:00 am
1–4																10	

Is activity recorded? Consider its impact.

Are carbs or food intake included and consistent?

Identify 2–3 day patterns of high or low BGs

Are BGs included post-meal and pre-meal if indicated?

FIGURE 11.1 Sample blood glucose log. Insulin plan: 5 units Humalog (lispro; Eli Lilly & Company, Indianapolis, IN 46285) premeals; 20 units glargine at bedtime. Abbreviations: BG, blood glucose value (mg/dL); carb, carbohydrate (g); G, glargine; H, Humalog; Med, medication; pre-BG, blood glucose value (mg/dL) before meal; post-BG, blood glucose value (mg/dL) after meal.

glucose patterns. Individuals can also develop their own record forms for use on their computer or personal data analyzer. Achievement of glycemic goals and the rewards that follow often help motivate individuals to continue recording monitoring data.

MANAGING PATTERNS

Steps

When beginning pattern management, individuals should maintain consistency in their schedule, carbohydrate intake, diabetes medication dosage, and activity level. Steps in pattern management are described in the following section (1).

Identification of Blood Glucose Goals

Standard glycemic goals have been established by the American Diabetes Association (see Chapter 10 on monitoring) as general guidelines; however, individual targets are influenced by age, presence of hypoglycemic unawareness, and other factors. The individual with diabetes should be involved in setting personal glycemic goals (both premeal and postmeal).

Testing and Recording of Blood Glucose, Food and Carbohydrate Intake, Physical Activity, Diabetes Medication, and Schedule

Pattern management is impossible with inadequate data. Frequency and timing of blood glucose tests depend on the management plan and goals.

Identification of Patterns

The RD should look for a pattern of high readings at the same time of day for at least three consecutive days or a pattern of low readings on at least two consecutive days. The goal is to keep blood glucose results within the target blood glucose range 75% to 85% of the time for individuals with type 1 diabetes and 95% to 100% of the time for individuals with type 2 (5).

Assessment of Influencing Factors

Once the patterns have been identified, the health practitioner should determine which factors appear to be influencing the pattern(s). Knowledge of the action, peak, and duration of insulins is important for insulin users (see Chapter 9). The impact of food, daily schedule, physical activity, illness, and stress should be addressed in the problem-solving process. Box 11.1 lists some of the primary factors that affect blood glucose results.

BOX 11.1

Factors That Affect Blood Glucose

Low Blood Glucose
- Too much time between meals
- Inadequate food intake at previous meal
- Unusual or inconsistent exercise/physical activity
- Too much insulin
- Inappropriate insulin/food adjustment for exercise

High Blood Glucose
- Increased carbohydrate intake at previous meal/snack
- Illness or infection
- Unusual inactivity
- Omission of insulin/diabetes medication
- Inappropriate adjustments in insulin/medication
- Insulin ineffective (outdated or improperly stored)
- Inappropriate timing of insulin injection
- Other medications that affect blood glucose levels

Inconsistent Lows and Highs
- Consistency in carbohydrate intake
- Sporadic exercise/physical activity
- Inconsistent timing of medication and meals
- Swing shifts
- Travel across time zones

Taking Action

If consistency is a problem, this should be addressed first, along with any additional educational needs. Situations that pose greater challenges to glycemic control because of inconsistency include swing shifts, college or student schedules, travel across time zones, sporadic physical activity, and frequent dining out. If clear patterns and influencing factors have been identified, adjustments should be made in medication, food, activity, and/or the schedule.

Insulin-to-Carbohydrate Ratios

When individuals on multiple injections are competent with identifying and evaluating blood glucose patterns, they can proceed with establishing insulin-to-carbohydrate ratios to cover anticipated food intake. The insulin-to-carbohydrate ratio will depend on the individual's sensitivity to insulin. The more sensitive one is to insulin, the larger the amount of carbohydrate covered by a unit of insulin. A common starting point for adults is 1 unit of short or rapid-acting insulin per 15 g of carbohydrate consumed. As insulin sensitivity may vary with the time of day, insulin-to-carbohydrate ratios may differ for different meals (5). (See Chapter 18 for more information on establishing insulin-to-carbohydrate ratios).

Supplemental Insulin Therapy

A variety of methods for determining insulin supplementation are used to correct an unanticipated high or low blood glucose at a particular moment in time. Formulas may be used that determine an insulin sensitivity factor, such as the "1500 rule" for regular insulin or the "1800 rule" for rapid-acting insulin (5). For example, 1,500 divided by the total daily insulin dose equals the mg/dL drop in blood glucose from 1 unit of short-acting insulin, and 1,800 divided by the total daily insulin dose equals the mg/dL drop in blood glucose from 1 unit of rapid-acting insulin. The use of supplemental insulin or sliding scale insulin approaches provides a "quick fix" but does not correct the underlying problem and does not take the place of pattern management (1).

IMPROVING GLYCEMIA IN ACCORDANCE WITH LIFESTYLE

The RD should learn to evaluate all possible interpretations in order to help individuals with diabetes identify ways to improve glycemia that best match their lifestyle. Box 11.2 summarizes the basic steps needed to assist individuals with diabetes in evaluating blood glucose records. The case studies that follow are a practical application of these steps.

CASE STUDIES*

Case Study A: Effect of Dining Out and Carbohydrate on a Person With Type 2 Diabetes Who Takes No Diabetes Medications

BB was diagnosed with type 2 diabetes 2 years ago. Her height is 65 inches and her weight is 154 lb. BB does not take any diabetes medications. Although she counts carbohydrates, she does not maintain specific food records. She eats three meals a day and an occasional snack at night. BB checks blood glucose alternately before meals and 2 hours after meals. Her plasma blood

*Case studies A, C, E, and F are adapted with permission from reference 8.

BOX 11.2

Factors to Evaluate When Reviewing Records

1. Determine whether adequate data are available.
   a. Are there blood glucose values representing all times of day, including peak medication times?
   b. Are premeal blood glucose values within 20 to 40 mg of postmeal values based on the use of rapid-acting insulin?
   c. Are data included regarding food and carbohydrate intake, physical activity, and medication?
2. Look for 2- to 3-day blood glucose level patterns.
   a. Are there blood glucose values outside the target range at the same time of day for 2 consecutive days for lows and at least 3 consecutive days for highs?
3. Identify factors influencing blood glucose patterns.
   a. Evaluate the effect of medication (timing, missed doses, peak action, out-of-date medication).
   b. Evaluate the effect of food and carbohydrate intake (consistency, ability to correctly identify portions and grams of carbohydrate).
   c. Evaluate the effect of physical activity (type, intensity, duration).
   d. Evaluate the effect of schedule (timing of meals/snacks, medication, physical activity) (see Box 11.1).
4. Make recommendations for change.

---

glucose target ranges are 80 to 120 mg/dL before meals and less than 160 mg/dL after meals. See Table 11.2 for BB's blood glucose log and for the steps in pattern management and factors a dietitian should consider.

Case Study B: Use of Insulin-to-Carbohydrate Ratios by a Person With Type 1 Diabetes

PV has type 1 diabetes, is 66 inches tall, and weighs 128 lb. A recent A1C value was 7.5%. PV's insulin plan is as follows: 22 units glargine at bedtime. Insulin-to-carbohydrate ratio is 1:10 (1 unit of lispro for every 10 g of carbohydrate) for breakfast; 1:15 for lunch and dinner (1 unit of lispro for every 15 g of carbohydrate). PV's plasma blood glucose target ranges are 80 to 130 mg/dL before meals; within 20 to 40 mg/dL of premeal value for 2 hours postmeals; and 100 to 140 mg/dL at bedtime. See Table 11.3 for PV's blood glucose log and for the steps in pattern management and factors a dietitian should consider.

TABLE 11.2 Findings for Case Study A

Date	Breakfast			Lunch			Dinner			Bedtime		Notes
	Pre-BG, mg/dL	Carb, g	Post-BG, mg/dL	Pre-BG, mg/dL	Carb, g	Post-BG, mg/dL	Pre-BG, mg/dL	Carb, g	Post-BG, mg/dL	BG, mg/dL	Carb, g	
1–1	118	60	154		60		124	60	141	121	15	Ate dinner at home. No exercise.
1–2		60		121	60	141	121	70	198		0	Ate dinner at Italian restaurant. No exercise.
1–3	115	60	140	119	60	138	118	60	178		0	Ate dinner at Chinese restaurant. No exercise.
1–4	89	60	128	111	60	134	101	60	220		0	Had fast food for dinner. Walked dog after dinner.

Step	Consider
1. Obtain sufficient, accurate data.	• Food: carb grams recorded; no specific food records other than notes about dining out. • Activity: information available. • Medication: none for diabetes. • SMBG: alternating premeal and 2 h postmeal.
2. Identify blood glucose patterns.	• Pattern of high BGs 2 h after dinner.
3. Identify all possible influencing factors.	• Food: need some specific food records. Carb consumption may be underestimated when dining out. • Activity: physical activity could improve BGs. • Medication: none.
4. Make recommendations for change.	• Review basic carbohydrate counting and portion control. Recommend that BB record specific food intake along with estimated carbohydrate. Measure and weigh foods for next 2 wk, to improve accuracy of portion estimates. • Discuss effect of physical activity (eg, walking) on BG and possible options for her. • Weight loss may be considered as an option on which to focus, to improve BGs depending on her past experience and stage of readiness. Set realistic goals so she can be successful. • Oral diabetes medication is an option for the future, based on success of lifestyle interventions.

Abbreviations: BG, blood glucose value; carb, carbohydrate; pre-BG, blood glucose value before meals; post-BG, blood glucose value 2 hours after meal; SMBG, self-monitoring of blood glucose.

Source: Adapted with permission from Austin MA, Kulkarni K, Powers MA. *Blood Glucose Monitoring: Essential Skills for Health Care Professionals.* 3rd ed. St. Paul, Minn: PP Publications; 2003:64–69.

TABLE 11.3 Findings for Case Study B

	Breakfast				Lunch				Dinner				Bedtime		
Date	Pre-BG, mg/dL	Ins, units	Carb, g	Post-BG, mg/dL	Pre-BG, mg/dL	Ins, units	Carb, g	Post-BG, mg/dL	Pre-BG, mg/dL	Ins, units	Carb, g	Post-BG, mg/dL	BG, mg/dL	Ins, units	Activity
1–1	79	6 LP	60	115	95	3 LP	45	**145**	134	5 LP	75	148	140	22 G	Walked before dinner for 30 min.
1–2	74	3 LP	30	109	120	4 LP	60	**165**	121	6 LP	90	119	135	22 G	Walked before dinner for 30 min.
1–3	68	4 LP	40	98	110	3 LP	45	**162**	136	5 LP	75	142	129	22 G	No exercise.

Step	Consider
1. Obtain sufficient, accurate data.	• Food: carb intake provided. • Activity: available. • Medication: insulin as shown. • SMBG: as shown above.
2. Identify blood glucose patterns.	• Low BG before breakfast. • High BG 2 h after lunch.
3. Identify all possible influencing factors.	• Food: using insulin:carbohydrate ratios. • Activity: no effect noted. • Insulin: ratio at lunch needs adjusting, because 2 h postmeal is greater than 20–40 mg/dL above premeal BGs. Evening glargine needs to be decreased because of pattern of lows before breakfast.
4. Make recommendations for change.	• Consider increasing the insulin:carbohydrate ratio at lunch because of higher 2-h postmeal BGs. • Decrease evening dose of glargine by 2 units (to 20 units), to increase fasting BG.

Abbreviations: BG, blood glucose value; carb, carbohydrate; G, glargine insulin (long-acting); Ins, insulin; LP, lispro insulin (rapid-acting); Post-BG, blood glucose value 2 hours after meals; Pre-BG, blood glucose value before meals; SMBG, self-monitoring of blood glucose.

Case Study C: Progression of Type 2 Diabetes in a Person Using Oral Diabetes Medication

ML has had diabetes for 7 years. His height is 69 inches, and he weighs 210 lb. ML's diabetes medication includes glyburide 10 mg twice daily. ML has been instructed to check blood glucose fasting and 2 hours after meals at alternate times. He has been instructed in basic carbohydrate counting. ML's plasma blood glucose target ranges are 80 to 130 mg/dL fasting and before meals and less than 150 mg/dL 2 hours after meals. For ML's blood glucose log and the steps in pattern management and factors a dietitian should consider, see Table 11.4.

Case Study D: Exercise and Insulin in a Person With Type 2 Diabetes

LS has type 2 diabetes and is 43 years old. Her height is 64 inches, and her weight is 138 lb. She is interested in

TABLE 11.4   Findings for Case Study C

Date	Breakfast Pre-BG, mg/dL	Carb, g	Post-BG, mg/dL	Lunch Pre-BG, mg/dL	Carb, g	Post-BG, mg/dL	Dinner Pre-BG, mg/dL	Carb, g	Post-BG, mg/dL	Bedtime BG, mg/dL	Carb, g	Notes
1–1	210	75			75			75	116		30	Swam 30 min before dinner.
1–2	189	75	138		68	141		82	129		30	No exercise.
1–3	214	64			70			75	131		30	Walked 30 min before dinner.

Step	Consider
1. Obtain sufficient, accurate data.	• Food: carbs recorded. • Activity: information recorded. • Medication: maximum dose of glyburide. • SMBG: information provided; checking fasting and 2 h postmeal; appropriate for use of oral diabetes medication.
2. Identify blood glucose patterns.	• Pattern of high fasting BGs.
3. Identify all possible influencing factors.	• Food: food not likely to affect fasting BGs. • Activity: exercise not having significant impact on fasting BGs. • Medication: needs may change with the natural progression of his diabetes. He needs to add a different type of diabetes medication at this time. Because his fasting BGs are high and 2-h postmeal BGs are within the goal, the addition of metformin would be a good choice, because the primary action is to decrease nocturnal hepatic glucose release, which would impact the fasting glucose value.
4. Make recommendations for change.	• Discuss recommendation to add metformin with diabetes care team. Discuss with CP the effect of hepatic glucose release on fasting blood glucose values.

Abbreviations: BG, blood glucose value; carb, carbohydrate; Post-BG, blood glucose value 2 hours after meals; Pre-BG, blood glucose value before meals; SMBG, self-monitoring of blood glucose.
Source: Adapted with permission from Austin MA, Kulkarni K, Powers MA. Blood Glucose Monitoring: Essential Skills for Health Care Professionals. 3rd ed. St. Paul, Minn: PP Publications; 2003: 64–69.

losing some weight. For activity, LS walks on her tread-mill for 30 minutes midmorning 5 or 6 days a week. LS's medications for diabetes include 20 units glargine at bedtime, 7 units lispro before breakfast, and 6 units lispro before lunch and before dinner. LS's plasma blood glucose target ranges are 80 to 120 mg/dL before meals and within 20 to 40 mg/dL of premeal blood glucose 2 hours after meals. For LS's blood glucose log and the steps and factors in pattern management a dietitian should consider, see Table 11.5.

Case Study E: Changing Split/Mixed Plan to Basal/Bolus Plan in a Person With Type 1 Diabetes

DR is 34 years old and has had type 1 diabetes for 27 years. DR's height is 69 inches and his weight is 163 lb. DR eats three meals and two snacks with consistent carbohydrate intake every day: 90 g for each meal and 30 g for each snack. For activity, DR swims 1 mile daily before dinner. DR's medications for diabetes include 9 units lispro and 21 units NPH prebreakfast, and 6

TABLE 11.5 Findings for Case Study D

Date	Breakfast Pre-BG, mg/dL	Ins, units	Carb, g	Post-BG, mg/dL	Lunch Pre-BG, mg/dL	Ins, units	Carb, g	Post-BG, mg/dL	Dinner Pre-BG, mg/dL	Ins, nits	Carb, g	Post-BG, mg/dL	Bedtime BG, mg/dL	Ins, units	Carb, g	Activity
1–1	110	7 LP	75	130	**63**	6 LP	70	99	134	6 LP	75	132	140	20 G	15	Walk, 10:00–10:30 am.
1–2	125	7 LP	68	129	**53**	6 LP	75	105	121	6 LP	90	119	135	20 G	0	Walk, 10:00–10:30 am.
1–3	131	7 LP	79	151	**69**	6 LP	78	89	136	6 LP	82	128	129	20 G	0	Walk, 10:00–10:30 am.
1–4	116	7 LP	80	119	**71**	6 LP	65	81	99	6 LP	74	115	138	20 G	10	Walk, 10:00–10:30 am.

Step	Consider
1. Obtain sufficient, accurate data.	• Food: carb information available. • Activity: information available. • Medication: information available. • SMBG: sufficient information.
2. Identify blood glucose patterns.	• Pattern of low BGs prelunch.
3. Identify all possible influencing factors.	• Food: carb intake appears consistent and spaced well throughout day. • Activity: daily walking midmorning contributes to low BG prelunch. • SMBG: most are well within target range. Postmeal BGs are within 20–40 mg of premeal. • Insulin: morning lispro affects mid- to late-morning BG.
4. Make recommendations for change.	• Plan: Discuss possible solutions—add snack midmorning or reduce prebreakfast lispro insulin. Because weight loss is a goal, negotiate a plan to reduce lispro by 20% (1 unit) prebreakfast. Follow up in 2 wk.

Abbreviations: BG, blood glucose value; Carb, carbohydrate; G, glargine insulin (long-acting); Ins, insulin; LP, lispro insulin (rapid-acting); Post-BG, blood glucose value 2 hours after meals; Pre-BG, blood glucose value before meals; SMBG, self-monitoring of blood glucose.

units lispro and 15 units NPH predinner. DR's plasma blood glucose target ranges are 80 to 130 mg/dL before meals and less than 150 mg/dL after meals. See Table 11.6 for DR's blood glucose log and for the steps in pattern management and factors a dietitian should consider.

Case Study F: Prepregnancy in a Woman With Type 1 Diabetes

SL is 27 years old. She has had type 1 diabetes for 12 years and is interested in becoming pregnant. Her recent A1C value was 7.6%. Her food intake consists of three meals per day with no snacks except to treat hypo-

TABLE 11.6 Findings for Case Study E

	Breakfast				Lunch				Dinner				Bedtime		
Date	Pre-BG, mg/dL	Ins, units	Carb, g	Post-BG, mg/dL	Pre-BG, mg/dL	Ins, units	Carb, g	Post-BG, mg/dL	Pre-BG, mg/dL	Ins, units	Carb, g	Post-BG, mg/dL	BG, mg/dL	Ins, units	Carb, g
1–1	192	9 LP 21 NPH	90		175		90		100	6 LP 15 NPH	90		153		30
1–2	68	9 LP 21 NPH	90		164		90		185	6 LP 15 NPH	90		100		30
1–3	223	9 LP 21 NPH	90		192		90		122	6 LP 15 NPH	90		116		30

Step	Consider
1. Obtain sufficient, accurate data.	• Food: information available. • Activity: information available. • Medication: information available. • SMBG: premeal/snack checks, as shown above.
2. Identify blood glucose patterns.	• Pattern of high BGs prelunch.
3. Identify all possible influencing factors.	• Carb intake record reveals good carbohydrate consistency and distribution, but no specific food records available to determine ability to accurately estimate carb intake. • Activity: swimming before dinner not likely to influence out-of-range BG values. • Medication: split mixed dose of insulin could be replaced with basal/bolus plan, to allow more flexibility and improve BGs.
4. Make recommendations for change.	• Consider glargine at bedtime and discontinue the NPH prebreakfast and predinner, beginning with 20% less glargine as compared to the total daily dose of NPH. Begin with fixed dose of lispro before each meal, to match fixed amount of carbs. • Consider learning carbohydrate counting and trying an insulin:carbohydrate ratio. • Negotiate a 3 am BG check. Add 2-h postmeal checks, with a goal of 20–40 mg of premeal BG.

Abbreviations: BG, blood glucose value; carb, carbohydrate; Ins, insulin; LP, lispro insulin (rapid-acting); NPH, NPH insulin; Post-BG, blood glucose value 2 hours after meals; Pre-BG, blood glucose value before meals; SMBG, self-monitoring of blood glucose.
Source: Adapted with permission from Austin MA, Kulkarni K, Powers MA. *Blood Glucose Monitoring: Essential Skills for Health Care Professionals.* 3rd ed. St. Paul, Minn: PP Publications; 2003: 64–69.

glycemia, which she usually treats with 4 ounces of fruit juice. SL drinks 8 ounces of nonfat milk at breakfast and at dinner. For physical activity, SL attends an aerobics class 4 days per week before breakfast. SL's diabetes medications include 20 units of glargine at bedtime and 5 units of aspart before each meal. SL's plasma blood glucose target ranges are 80 to 140 mg/dL before meals and < 180 mg/dL after meals. For SL's blood glucose log and for the steps in pattern management and factors a dietitian should consider, see Table 11.7.

TABLE 11.7 Findings for Case Study F

	Breakfast				Lunch				Dinner				Bedtime		
Date	Pre-BG, mg/dL	Ins, units	Carb, g	Post-BG, mg/dL	Pre-BG, mg/dL	Ins, units	Carb, g	Post-BG, mg/dL	Pre-BG, mg/dL	Ins, units	Carb, g	Post-BG, mg/dL	BG, mg/dL	Ins, units	Activity
1–1	103	5 Asp			84	5 Asp			267	5 Asp			194	20G	Aerobics before breakfast.
1–2	237	5 Asp			126	5 Asp			188	5 Asp			145	20G	Aerobics before breakfast.
1–3	71	5 Asp			131	5 Asp			196	5 Asp			118	20G	Aerobics before breakfast.

Step	Consider
1. Obtain sufficient, accurate data.	• Food: some information available. • Activity: some information available. • Medication: information available. • SMBG: premeal/bedtime checks, as shown above. Need to provide some postmeal BG checks, to evaluate the dose of aspart premeals.
2. Identify blood glucose patterns.	• The only identifiable pattern is high BG before dinner, although goals will need to be renegotiated for preconception planning.
3. Identify all possible influencing factors.	• Food: inadequate data to evaluate effect. • Medication: need additional BG data to evaluate current insulin plan.
4. Make recommendations for change.	• Negotiate glycemic goals for preconception, ideally maintaining A1C < 7%. Encourage premeal and 1-h postmeal BG checks. • Possible increase in basal insulin dose—insulin plans frequently start at 50% of total daily dosage for basal needs and 50% for bolus. Possible candidate for future insulin pump. • Discuss carbohydrate counting and record carb intake.

Abbreviations: Asp, aspart insulin (rapid-acting); BG, blood glucose value; carb, carbohydrate; G, glargine insulin (long-acting); Ins, insulin; Post-BG, blood glucose value 2 hours after meals; Pre-BG, blood glucose value before meals; SMBG, self-monitoring of blood glucose.
Source: Adapted with permission from Austin MA, Kulkarni K, Powers MA. *Blood Glucose Monitoring: Essential Skills for Health Care Professionals.* 3rd ed. St. Paul, Minn: PP Publications; 2003: 64–69.

SUMMARY

The effective use of blood glucose information in making clinical decisions leads to improvements in diabetes control. Proficiency in interpreting blood glucose results takes time and practice. The RD can play an important role in educating individuals with diabetes about the effects of food, physical activity, medication, and other factors on blood glucose; in assisting in interpretation of blood glucose patterns; and in providing ongoing support and motivation to improve self-management skills.

REFERENCES

1. Pearson J, Bergenstal R. Fine-tuning control: pattern management versus supplementation. View 1. Pattern management: an essential component of effective insulin management. *Diabetes Spectrum.* 2001;14:75–78.

2. The Diabetes Control and Complications Trial Research Group. The effect of intensive treatment of diabetes on the development and progression of long-term complications in insulin dependent diabetes mellitus. *N Engl J Med.* 1993;329:977–986.

3. UK prospective Diabetes Study (UKPDS) Group. Intensive blood glucose control with sulfonylureas or insulin compared with conventional treatment and risk of complications in patients with type 2 diabetes (UKPDS 33). *Lancet.* 1998;352:837–853.

4. Ohkubo Y, Kishikawa H, Araki E, Miyata T, Isami S, Motoyoshi S, Kojima Y, Furuyoshi N, Shichiri M. Intensive insulin therapy prevents the progression of diabetic microvascular complications in Japanese patients with non-insulin dependent diabetes mellitus: a randomized prospective 6-year study. *Diabetes Res Clin Pract.* 1995; 28:103–117.

5. Hinnen DA, Guthrie DW, Childs BP, Friesen J, Rhiley DS, Guthrie RA. Diabetes management therapies. In: Franz M, Kulkarni K, Polonsky W, Yarborough P, Zamudio V. *A Core Curriculum for Diabetes Educators.* 5th ed. Chicago, Ill: American Association of Diabetes Educators; 2003:215–246.

6. Blonde L, Ginsberg BH, Horn S, Hirsch IB, James B, Mulcahy K, Nettles A, Smout R, Wright H. Frequency of blood glucose monitoring in relation to glycemic control in patients with type 2 diabetes. *Diabetes Care.* 2002;25: 245–246.

7. Kulkarni K, Tomky D, Mulcahy K, Rosenstock J. Monitoring to target. Workshop presented at: Annual Meeting of American Association of Diabetes Educators; August 2002; Philadelphia, Pa.

8. Austin MA, Kulkarni K, Powers MA. *Blood Glucose Monitoring: Essential Skills for Health Care Professionals.* 3rd ed. St. Paul, Minn: PP Publications; 2003: 64–68.

ADDITIONAL RESOURCES

Avignon A, Radauceanu A, Monnier L. Non fasting plasma glucose is a better marker of diabetic control than fasting plasma glucose. *Diabetes Care.* 1997;20:1822–1826.

Davidson J, Reader D, Rickheim P. *Blood Glucose Patterns: A Guide to Achieving Targets.* Minneapolis, Minn: IDC Publishing; 2003.

Farkas-Hirsch R, ed. *Intensive Diabetes Management.* 3rd ed. Alexandria, Va: American Diabetes Association; 2004.

12

Hypoglycemia and Hyperglycemia

Marilynn S. Arnold, MS, RD, CDE

CHAPTER OVERVIEW

- Hypoglycemia (low blood glucose level) and hyperglycemia (high blood glucose level) are frequent and common side effects of diabetes and/or its treatment (1,2). The acute complications of these conditions range from minor variations in blood glucose to a potentially life-threatening emergency (1).
- Education provided by dietetics professionals to individuals with diabetes about the balance of food intake, physical activity, and diabetes medications can minimize fluctuations in blood glucose.
- Individuals with diabetes can develop the knowledge and skills necessary to prevent and appropriately treat acute complications, to substantially reduce their negative impact and help prevent serious side effects (2–5).

HYPERGLYCEMIA DEFINED

Hyperglycemia refers to any preprandial blood glucose level higher than 130 mg/dL or postprandial blood glucose higher than 180 mg/dL, for men and nonpregnant women (6). Anyone living with diabetes will at times experience a blood glucose level higher than normal. Risks for chronic complications (see Chapter 13) are greater with increases in blood glucose level, regardless of whether the individual with diabetes is symptomatic

(6,7). The level at which individuals are symptomatic varies. Individuals with diabetes can better participate in self-care if they learn to recognize the symptoms and causes of hyperglycemia and understand the role that food intake, physical activity, and medications have in glycemic control.

MILD HYPERGLYCEMIA

Definition

Mild hyperglycemia is a blood glucose level above normal range but not acutely dangerous. Individuals may not feel or function optimally, but they generally continue with usual responsibilities (8).

Causes

The primary causes of hyperglycemia are related to the balance of food intake, physical activity, therapy for insulin deficiency and/or insulin resistance, and the level of physiologic stress (4) (see Chapter 4). The reasons for a variable blood glucose level are more challenging to identify. Overeating can be, but is not necessarily, the culprit. The inappropriate timing of food and medications is a common contributor (especially after a medication adjustment) (4). For example, a meal plan with three meals and three snacks might work well with

70/30 insulin taken at breakfast and dinner, but not with bedtime insulin glargine and rapid-acting insulin before each meal. Illness, surgery, hormonal changes, and intense emotions are among the physiologic stressors that can elevate a blood glucose level (6).

Symptoms

Most but not all individuals with diabetes experience some symptoms of hyperglycemia. The most common symptoms are polyuria, polydipsia, blurred vision, polyphagia, and weight loss when insulin deficiency is present long enough (8). Additional symptoms include fatigue, low energy, delayed healing, and irritability (8). Acute episodes of hyperglycemia may reduce cognitive function and increase anxiety (9,10).

Individuals may attribute symptoms such as fatigue to getting older or to stress. Often one symptom causes or exacerbates another. Osmotic diuresis from hyperglycemia may lead to dehydration. Polyuria that interrupts sleep may contribute to fatigue. Low energy due to inadequate sleep may appear as or may exaggerate depression. Self-monitoring of blood glucose can help individuals with diabetes to recognize their own individual signs of an elevated blood glucose level (8). Awareness of hyperglycemia is a powerful first step toward improving metabolic control.

Treatment

Options for short-term treatment of hyperglycemia are usually limited to (*a*) injecting a correction dose of rapid-acting insulin or increasing oral diabetes medications; (*b*) modifying food intake; and/or (*c*) increasing activity level (4,11). When blood glucose level is chronically elevated, changes in the diabetes plan are needed. It is time to review and to individualize the type and amount of medication, as well as to discuss plans for food and activity.

Prevention

Identifying the cause of hyperglycemia helps identify a strategy to prevent the problem. See Table 12.1 for prevention strategies (6,7,12–14).

TABLE 12.1 Causes and Prevention of Mild to Moderate Hyperglycemia

Causes	Prevention
Lack of blood glucose monitoring	Regular self-monitoring of blood glucose.
Inadequate diabetes medication	Add, adjust, or change diabetes medication(s).
Inappropriate timing of diabetes medication(s)	Coordinate timing of diabetes medication(s) and food.
Overtreatment of hypoglycemia	Use appropriate amounts of carbohydrate sources.
Excess food and/or carbohydrate	Eat less food and/or carbohydrate.
Large meal or excess snacking	Distribute food/carbohydrate appropriately.
Physical inactivity	Gradually increase physical activity.
Adverse effect of nondiabetes medications	Read package insert on prescription and over-the-counter medication to learn about the effect of the medication on glucose.
Illness	Know how to manage diabetes during illness.
Variability in insulin absorption	Proper site rotation; proper insulin storage (ie, store at appropriate temperature and pay attention to expiration date).
Variability in rates of digestion/absorption of food	Address issues related to gastroparesis (eg, eat small meals, know what types of foods are tolerated).*
Stress	Learn relaxation techniques.

*See Chapter 13.
Source: Data are from references 6, 7, and 12–14.

The changes necessary to reduce risks may be unique to the individual. For example, if hyperglycemia follows meals consumed in restaurants, changing the frequency of eating out, portion size of foods eaten, or food choices made may help. Similarly, if the fasting blood glucose level is consistently elevated after late-evening meals or all-night grazing, eating meals earlier or choosing fewer snacks may help.

If the individual's blood glucose level is consistently elevated on weekends but not during the workweek, less food or more activity on the weekend may solve the problem. If his or her blood glucose level is elevated after episodes of hypoglycemia, appropriate treatment of reactions (ie, types and amounts of food) may minimize rebound highs. If blood glucose is elevated due to illness, it can improve when the cause of the illness is treated. If elevation of blood glucose level is due to stress, it may be resolved with a lifestyle change, such as changing jobs or learning relaxation techniques.

Some individuals need help to identify the cause of hyperglycemia and to determine action steps for their efforts to be effective. Causes for episodic hyperglycemia are not always clear, but keeping records and applying pattern management strategies (see Chapter 11) provide useful clues.

DIABETIC KETOACIDOSIS

Both diabetic ketoacidosis (DKA) and hyperglycemic hyperosmolar syndrome (HHS) are considered severe forms of hyperglycemia. These conditions are life threatening and require prompt medical attention to avoid adverse health outcomes (1).

A blood glucose level greater than 250 mg/dL and the presence of urinary ketones (ketosis) are characteristic of DKA. DKA occurs more often in people with type 1 diabetes but is also a risk for individuals with type 2 diabetes during acute illness and/or when they have become insulin deficient (5).

Causes

DKA evolves when insulin is so deficient that little, if any, glucose can enter cells. Counterregulatory hormones stimulate glucose production via gluconeogenesis and lipolysis, in an effort to avoid starvation. In addition to glucose production, lipolysis generates ketones as a by-product. Accumulating glucose and ketones causes osmotic diuresis, which results in dehydration and subsequent electrolyte imbalances. Electrolytes control key biological functions, such as potassium regulation of heart rhythm, which makes losses life threatening. Dehy-

dration further concentrates and therefore increases blood glucose level. Treatment is essential to reverse escalating risks for mortality.

The risk for DKA increases during infection, illness, or emotional stress. Insulin omission is a frequent cause of DKA; people may skip insulin when they feel too sick to eat or because they are afraid of having an insulin reaction (hypoglycemia). Intentionally omitting insulin for weight loss may signal an eating disorder (1,5).

Symptoms

Symptoms of DKA include the following (5):

- Nausea and/or vomiting
- Stomach pain
- Fruity or acetone breath
- Heavy or Kussmaul breathing
- Mental status changes

Treatment

Treatment of severe DKA typically requires hospitalization, so that intravenous fluids, insulin, and electrolyte levels can be assessed and/or administered and supplemental doses of insulin can also be administered until metabolic stability returns (12). Potassium is the electrolyte most often deficient due to osmotic losses. Although techniques to treat DKA resolve most cases, 2% to 5% of cases are fatal (1).

Prevention

Identifying the cause or causes for DKA helps to determine approaches to prevention. Table 12.2 (1,5,7) identifies causes and appropriate prevention measures.

HYPERGLYCEMIC HYPEROSMOLAR SYNDROME

A blood glucose level greater than 600 mg/dL without ketones characterizes HHS (1). HHS occurs primarily in undiagnosed or elderly individuals with type 2 diabetes and is especially common in residents of long-term-care facilities. HHS can occur whether or not diabetes medications are part of usual treatment (1).

Causes

Dehydration is the primary precipitating factor for HHS. Those with inadequate fluid intake or excess fluid losses

TABLE 12.2 Causes and Prevention of Diabetic Ketoacidosis

Causes	Prevention
Lack of blood glucose self-monitoring	Regular self-monitoring of blood glucose; test for ketones if glucose > 250 mg/dL.
Severe illness or infection	Monitor closely the effects of illness on blood glucose; treat illness if indicated; take diabetes medications even when eating less; have a plan for sick-day management.
Inappropriately stored insulin	Discard expired insulin; protect insulin from excess heat and cold.
Insulin omitted	Probe rationale.
Increased insulin needs with growth spurts	Frequent blood glucose monitoring.

Source: Data are from references 1, 5, and 7.

over several days or weeks are at risk for HHS (1). Because symptoms progress slowly, they are less noticeable and more easily missed than those of DKA. Without careful monitoring, elderly individuals with an inability to self-hydrate may slide into a cyclical process of gradual but steady fluid losses and rising blood glucose level, which can lead to severe dehydration (1). Common situations that contribute to fluid depletion are listed, along with suggested preventive measures, in Table 12.3 (7).

Symptoms

Symptoms of HHS are similar to those of moderate hyperglycemia and include polyuria, polydipsia, polyphagia, and weight loss. HHS symptoms persist and worsen over several days or weeks as glucose level exceeds 600 mg/dL and hydration status deteriorates. The mortality rate for HHS is approximately 15%, which is much higher than for DKA (5).

Treatment

HHS requires hospitalization for slow rehydration as well as treatment for complications and underlying medical problems (7). Insulin may or may not be required to adequately reduce blood glucose level.

Prevention

Frequent monitoring of fluid status and blood glucose level helps prevent HHS. Constructing the individual environment to support routine hydration and adequate

monitoring is important, especially when the individual lives alone or in a long-term-care facility. See Table 12.3 for action steps to reduce risks for HHS.

HYPOGLYCEMIA DEFINED

Hypoglycemia (low blood glucose level) occurs when blood glucose drops below optimal levels. It is the limiting factor to reaching euglycemia in the treatment of diabetes with insulin or an oral insulin secretagogue

TABLE 12.3 Risks and Prevention for Hyperglycemic Hyperosmolar Syndrome

Risk	Prevention
Inadequate fluid intake*	Monitor fluid intake, evaluate fluid status, and establish plan to offer fluids regularly.
Excessive fluid losses†	Monitor fluid status, address contributing causes, and replace fluids.
Prolonged hyperglycemia	Monitor blood glucose regularly; treat mild hyperglycemia.

*Risk is greater for individuals (a) with impaired thirst mechanism; (b) who have difficulty communicating; (c) who live alone; (d) who are hospitalized; (e) who are nursing home residents.
†Excessive fluid losses may be caused by severe diarrhea, diuretics, dialysis, or illness/fever.
Source: Data are from reference 7.

(sulfonylurea or meglitinides). There have even been documented occurrences of hypoglycemia with metformin (2). Symptoms of iatrogenic hypoglycemia occur at varying levels, but it is defined as a blood glucose level less than 72 mg/dL (2). Minimal targets and the threshold for intervention will vary among those who are young, elderly, pregnant, ill, or unaware when hypoglycemic.

MILD HYPOGLYCEMIA

Causes

The cause of hypoglycemia is insulin—more is available than needed relative to food intake and physical activity (1). When the dose(s) of insulin or insulin secretagogue are consistent and food intake and/or exercise are not, blood glucose level varies (2).

The lower the blood glucose targets, the more likely that hypoglycemia will occur (2). Stress, variability in the absorption of diabetes medications, and the action of nondiabetes drugs can also contribute to inconsistent blood glucose level and the risk for hypoglycemia (2,7). For example, drugs such as alcohol and beta blockers reduce awareness of hypoglycemic symptoms and cause the individual to delay treatment of the low blood glucose level.

Symptoms

Symptoms of hypoglycemia are highly individualized but may include weakness, shakiness, perspiration, hunger, and a rapid heart beat (2,3). See Box 12.1 (2,3) for a more complete list of symptoms. People experience symptoms of hypoglycemia at varying levels. Study results from the use of a continuous glucose-monitoring sensor (CGMS) device in persons with type 1 diabetes show that subjects were unaware of 40%–60% of hypoglycemic episodes (12). More frequent and severe hypoglycemia reduces the threshold for experiencing symptoms (also called hypoglycemia unawareness) (3,15). Because the consequences of reduced blood glucose to the brain and other organs occur regardless of symptoms, learning to recognize one's individual symptoms is a valuable self-care tool. Dietetics professionals who work with people who have diabetes will need to address this problem.

Treatment

Mild hypoglycemia can be self-treated. Treatment involves several steps:

BOX 12.1

Symptoms and Treatment for Hypoglycemia

Mild/Moderate Hypoglycemia

Symptoms
Trembling, nervousness, trouble concentrating, anxiety, blurred vision, sweating, irritability, rapid heart beat, inability to think clearly, tingling in extremities, dizziness, hunger, nausea, fatigue, weakness, headache

Treatment
- If glucose level is 51–70 mg/dL, consume 15 g carbohydrate (eg, ½ cup juice or regular soft drink, 3–4 glucose tabs, or 3–8 hard candies). If glucose level is ≤ 50 mg/dL, consume 20–30 g carbohydrate.
- Repeat if glucose does not return to normal range after 15 minutes.
- Follow with snack after exercise, during the night, or more than 60 minutes before the next meal. Even if glucose level is normal after treatment, individual is at risk for repeat hypoglycemia in these circumstances.

Severe Hypoglycemia

Symptoms
Mental confusion, argumentativeness, combativeness, lethargy, seizures, unconsciousness

Treatment
Glucagon, intravenous glucose

Source: Data are from references 2 and 3.

---

1. Consume 10 to 15 g of any form of carbohydrate that contains glucose. If the individual's blood glucose level is less than 50 mg/dL, he or she should eat 20 to 30 g of carbohydrate (15). Theoretically, 10 to 15 g of carbohydrate will elevate blood glucose 30 to 45 mg/dL (15). A form of glucose (eg, glucose tab) or a carbohydrate-containing food is used to treat hypoglycemia, so that blood glucose level rises quickly. Food or beverages high in fat content can slow gastric emptying and absorption of carbohydrate, which causes blood glucose level to rise more slowly (15). Adding protein to the treatment of hypoglycemia does not raise blood glucose level and does not prevent subsequent hypoglycemia (16).

2. After treating, wait 15 minutes and recheck blood glucose to determine whether glucose has returned to the normal range. If not, repeat process (15).

3. Determine whether additional snacks are needed. If blood glucose normalizes but the individual (*a*) will not eat for an hour or more, (*b*) has recently exercised, or (*c*) is going to bed, an additional snack may be necessary to prevent repeated hypoglycemia. Test blood glucose level and treat as appropriate (15). Treatment information is summarized in Box 12.1 (2,3). In individuals treated with a combination of an oral insulin secretagogue and an alpha-glucosidase inhibitor, such as acarbose or miglitol (which interferes with the digestion of disaccharide), only glucose or lactose (glucose tablets or milk) will resolve hypoglycemia quickly.

Individuals with diabetes may be tempted to use hypoglycemia as an opportunity to eat something sweet if they typically avoid these foods. The urgent drive to relieve hypoglycemic symptoms, combined with a perceived opportunity to indulge, can easily lead to overtreatment; thus, hypoglycemia may be followed by hyperglycemia (15). Some educators recommend using commercially available glucose tablets or a glucose gel that are portion controlled and convenient to carry, for treating hypoglycemia. Frequent treatments for hypoglycemia are a common source of extra or excess calories (15). The dietetics professional can teach individuals with diabetes to include sweets in their meal plan, so that they are less likely to overindulge during hypoglycemic reactions.

To minimize adverse effects, hypoglycemia should be treated immediately when it is recognized. When treatment is within reach, such as on the nightstand or carried in a purse or pocket, this goal can be more readily achieved.

Prevention

Identifying the cause of a hypoglycemic reaction suggests a strategy for preventing it. Table 12.4 lists factors that contribute to hypoglycemia with corresponding preventive measures (2,3). Because the consequences of reduced blood glucose to the brain and other organs occur regardless of symptoms, learning to recognize one's individual symptoms is a valuable self-care tool. Prevention of hypoglycemia limits calories used to treat reactions and thereby assists individuals in achieving

TABLE 12.4 Causes, Treatment, and Prevention of Hypoglycemia

Cause	Treatment/Prevention
Excess diabetes medication	Adjust amount and/or type of diabetes medication(s).
Inappropriate timing of diabetes medications	Coordinate timing of diabetes medication(s), food, and activity.
Overcorrection with insulin for hyperglycemia	Use appropriate correction factor.
Too little food and/or carbohydrate	Eat all planned food and/or carbohydrate.
Skipped or delayed meal	Eat meals on time, or snack if meal will be late.
Increased activity	Increase food or reduce insulin when more active than usual.
Side effects of nondiabetes medication	Check effect of medication on glucose, whether or not formula includes sugar.
Variability in insulin absorption	Proper site rotation; store insulin appropriately and check insulin expiration date.
Variability in rates of digestion/absorption	Address issues related to gastroparesis (eg, food frequency; macronutrient composition, timing of medications).*
Alcohol consumption	Consume food when drinking alcohol. Limit amount of alcohol consumed.

*See Chapter 13.
Source: Data are from references 2 and 3.

their weight-management goals. Dietetics professionals have the opportunity to evaluate and reinforce prevention and prompt, appropriate treatment of mild hypoglycemia, which can deter the onset of severe hypoglycemia.

SEVERE HYPOGLYCEMIA

Severe hypoglycemia is defined as hypoglycemia that cannot be self-treated (2). A trained friend, family member, or emergency medical services must inject glucagon or glucose, to restore glucose to a normal level.

Causes

More-intensive insulin plans and lower A1C targets increase the risk for severe hypoglycemia (2). Causes or risk factors for severe hypoglycemia are included in Box 12.2 (3). Severe hypoglycemia occurs in type 1 and type 2 diabetes (advanced progression) due to the combination of absolute or relative insulin excess and compromised glucose counterregulation (2). Neuropathy, frequent reactions, and some medications, such as beta blockers, mask symptoms and further increase the risk (15).

Symptoms

With severe hypoglycemia, a person becomes unconscious or so confused that he or she is incapable of reasonable thinking. The blood glucose level at which this occurs varies between and within individuals. If conscious, an individual may appear lethargic or combative. Conscious or unconscious, the individual may not appreciate help but require it. See Box 12.1 to compare symptoms for mild and severe hypoglycemia.

Treatment

Outpatient treatment for severe hypoglycemia is glucagon, a hormone that elevates blood glucose by stimulating hepatic gluconeogenesis (15). Glucagon comes as a powder that must be reconstituted just before injecting. All persons at risk for severe hypoglycemia should have a glucagon emergency kit available and should train significant others to administer it. If hypoglycemia is alcohol induced or if the patient has inadequate glycogen stores (as with hepatic disease, starvation, or chronic hypoglycemia), glucagon is ineffective (15). The alternative is to call emergency medical services (911), so that intravenous glucose can be administered.

Prevention

Researchers have shown that it is possible to decrease A1C and still reduce the risk of severe hypoglycemia by as much as 60 times less than that reported in earlier trials (2). See guidelines suggested in Box 12.2. Note that specifics of the insulin plan have clear implications for meal planning. More physiologic insulin plans and matching diabetes medication(s) with food intake reduce risks for hypoglycemia and help limit glucose excursions (12).

QUALITY OF LIFE

An unstable blood glucose level can impact quality of life even when A1C results meet recommended goals. Negative consequences include the following:

BOX 12.2

Causes and Prevention of Severe Hypoglycemia

Causes

- Unrecognized or untreated mild hypoglycemia
- History of frequent and severe hypoglycemia
- Intensive insulin therapy
- Near normal A1C
- Autonomic neuropathy
- Defective hormonal regulation

Prevention

- Monitor frequently.
- Use physiological models of insulin replacement:
  - Pump
  - Rapid-acting (vs regular) insulin before meals and NPH or insulin glargine before bed (vs NPH at evening meal)
- Add between-meal snacks and/or change diabetes medications.
- Use information from continuous glucose monitoring.
- Obtain adequate diabetes self-management training.
- Revise target glucose ranges.
- If frequent lows, avoid alcohol.
- Carry treatment.

Source: Data are from reference 3.

- Reduced function—both physically and mentally (2)
- Reduced emotional stability (2)
- Increased caloric consumption as a result of overtreating reactions, which can result in weight gain or can prevent weight loss (4)
- Increased blood glucose level as a result of overtreating hypoglycemia (15)
- Hypoglycemic unawareness resulting from increased severity and frequency of reactions (2)
- Limited ability to participate in some activities (15)
- Brain damage or even death from severe hypoglycemia (2)

ASSESSING ACUTE COMPLICATIONS

The following questions can be used to explore how acute complications may affect an individual's life:

- Does your blood glucose level ever get too low/high? How often?
- What symptoms do you have?
- Is there a time of day you seem most likely to have low/high blood glucose?
- What do you do to treat low/high blood glucose?
- How long does it take for you to feel better?
- How low/high does your blood glucose go before you recognize it is low/high?
- How much does having low/high blood glucose interfere with your daily life?
- What clues, if any, do you have as to the causes of your low/high blood glucose?
- Tell me about your schedule. When do you eat and when do you take your diabetes medications? How much does it vary from day to day and from weekday to weekend?
- Have you trained family members on how to use glucagon? Do you have a glucagon emergency kit?

ESSENTIAL TOPICS FOR EDUCATING INDIVIDUALS WITH DIABETES

The risk for acute complications can be greatly reduced by understanding how medications work, by recognizing symptoms of hyper- and hypoglycemia, by knowing treatments for hyper- and hypoglycemia, and by regular monitoring of blood glucose levels.

How Medications Work

Individuals with diabetes need to know how their diabetes medications work and when to take them for maximum benefit. For example, they need to know whether their medication may cause hypoglycemia and, if so, what they can do to minimize the risk. An individualized approach to coordinating meal and snack times with a specific diabetes medication plan (eg, insulin) is essential (4). See Chapters 8 and 9 for more information on insulin and oral diabetes medications.

Teaching Point

Individuals with diabetes need to understand how their diabetes medications work, as well as the rationale for meal plan changes when they have medication changes.

Case Study

EM is a 32-year-old man with type 1 diabetes who has been treated with a mixed dose of NPH and regular insulin before breakfast and dinner for the past 8 years. During that time, he saw a dietetics professional a couple times and was using a meal plan developed for him that included three meals and three snacks each day. In a recent physical, his physician switched him to a more intensive therapeutic plan of insulin glargine at bedtime and rapid-acting insulin before each meal.

EM was unhappy with the new insulin plan because his blood glucose level seemed worse since the medication change. He reported persistent hyperglycemia before lunch and dinner, although he was very careful to follow his meal plan.

A solution for EM consists of reviewing the action times of the various insulins. Because rapid-acting insulin does not act as long as regular, and only insulin glargine provided basal insulin, EM's new insulin plan did not benefit from between-meal snacks. In fact, there was very little insulin available to provide coverage for snacks. His blood glucose level improved markedly when he stopped the snacks and instead consumed larger meals.

Symptoms of Hyper- and Hypoglycemia

People with diabetes need to know the symptoms for hyper- and hypoglycemia and be able to recognize their individual symptoms. If they develop hypoglycemia unawareness, they may need to learn to detect the more subtle neurological cues, such as numbness and blurred vision (3).

Teaching Point

Knowledge of how medications work, coupled with knowledge of the symptoms of hyper- and hypoglycemia, can help individuals with diabetes solve problems.

Case Study

AB is a 16-year-old female (body mass index = 22) with type 1 diabetes, which was recently diagnosed during a visit to her grandparents' farm during spring break. She gives herself an injection of NPH insulin at breakfast and at dinner, and uses a pen with rapid-acting insulin per sliding scale when blood glucose results are greater than 150 mg/dL before a meal. When she returned home, her local physician changed her insulin plan to NPH insulin at breakfast and bedtime, with rapid-acting insulin before each meal.

When AB went back at school, she felt dizzy and had trouble concentrating every day after lunch. AB ate a substantial lunch, choosing a large vegetable salad with generous portions of meat, cheese, and egg from the cafeteria salad bar. AB's rapid-acting insulin quickly entered her bloodstream. Although she did not skimp on the amount of food she ate at lunch, AB included insufficient carbohydrate to match the rapid-acting insulin.

Solutions for AB include teaching her about the new insulin plan and explaining how to recognize and treat hypoglycemia. Now AB makes a slightly smaller salad but adds crackers and fresh fruit to her salad bar lunch and rarely experiences symptoms of hypoglycemia after lunch.

Treatments for Hyper- and Hypoglycemia

Individuals with diabetes need to know how to appropriately treat hyper- and hypoglycemia, regardless of whether they have symptoms. Dietetics professionals should review this information, including instruction on glucagon when appropriate, with individuals as a normal part of the education process (2). Individuals with diabetes should be able to demonstrate application of the information.

Teaching Point

Individuals with diabetes need to know how to treat symptoms of hypoglycemia, but they also need to know that resolution of symptoms does not mean resolution of the problem.

Case Study

PQ had lived with diabetes for more than 20 years and was pleased with his recent A1C of 6.2%. He was familiar with the problems of hypoglycemia. PQ always carried glucose tabs, promptly chewed a couple whenever he perceived symptoms, and quickly felt better. He was shocked and indignant when the police pulled him over on his way home from work one day and suggested he was driving under the influence of alcohol. It had been 8 years since he had consumed any alcohol.

PQ typically did not feel hypoglycemic symptoms until his glucose had fallen under 50 mg/dL. When he did not experience symptoms, he was not aware that he was not functioning at full capacity. Two or three tablets (8 to 12 g of carbohydrate) were insufficient to restore blood glucose to his target range.

When PQ began monitoring before driving and after treating for hypoglycemia, the physician adjusted his insulin plan to reduce hypoglycemia, and PQ treated symptoms with more glucose. His A1C increased slightly, but he has had no episodes of severe hypoglycemia during the past 2 months.

Monitoring of Blood Glucose Level

Regular self-monitoring of blood glucose level can help individuals evaluate blood glucose level, determine appropriate actions based on blood glucose results, and evaluate the outcomes of the actions they take to treat a high or low blood glucose level (4,12). Individuals with diabetes should be encouraged to keep their blood glucose monitor with them to use as needed.

Teaching Point

Individuals with diabetes should use blood glucose monitoring as a tool to assess problems that could be related to blood glucose level.

Case Study

KM is a 55-year-old woman who was diagnosed with type 2 diabetes 5 years ago. She is currently being treated with 20 mg of long-acting sulfonylurea and 2,000 mg of metformin. KM's new physician referred her to a diabetes education program, but KM insisted that she needed only a meal plan to lose weight. KM was familiar with diabetes from helping her mother who also has type 2 diabetes and from raising a daughter with type 1 diabetes.

Forty minutes late for her 1-hour appointment, KM described her life on the fast track, with an irregular schedule of meetings and gourmet restaurant meals. She complained of fatigue and frequently waking up with headaches. KM states that she stopped monitoring because she was too busy, but she agreed to check her fasting blood glucose during the coming week.

KM began monitoring her blood glucose level and discovered that she was waking up with a blood glucose level between 60 and 80 mg/dL, so she contacted her physician. Her physician reduced the sulfonylurea, after which her fasting blood glucose level increased to about 100 mg/dL and her morning headaches stopped.

SUMMARY

The dietetics professional who understands the action of diabetes medications and can interpret blood glucose monitoring results is in a unique position to identify how the interactions between food, activity, and diabetes medications contribute to hyper- and hypoglycemia. Education to prevent and appropriately treat acute complications can substantially reduce their negative impact and can help prevent serious side effects.

REFERENCES

1. Umpierrez GE, Murphy MB, Kitabchi AE. Diabetic ketoacidosis and hyperglycemic hyperosmolar syndrome. *Diabetes Spectrum.* 2002;15:28–36.

2. Cryer PE, Davis SN, Shamoon H. Hypoglycemia in diabetes (American Diabetes Technical Review). *Diabetes Care.* 2003;26:1902–1912.

3. Cryer PE, Childs BP. Negotiating the barrier of hypoglycemia in diabetes mellitus. *Diabetes Spectrum.* 2002;15:20–27.

4. Franz MJ. Medical nutrition therapy for diabetes. In: 'Franz MJ, ed. *Diabetes Management Therapies: A Core Curriculum for Diabetes Educators.* 5th ed. Chicago, Ill: American Association of Diabetes Educators; 2003:3–18.

5. American Diabetes Association. Hyperglycemic crises diabetes (position statement). *Diabetes Care.* 2004;27(Suppl 1):S94–S95.

6. American Diabetes Association. Standard of medical care for patients with diabetes mellitus (position statement). *Diabetes Care.* 2004;27(Suppl 1):S15–S35.

7. Davidson MB, Schwartz S. Hyperglycemia in diabetes. In: Franz MJ, ed. *Diabetes and Complications: A Core Curriculum for Diabetes Educators.* 5th ed. Chicago, Ill: American Association of Diabetes Educators; 2003: 21–42.

8. American Diabetes Association. Diagnosis and Classification of Diabetes Mellitus (position statement). *Diabetes Care.* 2004;27(Suppl 1):S5–S10.

9. Cox DJ, Kovatchev BP, Gonder-Frederick LA, Summers KH, McCall A, Grimm KJ, Clarke WL. Relationships between hyperglycemia and cognitive performance among adults with type 1 and type 2 diabetes. *Diabetes Care.* 2005;28:71–77.

10. Sommerfield AJ, Deary IJ, Frier BM. Acute hyperglycemia alters mood state and impairs cognitive performance in people with type 2 diabetes. *Diabetes Care.* 2004; 27:2335–2340.

11. Hinnen D, Guthrie DW, Childs BP, Friesen J, Speelman Rhiley D, Guthrie R. Pattern management, In: Franz MJ, ed. *Diabetes Management Therapies: A Core Curriculum for Diabetes Educators.* 5th ed. Chicago, Ill: American Association of Diabetes Educators; 2003: 215–246.

12. Saleh M, Grunberger G. Hypoglycemia: an excuse for poor glycemic control? *Clin Diabetes.* 2001;19:161–167.

13. Mullooly C, Hanson Chalmers K. Physical activity and exercise. In: Franz MJ, ed. *Diabetes Management Therapies: A Core Curriculum for Diabetes Educators.* 5th ed. Chicago, Ill: American Association of Diabetes Educators; 2003:61–92.

14. Pastors JG, Arnold MS, Daly A, Franz MJ, Warshaw HS. *Diabetes Nutrition Q & A for Health Professionals: 101 Essential Questions Answered by Experts.* Alexandria, Va: American Diabetes Association; 2003.

15. Gonder-Frederick LA, Zrebiec J. Hypoglycemia. In: *Diabetes Management Therapies: A Core Curriculum for Diabetes Educators.* 5th ed. Chicago, Ill: American Association of Diabetes Educators; 2003:279–310.

16. American Diabetes Association. Nutrition principles and recommendations in diabetes (position statement). *Diabetes Care.* 2004;27(Suppl 1):S36–S46.

ADDITIONAL RESOURCES

American Diabetes Association. Clinical practice recommendations (2004). Available at: http://www.diabetes.org/for-health-professionals-and-scientists/cpr.jsp. Accessed September 28, 2004.

American Diabetes Association. *Managing Diabetic Hypoglycemia* [video]. Alexandria, Va: American Diabetes Association; 2000.

Cox DJ, Gonder-Frederick L, Polonski W, Schlundt D, Kovatchev B, Clarke W. Blood glucose awareness training. *Diabetes Care.* 2001;24:637–642.

Cryer PE, Davis SN, Shamoon H. Hypoglycemia in diabetes. *Diabetes Care.* 2003;26;1902–1912.

Diabetes and Complications: A Core Curriculum for Diabetes Educators. 5th ed. Chicago, Ill: American Association of Diabetes Educators; 2003.

Franz MJ, Bantle JB, eds. *American Diabetes Association Guide to Medical Nutrition Therapy for Diabetes.* Alexandria, Va: American Diabetes Association; 1999.

Kitabchi AE, Umpierrez GE, Murphy MB, Barrett EJ, Kreisberg RA, Malone JI, Wall BM. Management of hyperglycemic crises in patients with diabetes (technical review). *Diabetes Care.* 1998;21:2161–2177.

Lincoln TA, Eaddy JA. *Beating the Blood Sugar Blues: Proven Methods and Wisdom for Controlling Hypoglycemia.* Alexandria, Va: American Diabetes Association; 2001.

Lowe E, Arsham G. *Diabetes: A Guide to Living Well.* Alexandria, Va: American Diabetes Association; 2004.

Michigan Diabetes Research and Training Center. *Life With Diabetes.* 2nd ed. Alexandria, Va: American Diabetes Association; 2000.

Powers, Margaret, ed. *Handbook of Diabetes Medical Nutrition Therapy.* Gaithersburg, Md: Aspen Publishers; 1996.

Walsh J, Roberts R. *Pumping Insulin.* San Diego, Calif: Torrey Pines Press; 2000.

13

Long-Term Complications

Madelyn L. Wheeler, MS, RD, FADA, CD, CDE

CHAPTER OVERVIEW

- Optimal blood glucose and blood pressure control are the primary treatment priorities for reducing risk, or slowing the progression, of long-term complications associated with diabetes (heart disease, stroke, hypertension, blindness, renal disease, neuropathy, and amputations).
- Medical nutrition therapy (MNT) provided by dietetics professionals is integral to the attainment of optimal blood glucose control, blood pressure control, lipid management, and cardiovascular risk reduction. MNT is also helpful in the risk reduction or treatment of other chronic complications, including renal disease and gastroparesis.

BACKGROUND

In the past decade, two landmark studies have proved that incidence and rate of progression of the chronic complications of diabetes can be reduced. Results of the Diabetes Control and Complications Trial (DCCT) (1) showed that intensive treatment (multiple daily injections or continuous insulin infusion, combined with intensive diabetes self-management education, including MNT and skills development such as self-monitoring of blood glucose, and regular follow-up) of individuals with type 1 diabetes resulted in significantly lower A1C

(approximately 7%) than the standard care group (9%). The intensive treatment also resulted in significant reductions in the incidence and rate of progression of retinopathy, albuminuria, and neuropathy in the intensively treated group.

Results from the United Kingdom Prospective Diabetes Study (UKPDS) (2) indicated that intensive treatment (insulin, sulfonylureas, or metformin) of people with newly diagnosed type 2 diabetes showed somewhat better A1C results than did standard treatment (lifestyle interventions). A 0.9% difference in A1C between the intensive and standard treatment groups was associated with significant reductions in all microvascular end points. Although the trend toward a reduction in cardiovascular events did not reach statistical significance, epidemiological analysis of the UKPDS cohort showed a statistically significant effect of A1C on cardiovascular disease (CVD) outcomes: 14% reduction in all-cause mortality and myocardial infarction for every 1% reduction in A1C (3).

Two multicenter randomized controlled trials are currently being conducted under the sponsorship of the National Institutes of Health (NIH). These trials may be future landmark studies in the area of diabetes and reduction of complications or risk of complications. Action for Health in Diabetes (Look AHEAD) is funded by the NIH's National Institute of Diabetes and Digestive and Kidney Diseases to investigate the long-term effects of weight loss in patients with type 2 diabetes (4). It began in 2001, and results will be available about 2013. Action to Control Cardiovascular Risk in Diabetes (ACCORD) is funded by the NIH's National Heart, Lung, and Blood Institute to test approaches to lowering the risk of heart disease and stroke in adults with type 2 diabetes (5). It began in 2003, and results should be available in 2009.

Following is a brief discussion of the major macrovascular and microvascular complications of diabetes and the role of MNT in prevention and treatment of these complications (6–8).

MACROVASCULAR COMPLICATIONS

Cardiovascular Disease

CVD is a major complication and the leading cause of death among people with diabetes. About 65% of deaths among people with diabetes are due to heart disease or stroke (9). Adults with diabetes have heart disease death rates about two to four times higher than adults without diabetes (9).

Risk Factors

People with diabetes, particularly those with type 2 diabetes, have an increased prevalence of lipid abnormalities (dyslipidemias), hypertension, and obesity, all of which contribute to higher rates of CVD. Table 13.1 (6,10) compares the lipid levels found in individuals with type 2 diabetes with the goals set forth in the American Diabetes Association's Standards of Medical Care in Diabetes position statement (6). Diabetes is an independent risk factor for coronary heart disease and other forms of CVD (11).

Treatment

The first priority for treatment of diabetic dyslipidemia is to reduce levels of low-density lipoprotein (LDL) cholesterol, the major atherogenic lipoprotein (12). Lowering LDL cholesterol levels is associated with a reduction in cardiovascular events. Table 13.2 (13–17) contrasts dietary changes against their expected changes in LDL cholesterol levels. Lowering triglycerides and increasing high-density lipoprotein (HDL) cholesterol levels are also associated with a reduction in cardiovascular events (6). See Table 13.3 (11,18–24) for a review of how MNT and therapeutic lifestyle changes affect HDL and triglyceride levels.

Improvement in glycemic control can also beneficially modify plasma lipids, especially triglycerides, and should be encouraged, along with intensive treatment of dyslipidemia. Statins (HMG CoA reductase inhibitors) are the preferred pharmacologic treatment to lower LDL cholesterol levels (6).

TABLE 13.1 Diabetes and Dyslipidemia

Lipid Component	Goal, mg/dL	Approximate Levels in Type 2 Diabetes, mg/dL
LDL	< 100	110
HDL	> 40*	20–30
Triglycerides	< 150	200–400

Abbreviations: HDL, high-density lipoproteins; LDL, low-density lipoproteins.
*Because women typically have higher HDL cholesterol levels than men, an HDL goal 10 mg/dL higher (> 50 mg/dL) should be considered for women (6).
Source: Data are from references 6 (goals) and 10 (levels in type 2 diabetes).

TABLE 13.2 Nutrition Management of Elevated LDL Cholesterol

Medical Nutrition Therapy	Change in LDL Cholesterol
Primary option	
Decrease consumption of foods high in saturated or *trans* fatty acids*	Decrease 12%–16%
Secondary options	
Consume 2–3 g/d of stanols/sterols	Decrease 6%–15%
Consume 25 g/d of soy protein	Decrease 10%
Consume 1 g viscous fiber†	Decrease 1%–2%
Other therapies	
Garlic	Inconclusive
Antioxidants	No significant benefit proven

Abbreviation: LDL, low-density lipoprotein.
*For example, dairy fats (high-fat cheese, whole milk, ice cream); animal fats (high-fat meats, fried foods, skin from poultry, lard); high-fat bakery products (pastries, pies); other fried or deep-fried foods.
†From oat products, psyllium, or pectin.
Source: Data are from references 13–17.

TABLE 13.3 Medical Nutrition Therapy and Other Therapeutic Lifestyle Changes to Increase HDL Cholesterol and Decrease Triglycerides

MNT/TLC	Lipid Component Changes
Weight loss	Decreased TG, increased HDL*
Increased physical activity	Increased HDL*
Increased consumption of fish, especially fatty fish (salmon), and n-3 vegetable sources (soybean and canola oil)	Decreased TG
Fish oil supplements	TG decreased by almost 30% but increased LDL[†]
Light to moderate alcohol consumption[‡]	Increased HDL
Smoking cessation	HDL increased 5%

Abbreviations: HDL, high-density lipoproteins; LDL, low-density lipoproteins; MNT, medical nutrition therapy; TG, triglycerides; TLC, therapeutic lifestyle changes.
*Weight loss combined with a program of regular exercise may increase HDL cholesterol levels by 10%-30%.
[†]The increase in LDL can be counteracted by increased physical activity.
[‡]Chronic intake of light-to-moderate amounts (5–15 g/day) of alcohol has been associated with decreased risk for coronary heart disease, presumably due to the concomitant increase in plasma HDL (23). Caution: high intakes of alcohol produce multiple adverse effects; people who do not drink should not be encouraged to initiate regular alcohol consumption; individuals with high TG levels should avoid excess alcohol intake.
Source: Data are from references 11 and 18–24.

Implications for MNT

To reduce elevated LDL cholesterol levels, MNT should target reduction of saturated and *trans* fatty acids to less than 7% to 10% of energy (7). An important point to consider is that when saturated fat is reduced, so is monounsaturated fat. This is because the major monounsaturated fat in the diet is oleic, and the major dietary sources of oleic are the same as for saturated fat (dairy, beef, pork, poultry, and lamb). More than 50% of the fat in meat is monounsaturated. Thus, when advising individuals to reduce saturated fats by reducing animal products, dietetics professionals should be aware that this also reduces the amount of monounsaturated fat eaten.

If weight loss is desired, the individual should not replace the energy deficit from the reduction of saturated and *trans* fats. If weight loss is not a goal, energy can be replaced with carbohydrates. The carbohydrate (mainly grain and whole-grain products, vegetables, fruits, and fat-free and low-fat dairy products) should be kept at less than 60% of energy. Energy also can be replaced with monounsaturated fatty acids (in essence, replacing what was taken away when saturated fat was reduced), but not to exceed the required energy intake.

MICROVASCULAR COMPLICATIONS

Nephropathy

Diabetic nephropathy occurs in 20% to 40% of patients with diabetes and is the single leading cause of end-stage renal disease (ESRD) (6). (ESRD is an administrative term indicating that a patient is treated with dialysis or transplantation.) Diabetes accounts for 44% of new cases of ESRD (9). Diabetic nephropathy has several stages (6,24).

- Microalbuminuria: albumin levels of 30 to 299 μg per mg of creatinine, a risk factor for developing macroalbuminuria.
- Macroalbuminuria: albumin levels of 300 μg per mg of creatinine or higher.
- Chronic kidney disease: glomerular filtration rate (GFR) less than 60 mL/min/1.73 m² body surface area for 3 months or longer.
- ESRD (kidney failure): GFR less than 15 mL/min/1.73m².

The following information concerns the first two stages, micro- and macroalbuminuria. For information on chronic kidney disease and ESRD, visit the National Kidney Foundation's Kidney Disease Outcomes Quality Initiative Web site (see Additional Resources at end of this chapter; see also Chapter 23).

Risk Factors

High blood pressure and high levels of blood glucose increase the risk that a person with diabetes will progress to kidney failure (1,2,25). Native Americans, Hispanics, and African Americans with type 2 diabetes have much higher risks (6 times, 1.8–2.6 times, and 2.6–5.6 times the risk, respectively) of developing ESRD than non-Hispanic whites with type 2 diabetes (26).

Treatment

Treatment includes the following:

- Optimization of glucose control (goal: preprandial plasma glucose = 90–130 mg/dL; postprandial plasma glucose < 180 mg/dL) (2,6,27).
- Aggressive blood pressure control (goal: < 130/80 mm Hg) (6). Treatment with angiotensin-converting enzyme (ACE) inhibitors and angiotensin receptor blockers (ARBS) can reduce the risk and/or slow the progression of nephropathy (28).
- Reduction in the amount of protein consumed may slow the progression of the disease (7,8).

Implications for MNT

MNT for the management of hypertension focuses on weight reduction and reducing sodium intake (see Box 13.1) (6,8,9,29–32). In individuals with diabetes and microalbuminuria, reduction of protein to 0.8 to 1.0 g per kg of body weight per day may slow the progression to macroalbuminuria (7,8,33). In individuals with overt nephropathy, reduction of protein to 0.8 g/kg/day (approximately 10% of energy intake, and the current adult recommended daily allowance for protein) may slow the progression of nephropathy (7,8,33).

There is as yet no compelling evidence that antioxidant supplementation, total or saturated fat reduction, or change in protein source (animal to plant, beef to chicken) will reduce the risk or slow the progression of diabetic renal disease (7,8).

Retinopathy

Diabetic retinopathy occurs when blood vessels in the retina are damaged; this can lead to the three major causes of severe vision loss from diabetes: macular

---

BOX 13.1

Medical Nutrition Therapy to Manage Hypertension

Goal
Blood pressure <130/80 mm Hg

Steps
Reduce weight
The loss of 1 kg body weight can reduce mean systolic blood pressure by approximately 2 mm Hg and mean diastolic blood pressure by approximately 1 mm Hg.

Reduce sodium intake
- A moderate sodium restriction (700–1,000 mg reduction in sodium/day, equivalent to 1,800–2,500 mg salt) may reduce systolic blood pressure by approximately 5mm Hg and diastolic by approximately 2 mm Hg in hypertensive individuals. A moderate sodium restriction may reduce systolic blood pressure by approximately 3 mm Hg and diastolic by approximately 1 mm Hg in normotensive subjects.
- In general, for every 10 mm Hg reduction in systolic blood pressure, the risk for any complication related to diabetes is reduced by 12%.

Reduce excessive alcohol intake
There is an association between high alcohol intake (> 3 drinks/day) and elevated blood pressure.

Supplementation
A beneficial effect of potassium supplementation on lowering blood pressure has been shown, whereas there is little to no evidence that blood pressure is lowered with calcium and magnesium supplementation.

Implement the Dietary Approaches to Stop Hypertension (DASH) diet
Increase intake of fruits, vegetables, and low-fat dairy products; restrict sodium intake.

Source: Data are from references 6, 8, 9, and 29–32.

---

edema, proliferative retinopathy leading to massive hemorrhage, and retinal detachment. Diabetic retinopathy causes from 12,000 to 24,000 new cases of blindness each year (9).

Risk Factors

The presence of retinopathy is strongly related to the duration of diabetes (34). Hyperglycemia and high blood pressure are also risk factors for retinopathy (1,2,35).

Treatment

Optimal glycemic control and optimal blood pressure control can both substantially reduce the risk for and progression of diabetic retinopathy (34). Laser therapy (particularly when macular edema is still mild or in the early stages of development of new vessels) can reduce the risk of vision loss in individuals with high-risk characteristics (34).

Implications for MNT

MNT for hypertension control should be implemented (see Box 13.1). Although there is little evidence that antioxidants are beneficial in treating diabetic retinopathy, there is some evidence that the carotenoids lutein and zeaxanthin in foods can prevent or delay the development of cataracts and age-related macular degeneration (36,37). This is another reason to encourage individuals to eat a healthful diet high in fruits and vegetables, especially those that are highly pigmented (eg, kale, spinach, and other greens).

NERVOUS SYSTEM DISEASE

About 60% to 70% of people with diabetes have mild to severe forms of nervous system damage (9).

Peripheral Neuropathy

Diabetic peripheral neuropathy refers to the inflammation and degeneration of peripheral nerves, with the most common location being the feet.

Risk Factors

The risk of ulcers or amputation is increased in people who have had diabetes for 10 years or longer, have poor glucose control, or have other diabetes-related complications (38).

Treatment

Optimal blood glucose control may decrease pain and other symptoms of neuropathy. Therapeutic lifestyle changes include daily foot care, walking, gentle stretching, and relaxation exercises. Medications for pain relief include topical capsaicin (from chili peppers), antidepressants, and anticonvulsants.

Implications for MNT

Helping the patient to better control the blood glucose level, and to implement other lifestyle changes, is a priority. There is, as yet, no compelling evidence that vitamin supplementation (eg, pyridoxine, folic acid, vitamin C, or vitamin E) will prevent or significantly reduce symptoms of peripheral neuropathy.

Autonomic Neuropathy

Diabetic autonomic neuropathy (39) can involve one or more components in the autonomic nervous system, including (a) cardiovascular, causing postural hypotension and "silent" heart disease, (b) genitourinary, causing sexual dysfunction and bladder-emptying problems, or (c) gastrointestinal (also known as diabetic gastropathy or gastroparesis), which is characterized by abnormally delayed emptying of foods, particularly solid foods, from the stomach. Diabetic gastropathy or gastroparesis occurs because of damage to the vagus nerve, which controls the muscles moving food through the digestive tract. Delayed gastric emptying can cause anorexia, nausea, vomiting, early satiety, and postprandial bloating and fullness. It can also produce wide (and otherwise unexplained) swings between severe hypoglycemia and hyperglycemia.

Risk Factors

About 50% of individuals with longstanding diabetes have delayed gastric emptying of solid and/or liquid nutrient meals (gastroparesis) (40). Treatment for gastroparesis includes glycemic control optimization, because hyperglycemia appears to slow the rate of gastric emptying). Use of insulin after a meal and use of insulin pumps are options.

Other treatment forms include dietary modifications and other therapeutic lifestyle changes (see Box 13.2)

BOX 13.2

Medical Nutrition Therapy and Other Lifestyle Modifications for Treatment of Diabetic Gastropathy

- Try small frequent meals: less bloating sensation, less early satiety, and less possibility of impaired nutritional status.
- Reduce fat intake: may produce less delay in gastric emptying.
- Reduce fiber intake: may decrease possibility of bezoar formation.
- Use foods with soft consistency; replace solid with liquid or blenderized meals: liquid but non-hypertonic meals appear to be digested normally.
- Exercise after meals: may increase solid-meal gastric emptying rates.
- Adjust insulin doses and timing.

Source: Data are from reference 41.

(41); various pharmacologic options, such as cholinergic drugs, dopamine antagonists, and motilin-receptor agonists; and surgical treatment (jejeunostomy enteral feeding, gastrectomy).

Implications for MNT

Dietary modifications and other lifestyle changes for diabetic gastropathy appear to be based on logical interpretation of gastric physiology and interpolation from gastrointestinal studies of other disease states (41).

SUMMARY

The risk of developing any of the chronic complications of diabetes can be reduced substantially through therapeutic lifestyle changes, including MNT and physical activity. In addition, when chronic complications have developed, MNT can reduce the rate of progression of the disease.

REFERENCES

1. Diabetes Control and Complications Trial Research Group. The effect of intensive treatment of diabetes on the development and progression of long-term complications in insulin-dependent diabetes mellitus. *N Engl J Med.* 1993;329:977–986.

2. UK Prospective Diabetes Study Group. Intensive blood-glucose control with sulphonylureas or insulin compared with conventional treatment and risk of complications in patients with type 2 diabetes (UKPDS 33). *Lancet.* 1998;352:837–853.

3. Stratton IM, Adler AI, Neil HA, Matthews DR, Manley SE, Cull CA, Hadden D, Turner RC, Holman RR. Association of glycaemia with macrovascular and microvascular complications of type 2 diabetes (UKPDS 35): prospective observational study. *BMJ.* 2000;321:405–412.

4. Look Ahead Study Web site. Available at: http://lookahead.phs.wfubmc.edu. Accessed January 5, 2005.

5. Action to Control Cardiovascular Risk in Diabetes Web site. Available at: http://www.accord-ne.org. Accessed January 5, 2005.

6. American Diabetes Association. ADA standards of medical care in diabetes (position statement). *Diabetes Care.* 2005;27(Suppl 1):S4–S36.

7. American Diabetes Association. Nutrition principles and recommendations in diabetes (position statement). *Diabetes Care.* 2004;27(Suppl 1):S36–S46.

8. Franz MJ, Bantle JP, Beebe CA, Brunzell JD, Chaisson J-L, Garg A, Holzmeister LA, Hoogwerf B, Mayer-Davis E, Mooradian A, Purnell JQ, Wheeler ML. Evidence-based nutrition principles and recommendations for diabetes and related complications (technical report). *Diabetes Care.* 2002;25:148–198.

9. Centers for Disease Control and Prevention. National estimates on diabetes. Available at: http://www.cdc.gov/diabetes/pubs/estimates.htm. Accessed January 6, 2005.

10. Haffner SM. Management of dyslipidemia in adults with diabetes (technical report). *Diabetes Care.* 1998;21:160–178.

11. National Cholesterol Education Program (NCEP) Adult Treatment Panel III Report. Available at: http://www.nhlbi.nih.gov/guidelines/cholesterol. Accessed January 6, 2005.

12. American Diabetes Association. Dyslipidemia management in adults with diabetes (position statement). *Diabetes Care.* 2004;27(Suppl 1):S68–S71.

13. Yu-Poth S, Zhao G, Etherton T, Naglak M, Jonnalagadda S, Kris-Etherton P. Effects of the National Cholesterol Education Program's step I and step II dietary intervention programs on cardiovascular disease risk factors: a meta-analysis. *Am J Clin Nutr.* 1999;69:632–646.

14. Food labeling: health claims; plant sterol/stanol esters and coronary heart disease; interim final rule. 65 *Federal Register* 54686–54739 (2000) (codified at 21 CFR 101).

15. Food labeling: health claims; soy protein and coronary heart disease; proposed rule. 63 *Federal Register* 62977–63015 (1998) (codified at 21 CFR 101).

16. Brown L, Rosner B, Willett WW, Sacks FM. Cholesterol-lowering effects of dietary fiber: a meta-analysis. *Am J Clin Nutr.* 1999;69:30–42.

17. Agency for Healthcare Research and Quality. Garlic: effects on cardiovascular risks and disease, protective effects against cancer, and clinical adverse effects. Evidence Report/Technical Assessment #20 (2000). Available at: htpp://www.ahcpr.gov/clinic/epcindex.htm#cardiovascular. Accessed January 6, 2005.

18. Djousse L, Hunt SC, Arnett DK, Province MA, Eckfeldt JH, Ellison RC. Dietary linolenic acid is inversely associated with plasma triacylglycerol: the National Heart, Lung, and Blood Institute Family Heart Study. *Am J Clin Nutr.* 2003;78:1098–1102.

19. Friedberg CF, Janssen MJFM, Heine RJ, Grobbee DE. Fish oil and glycemic control in diabetes, a meta-analysis. *Diabetes Care.* 1998;21:494–500.

20. Montori VM, Farmer A, Wollan PC, Dinneen SF. Fish oil supplementation in type 2 diabetes, a quantitative systematic review. *Diabetes Care.* 2000;23:1407–1415.

21. Harris WS. N-3 fatty acids and serum lipoproteins: human studies. *Am J Clin Nutr.* 1997;65(Suppl 5):1645S–1654S.

22. Dunstan DW, Mori TA, Puddey IB, Beilin LJ, Burke V, Morton AR, Stanton KG. The independent and com-

bined effects of aerobic exercise and dietary fish intake on serum lipids and glycemic control in NIDDM. *Diabetes Care.* 1997;20:913–921.

23. Rimm EB, Williams P, Fosher K, Criqui M, Stampfer MJ. Moderate alcohol intake and lower risk of coronary heart disease: meta-analysis of effects on lipids and haemostatic factors. *BMJ.* 1999;319:1523–1528.

24. National Kidney Foundation. Clinical Practice Guidelines for Chronic Kidney Disease: Evaluation, Classification, and Stratification. Part 4, Guideline 1. Available at: http://www.kidney.org/professionals/kdoqi/guidelines_ckd/p4_class_g1.htm. Accessed January 6, 2005.

25. American Diabetes Association. Nephropathy in diabetes (position statement). *Diabetes Care.* 2004;27(Suppl 1): S79–S83.

26. American Diabetes Association. *Diabetes 2001 Vital Statistics.* Alexandria, Va: American Diabetes Association; 2001.

27. The DCCT Research Group. Effect of intensive therapy on the development and progression of diabetic nephropathy in the Diabetes Control and Complications Trial (DCCT). *Kidney Int.* 1995;47:1703–1720.

28. The UK Prospective Diabetes Study Group. Tight blood pressure control and risk of macrovascular and microvascular complications in type 2 diabetes. UKPDS 38. *BMJ.* 1998;317:703–713.

29. Wylie-Rosett J. Hypertension and medical nutrition therapy. In: Franz MJ, Bantle JP, eds. *American Diabetes Association Guide to Medical Nutrition Therapy for Diabetes.* Alexandria, Va: American Diabetes Association; 1999:295–311.

30. Staessen J, Fagard R, Lijnen P, Amery A. Body weight, sodium intake, and blood pressure. *J Hypertens.* 1989; 7(suppl):S19–S23.

31. Cutler JA, Follmann D, Allender PS. Randomized trials of sodium reduction: an overview. *Am J Clin Nutr.* 1997;65(Suppl 1):643S–651S.

32. Sacks FM, Svetkey LP, Vollmer WM, Appel LJ, Bray GA, Harsha D, Obarzanek E, Conlin PR, Miller ER 3rd, Simons-Morton DG, Karanja N, Lin PH. DASH-Sodium Collaborative Research Group. Effects on blood pressure of reduced dietary sodium and the Dietary Approaches to Stop Hypertension (DASH) diet. *N Engl J Med.* 2001; 344:3–10.

33. Wheeler ML. Nephropathy and medical nutrition therapy. In: Franz MJ, Bantle JP, eds. *American Diabetes Association Guide to Medical Nutrition Therapy for Diabetes.* Alexandria, Va: American Diabetes Association; 1999:312–329.

34. Fong DS, Aiello L, Gardner TW, King GL, Blankenship G, Cavallerano JD, Ferris FL III, Klein R; for the American Diabetes Association. Retinopathy in diabetes (position statement). *Diabetes Care.* 2004;27(Suppl 1):S84–S87.

35. UK Prospective Diabetes Study Group. Tight blood pressure control and risk of macrovascular and microvascular complications in type 2 diabetes: UKPDS 28. *BMJ.* 1998;317:708–713.

36. Brown L, Rimm EB, Seddon JM, Giovannucci EL, Chasan-Taber L, Spiegelman D, Willett WC, Hankinson SE. A prospective study of carotenoid intake and risk of cataract extraction in US men. *Am J Clin Nutr.* 1999; 70:517–524.

37. Chasan-Taber L, Willett WC, Seddon JM, Stampfer MJ, Rosner B, Colditz GA, Speizer FE, Hankinson SE. A prospective study of carotenoid and vitamin A intakes and risk of cataract extraction in US women. *Am J Clin Nutr.* 1999;70:509–516.

38. American Diabetes Association. Preventive foot care in diabetes (position statement). *Diabetes Care.* 2004;27 (Suppl 1):S63–S64.

39. Vinik AI, Maser RE, Mitchell BD, Freeman R. Diabetic autonomic neuropathy (technical review). *Diabetes Care.* 2003;26:1553–1579.

40. Kong M-F, Horowitz M, Jones KL, Wishart JM, Harding PE. Natural history of diabetic gastroparesis. *Diabetes Care.* 1999;22:503–507.

41. Wheeler ML. Diabetic gastropathy and medical nutrition therapy. In: Franz MJ, Bantle JP, eds. *American Diabetes Association Guide to Medical Nutrition Therapy for Diabetes.* Alexandria, Va: American Diabetes Association; 1999:330–334.

ADDITIONAL RESOURCES

The DASH Eating Plan. Available at: http://www.nhlbi.nih.gov/health/public/heart/hbp/dash. Accessed January 5, 2005.

National Diabetes Education Program Web site. Available at: http://www.ndep.nih.gov. Accessed January 5, 2005.

National Diabetes Information Clearinghouse. Available at: http://diabetes.niddk.nih.gov. Accessed January 5, 2005.

National Kidney Foundation's Kidney Disease Outcomes Quality Initiative. Available at: http://www.kidney.org/professionals/kdoqi/index.cfm. Accessed January 5, 2005.

14

Depression, Celiac Disease, and Cystic Fibrosis–Related Diabetes

Cindy Halstenson, RD, CDE, and Carol Brunzell, RD, CDE

CHAPTER OVERVIEW

- Nutrition therapy for diabetes can be complicated by other diseases or conditions that strongly influence nutritional status and clinical outcomes.
- Depression is common among individuals with diabetes. Nutrition management and diabetes self-care depend on an appropriate depression diagnosis and effective intervention.
- Celiac disease is an inheritable autoimmune disorder characterized by an abnormal T-cell response against the gliadin fraction of gluten. Once an individual with diabetes is diagnosed with celiac disease and removes gluten from the diet, self-monitoring of blood glucose is essential.
- In cystic fibrosis (CF), the ability to transport chloride into epithelial cells is impaired and results in altered fluid and electrolyte levels and highly viscous cellular secretions in many organs. CF-related diabetes has emerged as a comorbidity in individuals with CF.

DEPRESSION

Pathophysiology

Depression results from a chemical imbalance in the brain and involves the body, thoughts, mood, and behavior. Depression can be triggered by genetic, psy-chological, or environmental factors, as well as by dealing with a chronic illness such as diabetes. Depression in people with diabetes is associated with poor metabolic control, poor nutrition, diminished adherence to the medical plan, and diminished quality of life (1).

Dietetics professionals rarely receive formal education on depression, but they should be alert to indicators of depression among the diabetes population for several reasons: (*a*) so the individual can be referred for and benefit from assessment and treatment; (*b*) because depression can make diabetes self-management more difficult; and (*c*) because individuals typically do not respond well to lifestyle interventions while depressed.

Diabetes and Depression

Having diabetes doubles the risk for depression (2). Approximately 30% of people with diabetes have depression. The rates are similar among individuals with type 1 and type 2 diabetes. Depression is more common in women than in men and tends to correlate with the number of diabetes complications (3). A meta-analysis showed that the relationship between diabetes and depression was defined as significant and consistent. Increased depression was associated with increased numbers of, severity of, and ratings of diabetes complications (2).

The relationship between diabetes and depression is not fully understood. The pathology is speculated to be complex and multifactorial (4). The immunosuppressive nature of depression may bring out diabetes in individuals who are prone to it, but this is poorly understood and calls for further research and explanation.

Talbot and colleagues (4) identified that type 1 diabetes precedes the diagnosis of depression, but type 2 diabetes follows the depression diagnosis. A review of previous medical histories in a study population of individuals newly diagnosed with type 2 diabetes demonstrated that 75% had depression in the 8 years before their diabetes diagnosis (4).

Diabetes and depression are both costly, to the individual and to the entire health care economy. Among the diabetes population, total health care expenditures for people with both diabetes and depression are 4.5 times that of those without depression (5).

Characteristics

It is common to occasionally feel stressed, sad, or "blue," but if these feelings last longer than 2 weeks and are not associated with personal loss or change, medical conditions, or medications, they can signal depression. Other "red flags" that may indicate depression include a significant increase in A1C, change in stress level, family distress, change in performance, loss of important relationship or job, or relocation. Additional "red flags" are crisis-oriented care, the use of food to deal with stress, and missed school or work due to diabetes. See Box 14.1 (6) for a comprehensive list of symptoms of major depression.

Individuals who rate their depression at the highest level of severity have twice the frequency of omitting their oral medications; report poorer physical and mental functioning; demonstrate a greater probability of having emergency room care, primary care, specialty care, medical inpatient care, and mental health care; and have higher health care costs—primary care (51% higher), ambulatory care (75% higher), and total care (86% higher) (7). Symptoms of depression may be difficult to notice, unless one has frequent encounters with the individual or the individual shares feelings freely. However, once identified, depression can most often be treated successfully. Identification of depression, followed by effective intervention, is essential for achieving nutrition management and maximal diabetes self-care.

Seventy-four percent of people seeking help for depressive symptoms go to primary care, yet the diagnosis of depression is missed half the time (3). In an analysis of several studies, Anderson et al (3) found that the

---

BOX 14.1

Symptoms of Major Depression

Not all people experience the same symptoms of depression. A client may be suffering from a depressive disorder if: (*a*) at least three of the following symptoms persist daily for 2 weeks or more in conjunction with one of the asterisked items below, and (*b*) symptoms negatively affect his or her life, work, and relationships.

- Depressed mood (feeling sad, "blue," cheerless)*
- Loss of interest in things usually enjoyed*
- Feeling of guilt or worthlessness
- Persistent anxiety, worry, or "empty" mood
- Increased/decreased appetite
- Decreased energy level
- Decreased ability to concentrate, make decisions
- Difficulty remembering things
- Sleeping too much/too little
- Feeling restless/irritable
- Thought of death or suicide
- Loss of self-esteem
- Withdrawal from friends/family
- Increased crying
- Substance abuse
- Persistent physical pains that don't go away

Source: Recognized symptoms of major depression (table) from Gehling E. The next step: depression. Copyright © Diabetes Care and Education, a Dietetic Practice Group of the American Dietetic Association. Adapted with permission from *Newsflash*, Vol. 22; Number 5, 2001.

---

identification of depression by diagnostic interviewing yielded a prevalence of less than half that identified through self-report. Two of every three cases of depression are left untreated by primary care physicians (3). Without treatment, depressive symptoms can last for months or years.

Simple screening for depression can be performed using informal, unstructured interviewing. Ask about the symptoms listed in Box 14.1, their impact on ability to perform usual activities of daily living, and their persistence. Then, referral(s) to primary care or a mental health professional for further evaluation and diagnosis may be appropriate. A variety of validated tools are available to screen for, or to identify, depression; several involve short self-assessment surveys (see Table 14.1). Figure 14.1 (8,9) shows a patient health questionnaire

PATIENT HEALTH QUESTIONNAIRE—PHQ-9
Nine-Symptom Depression Checklist

1. In the *last 2 weeks*, how often have you been bothered by any of the following problems?

	Not at all (0)	Several days (1)	More than half the days (2)	Nearly every day (3)
a. Little interest or pleasure in doing things	☐	☐	☐	☐
b. Feeling down, depressed, or hopeless	☐	☐	☐	☐
c. Trouble falling or staying asleep, or sleeping too much	☐	☐	☐	☐
d. Feeling tired or having little energy	☐	☐	☐	☐
e. Poor appetite or overeating	☐	☐	☐	☐
f. Feeling bad about yourself—or that you are a failure or have let yourself or your family down	☐	☐	☐	☐
g. Trouble concentrating on things, such as reading the newspaper or watching television	☐	☐	☐	☐
h. Moving or speaking so slowly that other people could have noticed? Or the opposite—being so fidgety or restless that you have been moving around a lot more than usual	☐	☐	☐	
i. Thoughts that you would be better off dead or of hurting yourself in some way	☐	☐	☐	☐

2. If you checked off *any* problems on this questionnaire so far, how *difficult* have these problems made it for you to do your work, take care of things at home, or get along with other people?

Not at all difficult (0)	Somewhat difficult (1)	Very difficult (2)	Extremely difficult (3)
☐	☐	☐	☐

Total Number of Symptoms _____   Score _____

Scoring Method for Diagnosis

Depression is suggested if:
- Either item 1a or 1b is selected as "More than half the days"; and
- Question 2 is answered "Somewhat difficult," "Very difficult," or "Extremely difficult."

Major depression is suggested if: Five or more problems in question 1 are marked as "More than half the days" or worse (count item 1 if problem is present at all).

Other depression is suggested if: Items 1b, 1c, or 1d are marked as "More than half the days" or worse.

FIGURE 14.1 Patient health questionnaire—PHQ-9, Nine-Symptom Depression Checklist. Adapted from the Primary Care Evaluation of Mental Disorders Patient Health Questionnaire (PRIME-MD PHQ), developed by Drs. Robert L. Spitzer, Janet B.W. Williams, Kurt Kroenke, and colleagues (8,9). PRIME-MD is a trademark of Pfizer Inc. Copyright 1999 Pfizer Inc. All rights reserved.

TABLE 14.1 Screening Tools for Depression	
Tool	*Description*
Beck Depression Inventory (BDI)	Self-report in a 21-question written tool. Can be self- or professionally scored; score > 16 suggests further evaluation
Patient Health Questionnaire (PHQ-9)	9-question self-administered survey; positive screen relies on at least the presence of prolonged sadness or "blues," for 2 weeks or longer, and a lack of interest in usual activities
Medical Outcomes Study Short-Form (SF 20)	20-question, self-administered survey
Zung Self Rating Depression Scale (also available from commercial sources under different names)	20-item survey, yielding a score from 20 through 80

and scoring form. As a general rule, screening tools do not replace the focused interview necessary for a physician or mental health care professional to make the diagnosis of depression. Treating either diabetes or depression benefits both conditions.

Intervention Strategies

When diabetes and depression are both present, the dietetics professional can play an important role in the identification of depression and referral for treatment. Key strategies for intervention by the dietetics professional include understanding signs and symptoms of depression and making referrals to the primary care physician for antidepressant medications or to a behavioral health specialist for behavioral health interventions. See Table 14.2 for a comparison of medications (10). Multiple trials have demonstrated the effectiveness of cognitive behavioral therapy alone, or in combination with medications, for the successful treatment of depression in people with diabetes (11).

Other strategies include assessing readiness to change, helping the individual set realistic self-management goals, and providing support. If depression is identified before it takes control, interventions should focus on those that affect the individual's comfort and quality of

TABLE 14.2 Medications Used for Management of Depression	
Category	*Drug (Brand Name, Manufacturer*)*
Selective serotonin reuptake inhibitors (SSRIs)	• Fluoxetine (Prozac, Eli Lilly) • Sertraline (Zoloft, Pfizer) • Fluvoxamine (Luvox, Solvay Pharmaceuticals) • Paroxetine (Paxil, GlaxoSmithKline) • Citalopram (Celexa, AstraZeneca)
Tricyclic antidepressants (TCAs)	• Imipramine (Tofranil, Novartis) • Amitriptyline (Elavil, Merck) • Nortriptyline (Aventyl, Eli Lilly) • Desiprimine (Paroxatene, Abbott Laboratories)
Monoamine oxidase inhibitors (MAOIs)	• Phenelzine (Nardil, Pfizer) • Tranylcypromine (Parnate, GlaxoSmithKline) • Isocarboxizid (Marplan, Oxford Pharmaceuticals)
Atypical antidepressants	• Sedating—mirtazepine (Remeron, Organon) • Activating—buproprion (Wellbutrin, GlaxoSmithKline)
Other	• Venlafaxine (Effexor, Wyeth-Ayerst)

*Manufacturers: Abbott Laboratories, Chicago IL 60064; AstraZeneca, Boston, MA 01581; Eli Lilly, Indianapolis, IN 46285; GlaxoSmithKline, Philadelphia, PA 19102; Merck, Whitehouse, NJ 08889; Novartis, East Hanover, NJ 07936; Oxford Pharmaceuticals, Totowa, NJ 07512; Organon, Roseland, NJ 07068; Pfizer, Inc. New York, NY 10017; Solvay Pharmaceuticals, Marietta, GA 30062; Wyeth-Ayerst, Collegeville, PA 19426.

life, such as preventing overt, prolonged hyperglycemia, to avoid polydipsia and polyuria.

Key messages to convey to the individual experiencing depression are that depression is not a sign of weakness or a character flaw. It is common and treatable. Treatment for depression should be initiated promptly. Both psychotherapeutic and psychopharmacologic interventions are useful in treating depression (11). Individuals who receive treatment for depression often experience improvement in their overall medical condition and quality of life, because they have an increased likelihood of being able to follow their medical and self-management treatment plan.

Nutrition therapy can be more effective in the person with treated and controlled depression (11). Health care professionals must be cognizant of the high likelihood of depression recurrence, and the need for repeated or ongoing intervention for depression in people with diabetes.

CELIAC DISEASE

Pathophysiology

Celiac disease (also known as gluten-sensitive enteropathy or celiac sprue) is an inheritable, autoimmune disorder characterized by an abnormal T-cell response against the gliadin fraction of many grains, including wheat, barley, rye, and cross-contaminated oats, collectively referred to as gluten (12). Ingestion of gluten results in small-bowel mucosal injury in genetically susceptible individuals. Damage to the intestinal epithelium can cause an array of symptoms and complications, including malnutrition secondary to malabsorption of many nutrients. Life-threatening complications include an increased risk of small bowel lymphoma or cancer (13). In people with diabetes, the malabsorption from celiac disease can interfere with blood glucose control (13).

Prevalence

The prevalence of celiac disease in North America and Europe in not-at-risk subjects has been estimated at approximately 1 in every 133 people, or 0.75%, with higher disease prevalence in at-risk populations (14). A higher prevalence of celiac disease has been noted in people with type 1 diabetes, at a rate of 2% to 5% (15). Proneness to autoimmune disease may explain this association. In a study by Page et al, the prevalence of celiac disease in type 2 diabetes was found to be 1 in 340 patients (16).

Diabetes and Celiac Disease

Although specific screening frequency recommendations have not been established, many diabetes centers test for celiac disease yearly for the first 3 years after diagnosis with diabetes, then every 3 to 5 years thereafter, or sooner if symptoms develop. Serologic testing for celiac disease in individuals with type 1 diabetes can allow diagnosis in a presymptomatic state. A positive serologic test alone is not sufficient for diagnosis; a small bowel biopsy is necessary to confirm diagnosis.

Once an individual with diabetes is diagnosed with celiac disease and removes gluten from the diet, self-monitoring of blood glucose is essential, to determine whether insulin dose adjustment is needed. Individuals who adhere to a strict gluten-free diet have not been found to experience any deleterious effects on blood glucose control (15). Kaukinen et al (17) found no change in metabolic control with treatment of celiac disease in adults with type 1 diabetes. In a study of individuals with type 1 diabetes, Acerini et al (18) found no difference in A1C or total insulin needs between the celiac and nonceliac study groups.

Characteristics

Children and adults with celiac disease can have an array of symptoms. See Box 14.2 (19) for a comprehensive list. Of note, a significantly increased incidence of hypoglycemia has been observed among individuals with type 1 diabetes who have untreated celiac disease, presumably

---

BOX 14.2

Symptoms of Celiac Disease

- Frequent episodes of hypoglycemia in the presence of diabetes
- Abdominal distention and pain, flatulence, vomiting, diarrhea, steatorrhea
- Short stature, failure to thrive, pubertal delay
- Weight loss
- Dermatitis herpetiformis (pruritic papular rash)
- Nutrient deficiencies: iron, folate, zinc, vitamin B-12, calcium, magnesium, and fat-soluble vitamins
- Lactose intolerance
- Osteopenia and osteoporosis
- Menstrual irregularities
- Infertility
- Dental enamel hypoplasia
- Chronic hepatitis/hypertransaminasemia
- Neurologic problems
- Arthritis and arthralgia
- Irritability
- Fatigue and weakness

Source: Data are from reference 19.

due to malabsorption from intestinal damage (13). Most individuals with celiac disease are asymptomatic or unaware of symptoms (20). Absence of detectable symptoms with gluten ingestion does not mean ongoing intestinal injury does not occur.

The clinical signs, symptoms, and malabsorption are reversible once gluten is removed from the diet. Most individuals see an improvement in symptoms after 3 to 6 days on a gluten-free diet (21). Symptoms will recur, however, with even minimal gluten consumption.

Intervention Strategies

Gluten-Free Diet

Successful treatment of celiac disease involves adopting a lifelong gluten-free diet. This can seem overwhelming to individuals with diabetes who have already changed their eating habits because of the diabetes. However, initiation of a gluten-free diet eventually reduces the incidence of hypoglycemic episodes as the intestinal injury heals (13).

Complete removal of gluten from the diet is challenging, because hidden sources of gluten occur in many processed foods, nonfood items, and medications. Intensive education on gluten-containing foods and products is essential. A nutrition therapy protocol for celiac disease has been developed and is a valuable reference for ensuring comprehensive education for individuals with celiac disease (22). See Table 14.3 (19) for medical nutrition therapy goals and recommendations. See Box 14.3 for a checklist of topics to cover when educating an individual with diabetes and celiac disease.

"Wheat-free" does not necessarily mean a food is gluten-free. Food labels should always be scrutinized for gluten-containing ingredients. For example, individuals with dermatitis herpetiformis need to check labels and/or check with manufacturers regarding gluten in topical products.

Cross-contamination of gluten-containing foods with gluten-free foods is common. Health care institutions, diabetes camps, day-care providers, schools, and other care providers must be educated about the diet and the potential for cross-contamination. Cross-contamination can occur during harvesting, processing, and shipping of grains; in grains sold in bulk—cross-use of bins and scoops with gluten-containing grains; through shared home-kitchen items, such as toasters, counters, and spreads; and when eating out. Deep-fat fryers, pans, grills, and other surfaces may contain gluten residue if gluten-containing food items were prepared in them and

TABLE 14.3 Medical Nutrition Therapy Recommendations for Individuals With Celiac Disease and Diabetes

Consideration	Recommendation
Macro- and micronutrient needs	Same as American Diabetes Association recommendations for other individuals with diabetes; attain/maintain good nutritional status.
Hypoglycemia treatment	Use only gluten-free sources.
Exercise and carbohydrate replacement	Use only gluten-free foods.
Sick-day management	Use only gluten-free foods.
Alcohol	Use only gluten-free alcoholic beverages.
Vitamin/mineral supplementation	May require supplements if deficiency noted. Use only gluten-free supplements. May require calcium, vitamin D, and vitamin K if lactose intolerant.
Carbohydrate counting	Use only gluten-free foods.

Source: Data are from reference 19.

not cleaned between food orders. Individuals who are sensitive to gluten need to ask detailed questions about menu items and preparation.

As a general rule, gluten-free foods are not always equivalent in carbohydrate to similar gluten-containing foods. Gluten-free foods may be lower in B vitamins, folate, iron, and fiber. Therefore, careful planning is necessary to ensure adequate intakes of these nutrients (23,24). Fortified, whole-grain, gluten-free foods should be selected more often than refined, unenriched products. A daily gluten-free multivitamin may be recommended for some people with celiac disease. If lactose intolerance persists once initial intestinal injury is healed, ongoing attention to calcium, vitamin D, and vitamin K may be necessary for prevention of osteopenia or osteoporosis (25).

The gluten-free diet is not without controversy. Recommendations regarding acceptability of some grains and additives vary from one organization to another. Valuable references for the individual with celiac disease include the following:

- Educational materials and extensive food and ingredient lists published by the American Dietetic Association and other celiac organizations and Web sites (see Additional Resources list at the end of the chapter).
- Food and product labels: individuals with celiac disease must become lifelong label readers because ingredients in food and nonfood items can change over time.
- Manufacturers: calling the manufacturer may be necessary to verify the safety of questionable ingredients.
- Support groups: joining a local or national support group provides valuable support and allows access to the latest information and educational materials.

BOX 14.3

Education Topics for Individuals With Celiac Disease and Diabetes

- Principles of a healthful diet
- Carbohydrate counting with gluten-free foods
- Hypoglycemia treatment with gluten-free foods
- Gluten-free carbohydrate sources for exercise
- Sick-day management with gluten-free foods
- Menu planning, food staples, meal and snack examples, recipe modifications
- Lactose intolerance, as necessary
- Food ingredient label reading
- Specialty food sources, mail order, Internet resources
- "Safe" and "unsafe" food and ingredient lists
- Gluten-free kitchen basics: cross contamination, utensils, storage
- Gluten-free cookbooks
- Information for caregivers
- Alternative plans for events that involve food—school, holidays, birthday parties, special occasions, church events, camp
- Restaurants and dining out, traveling, airline meals, hotels
- Guidelines for use of alcohol, including gluten-free alcoholic beverages
- Prescription and over-the-counter medications, vitamins and minerals
- Celiac organizations and support groups

CYSTIC FIBROSIS–RELATED DIABETES AND ABNORMAL GLUCOSE TOLERANCE IN CYSTIC FIBROSIS

Pathophysiology

CF is a genetic disease that occurs in approximately 1 in every 3,000 live births (26). The primary defect in CF is an impaired ability to transport chloride into epithelial cells, resulting in altered fluid and electrolyte levels and highly viscous cellular secretions in many organs. The increased viscosity of secretions leads to progressive obstruction, inflammation, scarring, and destruction of multiple organs (27). Improvements in the medical and nutrition care of individuals with CF have resulted in an increased median life expectancy of 32.9 years (28).

Prevalence

Cystic fibrosis–related diabetes (CFRD) has emerged as the leading comorbidity in the CF patient population, occurring in approximately 13.6% of all people with CF (28). The prevalence of CFRD is likely underestimated, because of the lack of routine screening for diabetes in the CF population. CFRD is typically diagnosed between 18 and 21 years of age (29,30).

Cystic Fibrosis and Cystic Fibrosis–Related Diabetes

CFRD evolves as the pancreatic ducts become obstructed by viscous secretions, causing fibrosis and fatty infiltration of the islets, resulting in insulin deficiency. Deposition of islet amyloid is a distinguishing feature in individuals with CFRD compared with those having CF without diabetes. Islet amyloid also accumulates in individuals with type 2 diabetes, suggesting that CFRD occurs in those who also have the type 2 diabetes gene defect (31). Additionally, glucose metabolism is influenced by other factors specific to CF.

Individuals with CF who exhibit impaired glucose tolerance are at high risk for progressing to CFRD and should be tested annually with an oral glucose tolerance test. They should also monitor blood glucose frequently during acute illness (27).

Screening for impaired glucose tolerance and diabetes is routinely recommended for individuals with CF age 14 years or older. If a fasting blood glucose value is 126 mg/dL or higher, then a second fasting glucose test should be repeated the next day. If that value is

126 mg/dL or higher, or a casual blood glucose value is 200 mg/dL or higher, then a diagnosis of CFRD can be made (27,28).

Characteristics

CFRD shares some characteristics of type 1 and type 2 diabetes but has important clinical distinctions, making medical treatment and nutrition therapy significantly different from that for type 1 and type 2 diabetes. For example, insulin deficiency has a profoundly negative impact on nutritional status in individuals with CF. Individuals with CFRD have poorer pulmonary function and are more underweight than those without diabetes, which leads to increased mortality rates (32,33). Normalization of blood glucose is essential to optimize nutrient metabolism and to improve weight and general nutritional status (34).

Treatment with insulin has been found to reverse clinical decline in CFRD, which suggests a cause-and-effect relationship between insulin deficiency and decline in clinical status (34). Insulin treatment results in improved pulmonary function and weight, although it does not completely reverse protein catabolism in individuals with abnormal glucose tolerance or CFRD (35).

Individuals with CFRD usually produce adequate or nearly adequate amounts of basal insulin during the day but may require rapid- or short-acting insulin for meals and large snacks. If basal insulin is necessary, only small amounts are typically required when individuals with CF are in their usual state of health. During sickness or steroid use, insulin needs increase greatly, often quadrupling. However, not all individuals with CFRD require insulin therapy. Those who do not exhibit fasting hyperglycemia are typically not treated with insulin, unless they are unable to maintain an appropriate weight or pulmonary function declines more rapidly than expected.

Hypoglycemia risk is not different from that of individuals with type 1 or 2 diabetes requiring insulin. Absorption of simple carbohydrate is not compromised as patients with CF are able to secrete amylase in their saliva (36). Therefore, low blood glucose should be treated with simple carbohydrate sources that do not require pancreatic enzyme replacement. Use of oral diabetes medications is not recommended until studies confirm their safety and effectiveness in this population (27).

Individuals with CFRD have been found to have microvascular complications similar to those seen in diabetes not complicated by CF (29,37,38), but development of macrovascular artery disease is not generally a concern in this population (39–41). Normalization of blood glucose is recommended to prevent microvascular complications, which do occur because individuals with CF are living longer.

Intervention Strategies

In caring for the individual with CFRD, the team approach is ideal, with the pulmonary team working with an endocrinologist and other team members familiar with the distinctive nature of CFRD. The following are key nutrition concerns with CF:

- Malnutrition and weight loss, which result from malabsorption, maldigestion, anorexia, gastroesophageal reflux leading to vomiting, and increased resting metabolic rate resulting from declining pulmonary function (42)
- Malabsorption due to pancreatic exocrine insufficiency, which is found in approximately 85% to 90% of all patients with CF (43)
- Protein catabolic state
- Excessive sodium loss via sweat, illness, and exercise

Lifestyle interventions generally used for the prevention of diabetes, such as weight loss or restricted fat and energy intake, are not recommended for individuals with impaired glucose tolerance and CF because of the significantly greater energy requirements of CF (27). Furthermore, some of the nutrition recommendations for type 1 and type 2 diabetes (particularly recommendations to limit fat and sodium) are generally not applicable to individuals with CFRD because of the prevalence of malnutrition and its consequences in CFRD.

Little data exist regarding the implementation of nutrition therapy in this population. However, the primary goal is to achieve and maintain optimal weight and nutritional status through a diet that is high in calories (120%-150% of the recommended dietary allowance), fat (40% of energy intake with no restriction of fat type), and sodium (> 4,000 mg/day) (27,42,43). Achieving and maintaining optimal weight and nutritional status has been shown to dramatically improve longevity (44,45).

Energy restriction is never appropriate for individuals with CF. Energy intake may vary widely from day to day, depending on clinical status. Many individuals require additional nutrition support, in the form of oral supplements or gastrostomy feedings, to meet the increased energy demands of CF. Individuals who exercise may require significantly more energy because of the increased workload of breathing (46).

Carbohydrate intake should be individualized. The CFRD consensus guidelines recommend using insulin-to-carbohydrate ratios, as opposed to a structured meal plan, as one practical approach to address variations in energy and carbohydrate intake (27). Typical insulin requirements are approximately 0.5 to 2.0 units of rapid- or short-acting insulin per 15 g carbohydrate. Reviewing blood glucose and food records can be useful in fine-tuning the insulin-to-carbohydrate ratio (47). Individuals who take fixed doses of insulin should focus on keeping carbohydrate intake consistent (47). If insulin is not used, the carbohydrate load can be minimized by spreading carbohydrate throughout the day (47).

Because of malabsorption, a daily multivitamin and mineral supplement and daily supplementation of fat-soluble vitamins A, D, E, and K are necessary (43). Additionally, pancreatic replacement enzymes must be taken with all meals and snacks containing fat, protein, and/or starch. Calcium, iron, and zinc status should be monitored and supplemented as necessary (43).

Alcohol should be consumed only if approved by the primary care provider. Alcohol may interfere with medications used for individuals with CF, and liver disease occurs in more than 40% of people with CF (47).

Blood glucose targets for CFRD are the same as those recommended by the American Diabetes Association for other individuals with diabetes. See Box 14.4 for a checklist of education topics for individuals with CFRD.

Nutrition Therapy in Pregnancy

Pregnancy in women with CF is now quite common-place and is generally considered safe, with good fetal and maternal outcomes in women with mild to moderate disease (48,49). Preconception counseling and normalization of blood glucose are necessary, as with type 1 and type 2 diabetes (27). Women with CF are also at higher risk for gestational diabetes because of underlying insulin deficiency (27). A baseline oral glucose tolerance test is recommended before pregnancy or once the pregnancy is confirmed. The test should be repeated in the second and third trimesters, or earlier if weight gain is problematic (27).

All pregnant women with CF and impaired glucose tolerance or diabetes require increased energy with worsening pulmonary function and require close monitoring of weight gain and nutritional status for best outcomes. The use of oral supplements may be necessary to

---

BOX 14.4

Education Topics for Individuals With Cystic Fibrosis–Related Diabetes

- Principles of a healthful diet in the context of the usual high-calorie, high-fat, high-sodium diet for cystic fibrosis and how it differs from typical recommendations for type 1 and type 2 diabetes
- Importance of attaining/maintaining a healthy body weight
- Carbohydrate counting
- Meal spacing and carbohydrate distribution for individuals not requiring insulin
- Menu planning
- Appropriate use of artificial sweeteners, not to be used at expense of total calories
- Hypoglycemia treatment using only simple carbohydrates not requiring enzymes
- Carbohydrate sources for exercise
- Use of alcohol, check with physician
- Carbohydrate content of oral supplements when necessary
- Sick-day management

---

promote adequate weight gain. Self-monitoring of blood glucose is imperative, and aggressive use of insulin is recommended to achieve blood glucose goals.

Because of the risk of suboptimal weight gain, current practice does not encourage the restriction of energy or carbohydrate during pregnancy. However, empty calories should be replaced with nutrient-dense foods. In pregnant women with CFRD or CF and gestational diabetes requiring insulin therapy, insulin should be matched to carbohydrate intake to optimize blood glucose control without restricting carbohydrate intake.

SUMMARY

- Dietetics professionals should be alert to symptoms of depression among people with diabetes and should make referrals for treatment as needed.
- Medical nutrition therapy is more effective once depression is treated.
- For celiac disease, a strict gluten-free diet maintained for life is currently the only treatment available to prevent serious medical consequences.
- Undiagnosed or untreated celiac disease results in more frequent episodes of hypoglycemia and

reduced insulin needs, most likely due to malabsorption from intestinal damage.

- Initiation of a gluten-free diet reduces the incidence of hypoglycemic episodes as the intestinal injury heals. Therefore, more frequent blood glucose monitoring is essential to determine whether insulin doses need adjustment.

- Individuals with celiac disease need extensive education and support for the best outcomes.

- Diabetes is common with CF and cannot be prevented.

- Individuals with CFRD are not at risk for macrovascular disease but are at risk for microvascular disease.

- Nutrition recommendations and medical management for CFRD differ from those for type 1 and type 2 diabetes.

- A high-energy, high-fat, high-sodium diet is critical for maintenance of a healthy body weight, which is imperative for survival of individuals with CF.

REFERENCES

1. Egede LE, Zheng D. Independent factors associated with major depressive disorder in a national sample of individuals with diabetes. *Diabetes Care.* 2003;26:104–112.

2. de Groot M, Anderson R, Freedland KE, Clouse RE, Lustman PJ. Association of depression and diabetes complications: a meta-analysis. *Psychosom Med.* 2000;63:619–630.

3. Anderson RJ, Freedland KE, Clouse RE, Lustman PJ. The prevalence of comorbid depression in adults with diabetes. *Diabetes Care.* 2001;24:1069–1078.

4. Talbot F, Nouwen A. A review of the relationship between depression and diabetes in adults. *Diabetes Care.* 2000;23:1556–1562.

5. Egede LE, Zheng D, Simpson K. Comorbid depression is associated with increased health care use and expenditures in people with diabetes. *Diabetes Care.* 2002;25:464–470.

6. Gehling E. The next step: depression. *Newsflash.* 2001;22:20.

7. Ciechanowski PS, Katon WJ, Russo JE. Depression and diabetes: impact of depressive symptoms on adherence, function and cost. *Arch Intern Med.* 2000;160:3278–3285.

8. Kroenke K, Spitzer RL, Williams JBW. The PHQ-9: validity of a brief depression severity measure. *J Gen Intern Med.* 2001;16:606–613.

9. Spitzer RL, Kroenke K, Williams JBW; and the Patient Health Questionnaire Primary Care Study Group. Validation and utility of a self-report version of PRIME-MD: the PHQ Primary Care Study. *JAMA.* 1999;282:1737–1744.

10. National Institute of Mental Health. Medications. 2002. Available at: http://www.nimh.nih.gov/publicat/medicate.cfm#ptdep7. Accessed January 11, 2005.

11. Jacobson A. The psychological care of patients with insulin-dependent diabetes mellitus. *N Engl J Med.* 1996;334:1249–1253.

12. Thompson T. Gluten contamination of commercial oat products in the United States. *N Engl J Med.* 2004;351:2021–2022.

13. Mohn A, Cerruto M, Lafusco D, Prisco F, Tumini S, Stoppoloni O, Chiarelli F. Celiac disease in children and adolescents with type 1 diabetes: importance of hypoglycemia. *J Pediatr Gastroenterol Nutr.* 2001;32:37–40.

14. Fasano A, Berti I, Gerarduzzi T, Not T, Colletti RB, Drago S, Elitsur Y, Green PH, Guandalini S, Hill ID, Pietzak M, Ventura A, Thorpe M, Kryszak D, Fornaroli F, Wasserman SS, Murray JA, Horvath K. Prevalence of celiac disease in at-risk and not-at-risk groups in the United States: a large multicenter study. *Arch Intern Med.* 2003;163:286–292.

15. Collin P, Kaukinen K, Valimaki M, Salmi J. Endocrinological disorders and celiac disease. *Endocr Rev.* 2002;23:464–483.

16. Page SR, Lloyd CA, Hill PG, Holmes GK. The prevalence of coeliac disease in adult diabetes mellitus. *QJM.* 1994;87:631–637.

17. Kaukinen K, Salmi J, Lahtela J, Siljamaki-Ojansuu U, Koivisto AM, Oksa H, Collin P. No effect of gluten-free diet on the metabolic control of type 1 diabetes in patients with diabetes and celiac disease: retrospective and controlled prospective survey. *Diabetes Care.* 1999;22:1747–1748.

18. Acerini CL, Ahmed ML, Ross KM, Sullivan PB, Bird G, Dunger DB. Coeliac disease in children and adolescents with IDDM: clinical characteristics and response to gluten-free diet. *Diabet Med.* 1998;15:38–44.

19. Schwarzenberg SJ, Brunzell C. Type 1 diabetes and celiac disease: overview and medical nutrition therapy. *Diabetes Spectrum.* 2002;15:197–201.

20. Cronin CC, Feighery A, Ferriss JB, Liddy C, Shanahan F, Feighery C. High prevalence of celiac disease among patients with insulin-dependent (type 1) diabetes mellitus. *Am J Gastroenterol.* 1997;92:2210–2212.

21. Bahna SL. Celiac disease: a food allergy? Contra! *Monogr Allergy.* 1996;32:211–215.

22. Inman-Felton AE. Overview of gluten-sensitive enteropathy (celiac sprue). *J Am Diet Assoc.* 1999;99:352–362.

23. Thompson T. Thiamin, riboflavin, and niacin contents of the gluten-free diet: is there a cause for concern? *J Am Diet Assoc.* 1999;99:858–862.

24. Thompson T. Folate, iron, and dietary fiber contents of the gluten-free diet. *J Am Diet Assoc.* 2000;100:1389–1396.

25. Farrell RJ, Kelly CP. Current concepts: celiac sprue. *N Engl J Med.* 2002;346:180–188.

26. FitzSimmons S. The changing epidemiology of cystic fibrosis. *J Pediatr.* 1993;122:1–9.

27. Moran A, Hardin D, Rodman D, Allen HF, Beall RJ, Borowitz D, Brunzell C, Campbell PW 3rd, Chesrown SE, Duchow C, Fink RJ, Fitzsimmons SC, Hamilton N, Hirsch I, Howenstine MS, Klein DJ, Madhun Z, Pencharz PB, Quittner AL, Robbins MK, Schindler T, Schissel K, Schwarzenberg SJ, Stallings VA, Zipf WB. Diagnosis, screening, and management of cystic fibrosis related diabetes mellitus: a consensus conference report. *Diabetes Res Clin Pract.* 1999;5:61–73.

28. Cystic Fibrosis Foundation. Patient Registry Annual Data Report 2003. Available at: http://www.cff.org/publications. Accessed January 5, 2005.

29. Lanng S, Thorsteinsson B, Lund-Andersen C, Nerup J, Schiotz PO, Koch C. Diabetes mellitus in Danish cystic fibrosis patients: prevalence and late diabetic complications. *Acta Paediatr.* 1994;83:72–77.

30. Rosenecker J, Eichler I, Kuhn L, Harms HK, von der Hardt H. Genetic determination of diabetes mellitus in patients with cystic fibrosis. Multicenter Cystic Fibrosis Study Group. *J Pediatr.* 1995;127:441–443.

31. Couce M, O'Brien TD, Moran A, Roche PC, Butler PC. Diabetes mellitus in cystic fibrosis is characterized by islet amyloidosis. *J Clin Endocrinol Metab.* 1996;81:1267–1272.

32. Finkelstein SM, Wielinski CL, Elliott GR, Warwick WJ, Barbosa J, Wu SC, Klein DJ. Diabetes mellitus associated with cystic fibrosis. *J Pediatr.* 1988;112:373–377.

33. Lanng S, Thorsteinsson B, Nerup J, Koch C. Influence of the development of diabetes mellitus on clinical status in patients with cystic fibrosis. *Eur J Pediatr.* 1992;151:684–687.

34. Lanng S, Thorsteinsson B, Nerup J, Koch C. Diabetes mellitus in cystic fibrosis: effect of insulin therapy on lung function and infections. *Acta Paediatr.* 1994;83:849–853.

35. Moran A, Milla C, Ducret R, Nair KS. Protein metabolism in clinically stable adult cystic fibrosis patients with abnormal glucose tolerance. *Diabetes.* 2001;50:1336–1343.

36. Carroll R, Hendeles L. Pancreatic enzyme supplementation in cystic fibrosis patients. *US Pharmacist.* 2002;27:1. Available at: http://www.uspharmacist.com/index.asp?show=search. Accessed January 10, 2004.

37. Sullivan MM, Denning CR. Diabetic microangiopathy in patients with cystic fibrosis. *Pediatrics.* 1989;84:642–646.

38. Rodman HM, Doershuk CF, Roland JM. The interaction of two diseases: diabetes mellitus and cystic fibrosis. *Medicine.* 1986;65:389–397.

39. Schlesinger DM, Holsclaw DS, Fyfe B. Generalised atherosclerosis in an adult with cystic fibrosis and diabetes mellitus (abstract). *Pediatr Pulmonol.* 1997;16(Suppl 14):365A.

40. Stewart C, Wilson DC, Hanna AK, Corey M, Durie PR, Pencharz PB. Lipid metabolism in adults with cystic fibrosis. *Pediatr Pulmonol.* 1997;16(Suppl 14):366A.

41. Figueroa V, Milla C, Parks E, Schwarzenberg SJ, Moran A. Abnormal lipid levels in cystic fibrosis. *Am J Clin Nutr.* 2002;75:1005–1011.

42. Pencharz PB, Durie PR. Pathogenesis of malnutrition cystic fibrosis, and its treatment. *Clin Nutr.* 2000;19:387–394.

43. Borowitz D, Baker RD, Stallings V. Consensus report on nutrition for pediatric patients with cystic fibrosis. *J Pediatr Gastroenterol Nutr.* 2002;35:246–259.

44. Corey M, McLaughlin FJ, Williams M, Levison H. A comparison of survival, growth, and pulmonary function in patients with cystic fibrosis in Boston and Toronto. *J Clin Epidemiol.* 1988;41:583–591.

45. Kraemer R, Rudeberg A, Hadorn B, Rossi E. Relative underweight in cystic fibrosis and its prognostic value. *Acta Paediatr Scand.* 1978;67:33–37.

46. Ward SA, Tomezsko JL, Holsclaw DS, Paolone AM. Energy expenditure and substrate utilization in adults with cystic fibrosis and diabetes mellitus. *Am J Clin Nutr.* 1999;69:913–919.

47. Moran A. Cystic fibrosis-related diabetes: an approach to diagnosis and management. *Pediatr Diabetes.* 2000;1:41–48.

48. FitzSimmons SC, Fitzpatrick S, Thompson B, Aitkin M, Fiel S, Winnie G, Hilman B. A longitudinal study of the effects of pregnancy on 325 women with cystic fibrosis. *Pediatr Pulmonol.* 1996;13:99–101.

49. Gilljam M, Antoniou M, Shin J, Dupuis A, Corey M, Tullis DE. Pregnancy in cystic fibrosis: fetal and maternal outcome. *Chest.* 2000;118:85–91.

ADDITIONAL RESOURCES

Depression

Anderson BJ, Rubin RR. *Practical Psychology for Diabetes Clinicians.* Alexandria, Va: American Diabetes Association; 2002.

National Institutes for Mental Health Web site. Available at: http://www.nimh.nih.gov. Accessed September 8, 2004.

National Institutes of Diabetes and Digestive and Kidney Disorders Web site. Available at: http://www.niddk.nih.gov. Accessed September 8, 2004.

Celiac Disease

American Celiac Society. 59 Crystal Ave. West Orange, NJ 07052. 973/325-8837.

Canadian Celiac Association. Available at: http://www.celiac.ca. Accessed January 11, 2005.

Case S. *Gluten-Free Diet: A Comprehensive Resource Guide.* Regina, Canada: Centax Books; 2001.

Celiac Disease and Gluten-Free Diet Support Center. Available at: http://celiac.com. Accessed January 11, 2005.

Celiac Disease Foundation. Available at: http://www.celiac.org. Accessed January 11, 2005.

Celiac Sprue Association/USA Inc. Available at: http://www.csaceliacs.org. Accessed January 11, 2005.

Dietitians in Gluten Intolerance Diseases listserve. To subscribe, contact DIGIDRDs@aol.com.

Fenster C. *Wheat-Free Recipes & Menus: Delicious Dining Without Wheat or Gluten.* Rev. ed. Centennial, Col: Savory Palate; 2000.

Gluten Intolerance Group of North America. Available at: http://www.gluten.net Accessed January 11, 2005.

Hagman B. *The Gluten-Free Gourmet: Living Well Without Wheat.* 2nd ed. New York: Henry Holt and Company; 2000.

Korn D. *Kids with Celiac Disease: A Family Guide to Raising Happy, Healthy, Gluten-Free Children.* Bethesda, Md: Woodbine House; 2001.

Milazzo M. *Celiac Sprue: A Guide Through the Medicine Cabinet.* Medford, NJ: Stokes Pharmacy; 2001.

Raising Our Celiac Kids Web site. Available at: http://www.celiac.com/cgi-bin/webc.cgi/st_main.html?p_catid=8. Accessed January 11, 2005.

Thompson T, Dobler ML. *Celiac Disease Nutrition Guide.* Chicago, Ill: American Dietetic Association; 2003.

University of Maryland Center for Celiac Research Web site. Available at: http://celiaccenter.org. Accessed January 11,2005.

Cystic Fibrosis–Related Diabetes and Abnormal Glucose Tolerance in Cystic Fibrosis

Cystic Fibrosis Foundation. Available at: http://cff.org. Accessed January 11, 2005.

Hardin D, Brunzell C, Schissel K, Schindler T, Moran A. *Managing Cystic Fibrosis Related Diabetes (CFRD).* Bethesda, Md: Cystic Fibrosis Foundation; 2002.

Part 4

Life Stages and Special Populations

15

Birth Through Adolescence

Alison Evert, RD, CDE, and Stephanie Gerken, MS, RD, CDE

CHAPTER OVERVIEW

- Diabetes is one of the most common chronic conditions among school-aged children in the United States. Approximately 13,000 are diagnosed with diabetes each year (1).
- Historically, type 1 diabetes was seen almost exclusively among US children and adolescents; however, with the increased prevalence of childhood obesity, type 2 diabetes, formerly seen only in adults, is now on the rise (2–6). It is estimated that 8% to 45% of children with newly diagnosed diabetes in large US pediatric centers are diagnosed with type 2 diabetes (7).
- Family involvement is an important element of optimal diabetes management.
- The nutrition needs of youths with diabetes appear to be similar to those without diabetes (8). The key to achieving optimal blood glucose control is effectively balancing food intake, diabetes medication, and physical activity.
- Dyslipidemia is a concern for youths, because the atherosclerotic process linked with cardiovascular disease begins in childhood and is associated with elevated blood cholesterol values.

TYPES OF DIABETES THAT OCCUR IN YOUTHS

The types of diabetes that occur in youths include the following:

- Type 1 diabetes
- Type 2 diabetes
- Maturity onset diabetes in youth (MODY), which is due to specific genetic defects of beta-cell function
- Secondary diabetes induced by certain drugs, infections, endocrine diseases, and genetic syndromes
- Gestational diabetes, which may occur in pregnant teens

This chapter focuses on the management of type 1 and type 2 diabetes in youths.

GOALS OF NUTRITION THERAPY

The nutrition needs of youths with diabetes appear to be similar to those of youths without diabetes (8). Nutrition recommendations should focus on achieving optimal blood glucose goals without excessive hypoglycemia, lipid and blood pressure goals, and normal growth and development (8). This can be accomplished through individualized meal planning, flexible insulin plans and algorithms, self-monitoring of blood glucose, and education that promotes decision-making based on documentation and review of previous results (9).

In addition to the goals of medical nutrition therapy (MNT) that apply to all persons with diabetes (see Chapter 6), there are goals specifically designed for youths (8). For youths with type 1 diabetes, MNT goals are to provide adequate energy to ensure normal growth and development, and to integrate the insulin plan into usual eating and physical activity habits. MNT goals for youths with type 2 diabetes include facilitating changes in eating and physical activity habits, to reduce insulin resistance and to improve metabolic status. MNT goals for youths at risk for type 2 diabetes include decreasing risk by encouraging physical activity and by promoting food choices that facilitate moderate weight loss or at least prevent weight gain. For youths with type 1 or type 2 diabetes treated with insulin, MNT goals are to provide self-management education about the prevention and treatment of hypoglycemia, acute illnesses, and exercise-related blood glucose problems.

ASSESSMENT

To develop an individualized nutrition plan, information should first be collected through assessment of physical data and diabetes self-care history. Before beginning the assessment, for best rapport, the dietetics professional should explain what will occur during the session and should allow time for getting acquainted with the youth.

Physical Data

Weight, Height, and Body Mass Index-for-Age

To assess growth and development, weight and height should be measured at every appointment. The American Academy of Pediatrics recommends that all children should have their height, weight, and body mass index (BMI)-for-age assessed annually, using the 2000 Centers for Disease Control and Prevention (CDC) growth charts to allow longitudinal tracking (10). The growth charts include BMI-for-age charts, which help identify the current health status as it correlates with body fatness (11). A series of measurements over years are more valuable than single measurements (10).

Children tend to grow consistently along a percentile, and any deviation from this should be assessed. If

growth becomes a concern, the diabetes management plan should be evaluated to determine whether energy, insulin, and blood glucose control are adequate or whether another disease state is present.

In youths 2 to 20 years old, overweight is defined as sex- and age-specific BMI-for-age at or above the 95th percentile; at risk for overweight as at the 85th up to the 94th percentiles; and underweight as less than the 5th percentile, based on the CDC growth charts (11).

Poor weight gain or slowed linear growth can result from an overly restrictive meal plan in an effort to control blood glucose, inadequate insulin, or chronic hyperglycemia. Continuous glucosuria deprives the body of calories that would otherwise support growth. The diabetes meal plan, as well as the insulin prescription, should grow with the child. Adolescents with type 1 diabetes may skip some insulin injections for the purpose of weight control. If such a practice is identified, the health care provider should be notified immediately; a mental health referral may be indicated.

Excessive weight gain can result from excessive energy intake, physical inactivity, overtreatment of hypoglycemia, and overinsulinization leading to continuous snacking to avoid hypoglycemia. If weight is a sensitive issue, a "blind" weight should be taken; this allows the youth to step on the scale backwards and avoid seeing the weight. Placing scales in examination rooms provides greater privacy than does keeping them in public areas.

Sexual Development

Adequate growth and appropriate pubertal development are important indexes of insulin sufficiency. The Tanner stages of sexual development can be used as a guide to the usual progression of puberty (12,13). Normal progression through these stages varies widely, depending on the individual and ethnicity.

Recent research has focused on puberty's stress on insulin resistance and the age at diagnosis with type 2 diabetes. Studies have shown that the pubertal transition from Tanner stage 1 to Tanner stage 3 is associated with a reduction in insulin sensitivity and an increase in fasting glucose, insulin, and acute insulin response (5,6,13).

Diabetes Self-Care History

The diabetes self-care history should include review of nutrition, medications, laboratory data, blood glucose monitoring information, physical activity, relationships, and other variables (14). Box 15.1 provides a complete list of all variables. Table 15.1 (15,16) lists age-related

BOX 15.1

Diabetes Self-Care Variables to Assess

1. Nutrition
   - Weight history*
   - Previous nutrition therapy
   - Current meal plan, if any, and whether the youth is following it
   - Length of time since last education session with a dietetics professional
   - Food preferences, intolerances, aversions, or allergies
   - Who purchases and prepares the food
   - Types and quantities of food and beverages consumed (obtained from a 24-hour food recall or a 3-day food record)*
   - Time/place of meals and snacks and people with whom the youth eats*
   - Snack choices/availability at school*
   - Frequency of dining out*
   - Presence of disordered eating (stress eating, binge eating, eating alone in bedroom)*
   - Recent life changes (aside from diabetes) that may have altered eating*
   - Awareness of hunger and fullness*
   - Effect of socio-economic status, culture, ethnic background, and religious beliefs on food choices*
2. Medications (diabetes-related and other)
   - Type of insulin(s) and/or oral diabetes medication taken, dose, and time
   - Who administers injections, if using insulin
   - Injection sites, if using insulin
   - Dose adjustments
   - Other medications or supplements, dose, and time
3. Laboratory data
4. Blood glucose monitoring
   - Type of monitor used
   - Who performs blood glucose monitoring
   - Site used to obtain the blood sample (fingertips or alternate site)
   - Frequency of blood glucose monitoring
   - Record keeping
   - Evaluation of blood glucose records
5. Physical activity
   - Type, time, and duration of regularly scheduled physical activity, including physical education classes, recess, sports practices, or other physical activity *
   - Time spent in sedentary activity*
6. Routine (consider that many youths do not have predictable schedules)
   - School/class or day-care schedule*
   - Transportation to/from school (bus, carpool, walking)
   - Weekend schedule and how it differs from the weekday schedule
7. Relationships with family, friends, and significant others
   - Identify the primary caregivers and whether the family is intact*
   - Time spent at different households*
   - Role of food in the social life*
8. Financial concerns/limitations*
9. Family's readiness to change*
10. Youth's independence*

*Particularly important to assess in individuals with type 2 diabetes.

TABLE 15.1 Approximate Age-Related Traits of Youths and Delegation of Responsibilities

Age, y	Age-Specific Developmental Traits of Youths*	Age-Specific Considerations in Youths with Diabetes	Youth's Level of Participation in Diabetes Self-Care	Caregiver Responsibilities
0–3	• Develops gross motor skills • Develops speech skills • Begins to develop sense of self • Always moving • Learns to trust • Responds to love • Uses imagination	• Unable to recognize hypoglycemia • May protest insulin administration and blood glucose monitoring • May fear health care professionals	• None to minimal participation in care	• Performs all care • Identifies hypoglycemia vs a "normal" tantrum • Varies treatment schedule to accommodate normal changes in feeding and sleeping patterns • Reads and responds to child's signals • Moves insulin injection after meals/snacks if necessary because of inconsistent food intake
3–5	• Thinks imaginatively and concretely • Can act in a self-centered manner; desires to make own choices • Begins to ask cause-effect questions • Learns by curiosity and exploration • Begins to socialize with others outside the family • Expresses feelings more openly	• Unable to understand the importance of eating, insulin administration, and blood glucose monitoring • Unable to recognize hypoglycemia	• Can help choose site for blood glucose monitoring or insulin administration • Can help select foods for meals and snacks from appropriate choices provided by caregiver	• Performs almost all diabetes tasks • Identifies hypoglycemia versus behavior issues • Moves insulin injection after meals/snacks if necessary because of inconsistent intake • Provides snacks and meals similar to those eaten by siblings and friends and at similar times, as possible; avoids becoming a short-order cook • Sets limits about timing of meals and snacks for entire family
5–8	• Builds physical, artistic, and verbal skills • Compares self to peers • Feels secure outside of home	• By age 8, begins to recognize symptoms of hypoglycemia • Needs full involvement of parents or caregivers	• Gathers and stores diabetes supplies • Selects finger for lancing; may be able to self-monitor blood glucose independently • Pinches up skin for injection • Pushes plunger on insulin syringe • Names foods on plate • Starts to identify the major nutrients • Provides input about food choices for meals and snacks • Is responsible for eating meals and snacks	• Begins to delegate some diabetes self-management tasks to the youth • Aids in identifying hypoglycemia • Does not fully expect child to understand importance of eating, insulin administration, and blood glucose monitoring • Determines timing of meals and snacks and the foods that are prepared and served with input from the child on occasion • Trains and delegates some diabetes management tasks to school personnel

(*continued*)

TABLE 15.1 *(Continued)*

Age, y	Age-Specific Developmental Traits of Youths*	Age-Specific Considerations in Youths with Diabetes	Youth's Level of Participation in Diabetes Self-Care	Caregiver Responsibilities
5–8 *(continued)*			• provided to them at appropriate times • Completes a urine ketone test • Records results in a log book	
8–12	• Thinks concretely • Is more logical, understanding, curious, social • Acts more responsibly	• Should be able to consistently recognize and treat hypoglycemia • Able to perform many diabetes self-management skills independently • Needs ongoing support and supervision from parents and caregivers	• Performs self-monitoring of blood glucose • By approximately 10 y should be able to draw up and inject insulin using a syringe, pen, or insulin pump • Makes own food choices and counts carbohydrates • With supervision, some youths can participate in insulin dose decision making based on blood glucose correction factor and carbohydrate intake • States type(s) and dose(s) of diabetes medications and time taken • Stores insulin properly	• May need to ask youth to confirm hypoglycemic episode by checking blood glucose • Delegates diabetes self-management tasks; parental involvement still critical • Plans and prepares food with family input • Determines timing of meals and snacks and the foods that are prepared and served with input from the child on occasion
12–15	• Is more independent • Behavior is variable • Feels body image is important • Is away from home more frequently • Can be influenced by peers • Becomes more responsible for actions • Thinks abstractly	• Gradually recognizes the importance of glycemic control to prevent chronic complications • May be willing to intensify treatment to either multiple daily injections or pump therapy	• Administers insulin; parental involvement and assistance in decision making still important • Knows what foods to eat; able to count carbohydrates and make own food choices	• Continues to delegate diabetes self-management tasks • Provides physical and mental health support, as needed
15–18	• Becomes increasingly independent • Variable behavior • Feels body image is still important • Becomes more responsible • Thinks abstractly	• Knows the importance of tight glycemic control • Deals with adult issues, such as driving, relationships, alcohol, drugs, etc	• Takes almost total care of self, with parental support and involvement	• Minimal; mainly in support role

*With or without diabetes.
Source: Data are from references 15 and 16.

traits of youths and delegation of responsibilities based on age. For more information on assessment, see Chapter 6.

INTERVENTIONS FOR THE MANAGEMENT OF TYPE 1 AND TYPE 2 DIABETES

For type 1 diabetes, key concerns are matching the time food and beverages are consumed and the quantity and type consumed, with insulin action to achieve blood glucose goals that maintain normal growth and development without excessive hypoglycemia. This can be accomplished through individualized meal planning, flexible insulin plans and insulin algorithms, self-monitoring of blood glucose, and education promoting decision making based on outcomes (8,16).

The treatment goals for youths with type 2 diabetes are the same as those for youths with type 1 diabetes. However, the treatment plan for achieving those goals is different. The treatment plan for type 2 diabetes focuses on weight management and lifestyle change, with the addition of metformin (in youths older than 10 years) and/or insulin if glucose levels remain elevated. An appropriate weight goal for overweight children is a BMI below the 85th percentile, although such a goal should be secondary to the primary goal of healthy eating and activity. Weight loss is recommended if complications such as hyperlipidemia or hypertension are identified, and for children 7 years or older with a BMI-for-age at or above the 95th percentile; otherwise, weight maintenance is recommended (11,17). If weight loss is deemed appropriate, weight loss goals should be established only under physician supervision. Successful treatment of children with type 2 diabetes with diet and exercise is defined by the American Diabetes Association as cessation of excessive weight gain with normal growth, and near-normal fasting blood glucose values and A1C (4).

Specific management interventions, including nutrition therapy, diabetes medications, physical activity, and self-monitoring of blood glucose, are outlined in the following sections. Specific risk factors and screening criteria for type 2 diabetes in youths are outlined in Chapter 4 on pathophysiology.

NUTRITION THERAPY

Nutrition therapy should be provided at diagnosis and at least annually thereafter (18). The nutrition plan should be individualized based on information obtained from the assessment and should address food preferences, family schedules and eating patterns, cultural influences, age, weight, physical activity, and insulin action. Care should be taken to avoid overly aggressive nutrition modifications in very young children (18). Insulin therapy can be integrated into usual eating and physical activity habits, so the meal plan should be determined before the insulin plan. Guidelines for estimating energy needs can be found in Box 15.2 (11,17,19).

BOX 15.2

Estimating Energy Needs for Youths

Energy needs can be based on nutrition assessment and validated by using one of the following formulas. Energy intake should be sufficient to attain and/or maintain a reasonable body weight in order to support normal growth and development for children and adolescents.

Method 1
Start with 1000 kcal for the first year

- 1 to 3 years of age—add 40 kcal/inch length
- 4 to 10 years of age—add 100 kcal/year
- Girls 11 to 15 years of age—add ≤ 100 kcal/year
- Girls > 15 years, calculate as an adult
- Boys 11 to 15 years—add 200 kcal/year
- Boys > 15 years, 23 kcal/pound if very active; 18 kcal/pound for moderate activity; 16 kcal/pound if sedentary

Method 2 (rough estimate)
Start with 1000 kcal for the first year

- Add 125 kcal × age (in years) for boys
- Add 100 kcal × age (in years) for girls
- Add up to 20% more kcal for activity

Overweight children 2–20 years of age (rough estimate based on clinical practice)

- Obtain a 3-day food and beverage record to estimate total average energy intake.
- Subtract 125–150 kcal from this average total energy intake to achieve a slow steady weight loss of ¼ to ½ pound per week.

Source: Adapted from *Maximizing the Role of Nutrition in Diabetes Management* (11,17,19), with permission from the American Diabetes Association. Copyright © 1994 American Diabetes Association.

Meal-Planning Approaches

The variety of meal-planning approaches reviewed in detail in Chapter 18 can be used with youths. See Table 15.1 for guidance in how much and when children can assist with meal-planning responsibilities.

For type 2 diabetes, other child-friendly approaches include categorizing food based on nutritional value with smiley faces (designating foods to choose more often and less often) or color codes (eg, red = stop, yellow = caution, green = go) or striving for a certain number of servings from food categories, such as in "Being Healthy Rocks," shown in Figure 15.1 (20). The National Diabetes Education Program (NDEP) has developed a series of fact sheets for children with type 2 diabetes: "Eat Healthy Foods," "Stay at a Healthy Weight," "Be Active," and "What Is Diabetes?" The fact sheets can be downloaded from the NDEP Web site (21–23). These approaches are often used in combination with setting measurable, achievable goals, not only for weight, food choices, physical activity, and blood glucose, but also for blood pressure and lipids, as appropriate.

For type 1 diabetes, carbohydrate counting is frequently the method of choice, because it allows for greater flexibility in food choices, timing and frequency of meals, and physical activity. Carbohydrate-counting principles are the same for children and teens as for adults.

Carbohydrate consistency is often the meal-plan approach of choice for youths on a fixed insulin plan. This involves keeping carbohydrate intake consistent at each meal and snack from day to day, to correlate with the fixed insulin dose. Fairly consistent meal and snack times are necessary. For a comparison of frequently prescribed insulin plans for youths, see Table 15.2 (15).

Insulin-to-carbohydrate ratios are often the choice for youths on a flexible insulin plan because of the greater flexibility. Typical insulin-to-carbohydrate ratios based on age can be found in Box 15.3. Young children need adult assistance or guidance in calculating carbohydrate and insulin boluses. For practice, the dietetics professional should help the caregiver and/or youth calculate the carbohydrate content of favorite meals and snacks. Caregivers and youths must realize that, although carbohydrate counting allows greater flexibility in food choices, the principles of good nutrition should not be sacrificed (see Chapter 18 for additional information on carbohydrate counting).

When discussing food choices with youths, refrain from referring to foods as "good" or "bad." Instead, use nonjudgmental terminology such as "everyday foods" and "once-in-a-while" foods.

Feeding Frequency and Related Concerns

Caregivers of infants and young children on a fixed insulin plan should be counseled about the onset, peak, and duration of the child's individualized insulin plan. (Refer to Chapter 9 for information on insulin action.) An effort should be made to schedule naps, meals, and snacks, to coordinate with the child's individualized insulin plan and the anticipated insulin action.

Although infants require a 3- to 4-hour flexible feeding schedule to maintain blood glucose, regular nighttime feedings for infants and very young children on a fixed insulin plan are important to prevent hypoglycemia. If nocturnal hypoglycemia is a problem, a flexible insulin plan using glargine basal insulin (see Table 15.2) may be indicated.

Toddlers usually need three meals and three snacks daily. However, additional food or beverages (such as milk or juice) may be necessary, to prevent hypoglycemia during extra active periods. Most children younger than 6 years, who have more than 4 hours between meals, generally require a snack (24).

Most children older than 6 years on a fixed insulin plan may require three meals, a midafternoon snack, and a bedtime snack. Youths on a flexible insulin plan need to take an injection of rapid-acting insulin each time they have a meal or snack of more than 10 to 15 g of carbohydrate (16). A youth using a fixed insulin plan who likes to sleep can return to bed after eating and taking the morning insulin. A youth using a flexible insulin plan incorporating a peakless basal insulin, such as glargine, (Table 15.2) can usually sleep late without worries of hypoglycemia.

When using a flexible insulin plan, the youth should be counseled to take the rapid-acting insulin at the beginning of the meal. Self-injecting older children and adolescents may forget to take it after the meal. To prevent hypoglycemia during periods of erratic eating (a common behavior among young children), the rapid-acting insulin can be given immediately after the meal or snack, based on the amount of carbohydrate actually consumed.

Additional Nutrition Concerns for Type 1 Diabetes

Dramatic weight loss frequently precedes diagnosis with type 1 diabetes. Once exogenous insulin therapy is

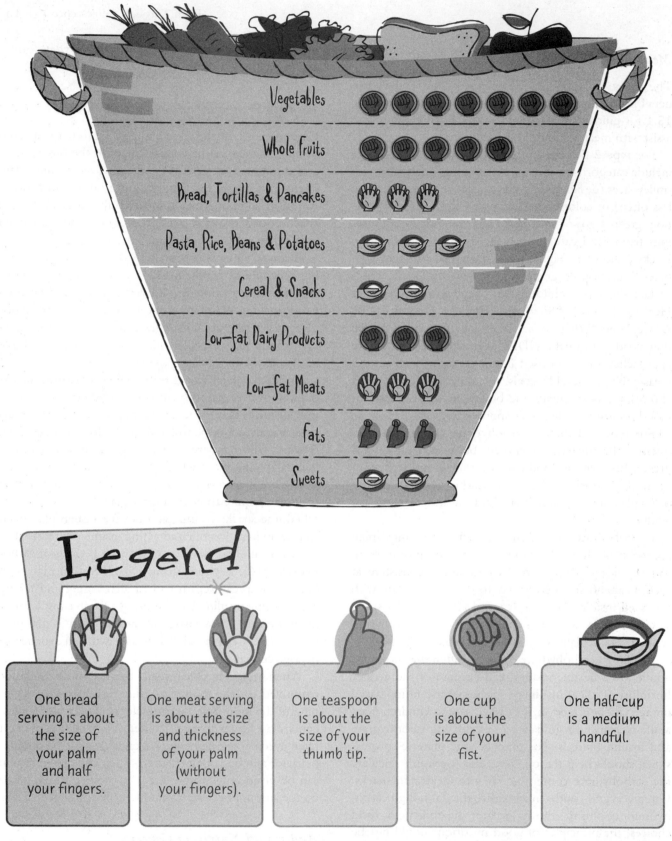

FIGURE 15.1 Healthy food basket and helping hand servings per day. Reprinted from: *Being Healthy Rocks* (20). Copyright ©2002 International Diabetes Center, Minneapolis, U.S.A. Used with permission. For ordering information, call 888/637-2675.

TABLE 15.2   Frequently Prescribed Insulin Plans for Youths

Insulin Plan	Pros	Cons	Nutrition Implications
Fixed			
OPTION 1: • RA or SA+ NPH or L before morning meal and before evening meal	• Requires the fewest injections. • May be desirable for a newly diagnosed individual or one resistant to injections.	• Does not allow for adjustments to match carbohydrate intake. • Timing of insulin and meal times are very important. • May not lead to adequate blood glucose control.	• Carbohydrate intake must be fairly consistent because of fixed insulin doses. • May require a morning snack to prevent hypoglycemia before mid-day meal. • May require a bedtime snack to prevent nocturnal hypoglycemia. • SA should be injected 30 minutes before meal is consumed for insulin effectiveness.
OPTION 2: • RA or SA+ NPH or L before morning meal • RA or SA before evening meal • NPH or L at bedtime	• Injecting NPH at bedtime reduces the likelihood of nocturnal hypoglycemia or insulin wearing off before morning.	• Requires a 3rd shot. • Does not allow for adjustments to match carbohydrate intake.	• Carbohydrate intake must be fairly consistent because of fixed insulin doses. • May require a mid-morning snack to prevent hypoglycemia before lunch. • SA should be injected 30 minutes before meal is consumed for insulin effectiveness.
Flexible			
OPTION 3: • RA or SA+ UL before morning meal and before evening meal • RA or SA before midday meal	• Allows for adjustments based on carbohydrate intake.	• Multiple injections—insulin injection is required before each meal or snack. • UL and RA or SA insulin must be mixed in the AM and PM. • UL may have variable duration and action.	• Ability to count carbohydrates is important to enable youths to "match" insulin with carbohydrate intake. • Most individuals must take an injection to "cover" the glycemic excursion of snack foods, unless consuming less than 5–10 g of carbohydrate. • Bedtime snack is not usually necessary.
OPTION 4: • RA or SA+ UL before morning meal • RA or SA before mid-day meal and before evening meal • NPH at bedtime	• Allows for adjustments based on carbohydrate intake.	• Multiple injections—insulin injection is required before each meal or snack. • Requires several different insulins, which can be confusing. • UL may have variable duration and action.	• Ability to count carbohydrates is important to enable youth to "match" insulin with carbohydrate intake. • Most individuals must take an injection to "cover" the glycemic excursion of snack foods, unless consuming less than 5–10 g of carbohydrate. • Bedtime snack is not usually necessary.
OPTION 5: • RA or SA before morning meal, before mid-day meal, and before evening meal • G at bedtime	• Allows for adjustments based on carbohydrate intake. • Most flexible insulin plan in terms of amount of food consumed and timing of meals. • Less risk of nocturnal hypoglycemia. • Many individuals use an insulin pen, which is quick and easy, for mealtime RA or SA.	• Multiple injections—insulin injection is required before each meal or snack. Most individuals take at least 4–5 injections per day. • Glargine cannot be mixed with other insulins. • If glargine is forgotten, must take multiple injections of rapid-acting insulin the following day.	• Ability to count carbohydrates is important to enable youths to "match" insulin with carbohydrate intake. • Most individuals must take an injection to "cover" the glycemic excursion of snack foods, unless consuming less than 5–10 g carbohydrate. • Bedtime snack is not usually necessary.

Abbreviations: G, glargine; L, lente; RA, rapid-acting (lispro or aspart); SA, short-acting (regular); UL, ultralente.
Source: Data are from reference 15.

BOX 15.3

Typical Insulin-to-Carbohydrate Ratios Based on Age*†

Carbohydrate Serving or Choice Approach

- 1 unit of bolus insulin is required to "cover" a specific number of carbohydrate servings or "choices"; the amount of bolus insulin required varies based on age and weight.
- 1 carbohydrate serving or choice (15 g carbohydrate) = 1 serving of grains, dried beans, starchy vegetable, fruit, milk, or sweet/dessert. (One serving of nonstarchy vegetable equals 5 g of carbohydrate, which would be considered free. If three or more servings are eaten in a meal, they can be counted as one carbohydrate serving.)

Age Group	Insulin:Carbohydrate Ratios
Toddler (0–3 y)	½–1 U insulin per 2–3 carbohydrate servings/choices
Preschool (3–5 y)	½–1 U insulin per 1–2 carbohydrate servings/choices
School-age (6–12 y)	½–1 U insulin per 1 carbohydrate serving/choice
Teenage (13–19 y)	1–2 U insulin per 1 carbohydrate serving/choice
Overweight Teen (13–19 y)	2–3 U insulin per 1 carbohydrate serving/choice

Gram Approach

1 unit of bolus insulin is required to "cover" a specific number of grams of carbohydrate; the amount of bolus insulin required varies based on age and weight. Using a gram approach may be particularly beneficial for toddlers and preschoolers.

Age Group	Insulin:Carbohydrate Ratios
Toddler (0–3 y)	½–1 U insulin:30–40 g carbohydrate
Preschool (3–5 y)	½–1 U insulin:20–30 g carbohydrate
School-age (6–12 y)	1 U insulin:15 g carbohydrate
Teenage (13–19 y)	1 U insulin:10–15 g carbohydrate
Overweight Teen (13–19 y)	1 U insulin:5–10 g carbohydrate

*Recommendations are based on clinical experience.

†To be used with multiple daily injection plans (or a flexible insulin plan).

initiated and the blood glucose level begins to normalize, huge appetite increases often follow with weight regain. Many children will request food every 2 to 3 hours during this period.

Polyphagia typically subsides 2 to 4 weeks after diagnosis. The dietetics professional should be aware that prescribing a food plan can be difficult until the appetite returns to normal. There are no specific guidelines in the scientific literature about how to deal with the period of polyphagia. The dietetic professional can suggest the inclusion of a source of protein at all meals during this period, to help sustain satiety for more than 1 to 2 hours. Approaches used in clinical practice to handle this situation include the following:

- Instructing the child or caregiver on a prescribed meal plan and offering low-carbohydrate foods, sugar-free beverages, and protein if still hungry at mealtime or between meals.
- Instructing the child or caregiver on a more liberal meal plan for 2 to 4 weeks and then adjusting the meal plan and insulin doses when appetite returns to the prediagnosis level.
- Allowing the child to eat larger portions of healthful foods and beverages. This option requires caregivers to be in frequent phone contact with the health care team for insulin dose adjustments, to correct the blood glucose levels until the appetite returns to normal. A meal plan is developed once the appetite returns to normal.

Nutrition Intervention Strategies for Youths With Type 2 Diabetes

Many of the eating and exercise habits of youths with type 2 diabetes are learned from their family, so behavior change often becomes a family affair. Specific nutrition intervention strategies are available for youths who have type 2 diabetes. A normal goal is to strive for balance and variety in food choices.

Decrease High-Calorie, High-Fat, and Low-Nutrition Food and Beverages

Dietetics professionals should encourage caregivers to provide lower-calorie drink and snack alternatives to help youths avoid feeling deprived of favorite higher calorie and fat foods, which in turn can decrease the desire to hide or sneak food. Similarly, youths with type 2 diabetes should be encouraged to drink only water between meals and snacks; this will decrease excessive empty calories (soda or fruit drinks).

Avoid Overconsumption

Youths with type 2 diabetes should be encouraged to eat only in designated dining areas (such as at the kitchen table) and to limit eating/drinking in bedrooms or in front of the television, which is often associated with overconsumption of high-calorie, high-fat foods. Plates or bowls should be used when eating all meals and snacks. Eating directly out of a box or bag is associated with overconsumption practices.

Reduce Fast Food, Carry-Out Meals, and Dining Out

If the youth cannot avoid eating out, the dietetics professional should discuss portion control and healthful alternatives to favorite selections, including condiments. With older adolescents, the dietetics professional should discuss how to make healthier choices from the food options at restaurants and school, especially a la carte items.

Increase Intake of Fruits, Vegetables, and Calcium-Rich Foods

The dietetics professional should encourage youths with type 2 diabetes to set a goal to consume at least five fruits and vegetables per day. Vegetables typically are not limited unless starchy vegetable consumption is excessive.

To control calories, youths should choose whole fruit rather than juice, because it is easy to drink juice in large quantities. Caretakers should be encouraged to offer new fruits or vegetables, and the youth should try at least two or three bites—they may be surprised to find that they actually like the fruit or vegetable. The family should be encouraged to consistently have fruits and vegetables available, because as foods become familiar, children are more apt to choose them. Dietetics professionals can help identify ways to incorporate more fruits and vegetables into meals and snacks for the whole family.

Youths with type 2 diabetes should strive for 3 to 4 servings per day of low-fat milk or low-fat, artificially sweetened yogurt. If calcium intake is minimal, supplementation may be warranted.

Strive for Regular Mealtimes

When possible, scattered eating patterns should be decreased. Dietetics professionals should encourage caregivers to establish specific meal and snack times, with a focus on sit-down family meals. Calories should be dis-

tributed between three meals, plus snacks if needed. Snacks may be necessary if there are more than 4 or 5 hours between meals. Breakfast should be encouraged for all family members because children model eating behaviors after older family members or caregivers.

Practice Portion Control

Youths with type 2 diabetes and their caregivers should be taught portion control based on the hand, with portion sizes measured in relation to the youth's hand (see Figure 15.1). Although not exact, this method is useful, particularly when away from home.

Get in Touch With Hunger Awareness and Fullness Cues

Getting in touch with one's hunger awareness takes time, but it helps children learn to eat only when truly hungry and to stop eating when full, rather than eating out of boredom, stress, or emotional refuge. The "clean plate club"—eating everything on the plate, even when full—should be discouraged.

Address Disordered Eating Patterns

Disordered eating patterns include closet eating or binge eating and can be triggered by emotional stressors, such as self-esteem issues or dealing with the diabetes diagnosis and associated weight issues. It is important to make youths feel that their self-worth has nothing to do with their weight status or diagnosis of diabetes. If disordered patterns are apparent, a mental health professional referral may be beneficial.

DIABETES MEDICATIONS

Insulin

Type 1 diabetes management depends on exogenous insulin injection because of cessation of endogenous insulin production. Insulin may be used to manage type 2 diabetes if blood glucose targets cannot be obtained through dietary modification, weight management, physical activity, and metformin (if appropriate). The insulin plan must be individualized based on weight, age, the meal plan and carbohydrate intake, physical activity, and blood glucose. For more information on insulin, see Chapter 9.

"Honeymoon" Period

After diagnosis with type 1 diabetes, approximately 70% of youths move into a remission phase, referred to as a "honeymoon" period, characterized by decreased insulin requirements (25). The honeymoon is highly variable in duration, lasting from a few weeks to 2 years. As endogenous insulin secretion declines, the amount of exogenous insulin required to maintain euglycemia steadily increases. Box 15.4 (25–27) outlines typical daily insulin doses. See Table 15.2 on frequently prescribed insulin plans in children. For more information on pathophysiology, see Chapter 4.

Insulin Adjustments With Growth and Development

During growth and development, frequent insulin adjustment is necessary. Younger, leaner children typically require less insulin to bring blood glucose levels into target ranges than older, heavier children. During adolescence, the hormonal and physiologic changes of puberty induce a state of insulin resistance (28). Metabolic control, as reflected by increasing A1C values, can deteriorate in some youths despite significantly higher insulin doses. Insulin requirements typically decrease after puberty.

As children grow, insulin and energy requirements grow as well. Some caregivers restrict energy in an effort to achieve desirable blood glucose control, when an insulin dose adjustment is often what's really needed. The dietetics professional should discourage energy restriction because it could affect linear growth. See Table 15.3 (29) on factors affecting total daily dose.

TABLE 15.3 Factors Affecting Total Daily Insulin Dose

Characteristic of Youth with Diabetes	Insulin Requirements
In honeymoon period	Decrease
Thin	Decrease
Obese	Increase
Athletic	Decrease
Sedentary lifestyle	Increase
On summer break	Decrease
When school is in session	Increase
Puberty	Increase
Steroid use	Increase

Source: Data are from reference 29.

Injection Sites

Injection sites for children are the same as those for adults. Caregivers of young children are often counseled to use the legs, arms, and upper/outer quadrant of the buttocks. Although youths with little adipose tissue may benefit from use of short needles, overweight children may receive better insulin absorption from half-inch needles.

Older children who self-inject should have their injection sites checked at every medical appointment. Self-injecting youths often do not rotate injection sites well because repeated injections in the same site do not hurt as much. However, overused injection sites that become thickened (hypertrophied) do not absorb insulin as effectively.

Insulin Pump Therapy

Because many young children and teens consume three meals and multiple snacks throughout the day, an insulin plan can consist of more than four injections per day (9). Many families are reluctant to commit to this many injections (9), and insulin pump therapy is becoming a popular alternative to multiple daily injections (30). (See Chapter 9 for further information on insulin pump therapy.) Adult support at home and school is essential for success with diabetes management in youths. This support is especially necessary with pump therapy until the youth is able to manage diabetes independently (31).

Hypoglycemia

Hypoglycemia is more difficult to predict, prevent, and recognize in young children than in adults. In infants, signs of hypoglycemia include crying, irritability, clammy

BOX 15.4

Typical Total Daily Insulin Dose

Most children:
approximately 1 U/kg body weight/day

A range of 0.5 to 1.5 U/kg body weight/day is acceptable and allows for individual differences based on eating habits, age, activity level, and metabolic requirements. After the honeymoon period has ended, typically 40%–60% of the total daily dose is used as basal insulin; the remainder is used for mealtime boluses.

Adolescents: 1.5–3.0 U/kg body weight/day

Honeymoon phase: 0.2 to 0.6 U/kg body weight/day

Source: Data are from references 25–27.

skin, pallor, sleepiness, restless sleep, listlessness, hunger, tachycardia, dilated pupils, and/or shakiness. In toddlers, common signs are stumbling, uncoordinated gate, and/or inactivity.

Treatment for hypoglycemia includes 10 to 15 g of carbohydrate, waiting 10 to 15 minutes, and repeating treatment if symptoms persist. Appropriate carbohydrate sources for hypoglycemia treatment in infants include 1 to 2 teaspoons Karo syrup (5 to 10 g carbohydrate); 4 oz undiluted baby fruit juice (15 g carbohydrate); and one tube cake gel (12 g carbohydrate). Appropriate carbohydrate sources for hypoglycemia treatment in children include ½ cup apple or orange juice (15 g carbohydrate); 3 teaspoons honey (15 g carbohydrate; note that honey is not recommended for use in children under the age of 2 years because of botulism risk); 2 tablespoons raisins (15 g carbohydrate); glucose gel tube (15 g carbohydrate); or three to four glucose tablets (15 g carbohydrate). Severe hypoglycemia should be treated with glucagon or intravenous glucose.

Oral Diabetes Medication

Metformin is the only oral diabetes medication approved for use in the United States in children older than 10 years (see Chapter 8) and is appropriate only for use in type 2 diabetes. Metformin can be added if blood glucose goals are not met through dietary modification, weight management, and physical activity. Treatment with both metformin and insulin can be used to target insulin resistance and insulin deficiency.

PHYSICAL ACTIVITY

Regular physical activity is an important component of diabetes management and long-term cardiovascular health, especially in type 2 diabetes, because activity helps to decrease insulin resistance, to increase insulin sensitivity, and to maintain a desirable weight. Youths with diabetes can participate fully in all types of physical activity. The key to long-term adherence to physical activity is finding an activity in which the child is interested. Aerobic exercise and flexibility for all youths, as well as strength training for older adolescents, can be part of a healthy exercise prescription.

For youths beginning an exercise program, particularly those who are overweight, the exercise prescribed should be suited to the physical ability of the child (32). Adolescents with a BMI in the 85th to 95th percentiles can participate in weight-bearing aerobic activities, such as walking, roller-blading, stair climbing, jumping rope, swimming, field sports, basketball, tennis, and martial arts (33). Adolescents with a BMI above the 95th percentile can engage in primarily non-weight-bearing aerobic activities, including strength-aerobic circuit training (done lying if needed), swimming, cycling (including recline bike), arm-ergometer (crank), and chair aerobics. These may be especially beneficial if the youths have joint problems. Some individuals may be able to participate in arm-specific aerobic dancing and interval walking (walking with rests as needed, working up to longer periods without rests) (33). Supervision by a trained exercise professional may be recommended.

Family support and commitment to physical activity reinforces its importance to youths. When regular physical activity is initiated early in life, there is a greater chance that it will become a lifelong habit (33,34).

Tips

Tips to help children and adolescents stay physically active include making the home environment suitable for active play, both inside and out. Caregivers should plan weekends around family fun and fitness. The youth will not feel that physical activity is a punishment if the whole family participates.

Dietetics professionals should find physical activities that the youth enjoys and should set goals for the type of activity, frequency, and length. Initial physical activity goals should be set at a minimum, to encourage feelings of success, then should be revised to increase time and intensity. Overall, any movement is better than none.

To increase willingness to participate, exercise should be mixed with another activity the youth enjoys. For instance, if the youth likes music, he or she may agree to walk the length of a favorite CD three times per week after school. Because a number of minutes is not attached to the physical activity, it is often better received.

Sedentary screen time (such as television, video games, or computer) should be limited to less than 2 hours per day. Interest in other hobbies and activities should be encouraged. When watching television, youths should be encouraged to be physically active during commercials (such as doing jumping jacks or jogging in place). If the home has exercise equipment, such as a treadmill or a stationary bicycle, the equipment can be placed in front of the television so that the youth can get physical activity while watching television.

Youths should walk briskly and use a pedometer to track steps per day, working to increase daily movement.

Caregivers should be encouraged to take a turn wearing the pedometer, too. Any involvement in activities, sports-related or not, can help the youth feel part of something, increase movement, and enhance self-esteem.

Risk for Hypoglycemia

Because hypoglycemia can result from physical activity in individuals treated with insulin, additional carbohydrate may be needed before exercise (see Chapter 7). Increased blood glucose monitoring during physical activity can help prevent exercise-induced hypoglycemia by alerting the individual to blood glucose changes, thereby allowing for appropriate adjustments in carbohydrate intake and/or insulin, to maintain blood glucose levels.

Individuals who are present during the youth's physical activity, whether it is gym class, recess, or sports, should be made aware of the symptoms and treatment of hypoglycemia (including glucagon). The youth should be encouraged to continue to wear a medical ID, such as a nylon bracelet, during exercise. A blood glucose monitor and hypoglycemia treatment should always be readily available during physical activity.

The youth and caregivers should be aware of the delayed blood glucose-lowering effect of physical activity. This is of particular concern after exercise in the late afternoon or evening, which can lead to increased risk for nocturnal hypoglycemia. Increased blood glucose monitoring at bedtime and at 2 or 3 am after physical activity may help prevent postexercise late-onset hypoglycemia. Additional carbohydrate at bedtime and/or at 2 or 3 am may be required. The physician can recommend insulin dose adjustments for extended sports practices or sports camps, to prevent hypoglycemia.

The dietetics professional should work with the youth, caregiver, and other members of the health care team to ensure that a plan for carbohydrate and insulin adjustment is in place for scheduled physical activity (such as gym days at school); during random, unplanned activity (such as playing hard at a friend's house); and during other physical activity scenarios (such as field day at school).

SELF-MONITORING OF BLOOD GLUCOSE

Blood glucose monitoring provides feedback on treatment effectiveness and guidance in balancing food intake, diabetes medication, and activity. Using the term blood glucose "checks" rather than blood glucose "tests" removes the perception that the individual is being "graded" on this aspect of diabetes management.

The dietetics professional should emphasize that a result is not "good" or "bad" but is simply an indication of the blood glucose level at a point in time.

Blood Glucose Goals

Blood glucose goals for youths are individualized based on age, ability to recognize hypoglycemic symptoms, history of severe hypoglycemia or seizures, and self-management skills. The overall goal is to achieve an A1C as close to normal as possible, without frequent or severe hypoglycemia. Children who are too young to recognize and report symptoms may have a higher target, such as 100 to 200 mg/dL, to prevent frequent or severe hypoglycemia (9,24). See Table 15.4 (9) for suggested blood glucose goals based on age.

Timing and Frequency

Timing and frequency of blood glucose monitoring should be tailored to the individual child. In general, the recommended frequency for blood glucose monitoring for children is before each meal and before the bedtime snack, with an increase in monitoring frequency during illness, ketosis, hyper- or hypoglycemia, and with changes in schedule or physical activity (24).

TABLE 15.4 Blood Glucose Goals Based on Age*

Age Group	Fasting Goal, mg/dL	Before Bed Goal, mg/dL	A1C, %
Toddlers and preschoolers (< 6 y)	100–180	110–200	< 8.5 (but > 7.5)
School age (6–12 y)	90–180	100–180	< 8
Adolescents and young adults (13–19 y)	90–150	90–150	< 7.5[†]

*Key concepts in setting glycemic goals:

- Goals should be individualized and lower goals may be reasonable on benefit-risk assessment.
- Blood glucose goals should be higher than those listed above in children with frequent hypoglycemia or hypoglycemia unawareness.
- Postprandial blood glucose values should be measured when there is a disparity between preprandial blood glucose values and A1C levels.

[†]A lower goal (< 7.0%) is reasonable if it can be achieved without excessive hypoglycemia.
Source: Data are from reference 9.

When evaluating postmeal glycemia, blood glucose should be checked 2 hours postprandial. Many adolescents consume high-fat foods frequently. The caregiver or youth should have an understanding of fat's effect of delaying gastric emptying, which can result in prolonged blood glucose elevation after a high-fat meal.

A blood glucose check at 2 or 3 am can be useful after hypoglycemia, if morning values are erratic, or if the typical physical activity or eating patterns have changed. Monitoring blood glucose around 3 am is often recommended on a weekly basis for youths in optimal glycemic control or who use pump therapy or multiple injections.

Caretakers of infants and toddlers must rely on frequent blood glucose monitoring to distinguish normal behaviors from symptoms of hypoglycemia. Adolescents who drive should always check their blood glucose before operating a vehicle and at 2-hour intervals while driving, keeping testing supplies and hypoglycemia treatment readily available.

Record Keeping

Blood glucose log books or computerized downloads help determine whether the youth is receiving a balance of food, physical activity, and medication, to achieve optimal blood glucose control (see Chapter 11). Many youths use more than one monitor (eg, one for school, one for home, and one in the sports duffle bag). Blood glucose values consistently out of range should be brought to the health care provider's attention, so that adjustments in food or insulin can be made.

MANAGEMENT OF DYSLIPIDEMIA

Research has shown that the atherosclerotic process linked with cardiovascular disease begins in childhood and is associated with elevated blood cholesterol values (35–38). Identified risk factors contributing to the early onset of coronary heart disease in youths include the following (35,39):

- Elevated low-density lipoprotein cholesterol levels
- Family history of premature coronary heart disease (younger than 55 years)
- Cardiovascular disease
- Peripheral vascular disease
- Smoking
- Hypertension
- High-density lipoprotein cholesterol levels below 35 mg/dL
- Overweight
- Physical inactivity

See Box 15.5 (35) for the screening and management of dyslipidemia in youths with diabetes.

BOX 15.5

Management of Dyslipidemia in Youth with Diabetes

Screening

After glycemic control is achieved

Type 1
   Obtain lipid profile at diagnosis and then, if normal, every 5 years
   Begin at age 12 years (or onset of puberty, if earlier)
   Begin prior to age 12 (if prepubertal) only if positive family history

Type 2
   Obtain lipid profile at diagnosis and then every 2 years

Goals
LDL < 100 mg/dL
HDL > 35 mg/dL
Triglycerides < 150 mg/dL

Treatment Strategies
   Diet
   Maximize glycemic control
   Weight reduction, if indicated
   Medications
      Age > 10 years
      LDL ≥ 160 mg/dL
      LDL 130–159 mg/dL: consider based on CVD risk profile
      Statins ± resins
      Fibric acid derivatives if triglycerides > 1,000 mg/dL

Manage Other Cardiovascular Risk Factors
Blood pressure
Tobacco
Obesity
Inactivity

Source: Copyright © 2003 American Diabetes Association. From American Diabetes Association. Position statement: management of dyslipidemia in children and adolescents with diabetes. *Diabetes Care.* 2003;26:2194–2197. Reprinted with permission from the American Diabetes Association.

SCHOOL RESOURCES

The NDEP has worked with several other diabetes, education, and health organizations to develop *Helping the Student With Diabetes Succeed: A Guide for School Personnel* (40). The guide is designed to educate school personnel about diabetes, particularly type 1 diabetes, and to share a set of practices that enable schools to provide a safe environment for students with diabetes. It includes a primer on the basics of diabetes management; it lays out the roles and responsibilities of key school personnel, parents, and students with diabetes; it includes tools to help implement effective diabetes management; and it offers an overview of federal laws that address school responsibilities to students with diabetes. The resource can be downloaded from the NDEP Web site (40) for use by school personnel, healthcare workers, and parents. All sections of the guide can be reproduced and distributed with no copyright restrictions.

SUMMARY

- In the past, young children and adolescents in the United States have been affected almost exclusively with type 1 diabetes. However, with the increased prevalence of childhood obesity, type 2 diabetes, formerly seen only in adults, is now on the rise.
- A comprehensive assessment, including an evaluation of growth and current diabetes self-care, is crucial on an ongoing basis for youths with type 1 or type 2 diabetes.
- Interventions for the management of youths with type 1 or type 2 diabetes include nutrition, physical activity, self-monitoring of blood glucose, and medication, if appropriate.
- The key to achieving optimal blood glucose control during the years of dramatic growth is effectively balancing fluctuating food intake, diabetes medication, and physical activity.
- Family involvement and school cooperation are important support systems for youths with diabetes.
- When developing an individualized food plan, the dietetics professional should attempt to engage the youth in the discussion, even though it may be easier to develop the food plans based on responses from the caregiver, without much input from the individual with diabetes.

REFERENCES

1. American Diabetes Association. Position statement: diabetes care in the school and day care setting. *Diabetes Care.* 2004;27(Suppl 1):S122–S128.

2. Rosenbloom AL, Joe JR, Young RS, Winter WE. Emerging epidemic of type 2 diabetes in youth. *Diabetes Care.* 1999;22:345–354.

3. Arslanian SA. Type 2 diabetes mellitus in children: pathophysiology and risk factors. *J Pediatr Endocrinol Metab.* 2000;13:1385–1394.

4. American Diabetes Association. Consensus statement on type 2 diabetes in children and adolescents. *Diabetes Care.* 2000;23:381–389.

5. Rocchini AP. Childhood obesity and a diabetes epidemic. *N Engl J Med.* 2002;346:854–855.

6. Shim M, Geffner M. Insulin resistance in children. *Endocrinologist.* 1999;9:270–276.

7. Fagot-Campagna A. Emergence of type 2 diabetes mellitus in children: epidemiological evidence. *J Pediatr Endocrinol Metab.* 2000;13(Suppl 6):S1395–S1402.

8. American Diabetes Association. Position statement: evidence-based nutrition principles and recommendations for the treatment and prevention of diabetes and related complications. *J Am Diet Assoc.* 2002;102:109–118.

9. American Diabetes Association. Position statement: care of children and adolescents with type 1 diabetes. *Diabetes Care.* 2005;28:186–212.

10. Krebs NF, Jacobson MS; American Academy of Pediatrics Committee on Nutrition. Prevention of pediatric overweight and obesity. *Pediatrics.* 2003;112:424–430.

11. Centers for Disease Control and Prevention. 2000 CDC growth charts. Available at: http://www.cdc.gov/growthcharts. Accessed October 26, 2004.

12. Barone MA, ed. *The John Hopkins University Harriet Lane Handbook: A Manual for Pediatric House Officers.* 14th ed. St Louis, Mo: Mosby; 1996:204–205.

13. Kreipe RE, Kodjo C. Adolescent medicine. In: Behrman RE, Kliegman RM, eds. *Nelson Essentials of Pediatrics.* 4th ed. Philadelphia, Pa: WB Saunders; 2002:226–262.

14. Green Pastors J, Holler H. Management of diabetes: different life stages. In: *Diabetes Medical Nutrition Therapy.* Chicago, Ill: American Dietetic Association; 1997: 61–73.

15. Chase P. Blood glucose testing and responsibilities of children at different ages. In: Chase P. *Understanding Insulin-Dependent Diabetes.* 9th ed. Denver, Colo: Children's Diabetes Foundation at Denver; 1999:31–34,161–168.

16. On the homefront: living with one another, living with diabetes. In: *Caring for Young Children Living With Diabetes.* Boston, Mass: Joslin Diabetes Center; 1996:53–56.

17. Barlow SE, Dietz WH. Obesity evaluation and treatment: expert committee recommendations. The Maternal and Child Health Bureau, Health Resources and Services Administration and the Department of Health and Human Services. *Pediatrics.* 1998;102:E29.

18. American Diabetes Association. Position statement: standards of medical care in diabetes. *Diabetes Care.* 2004; 27(suppl):S15–S35.

19. American Diabetes Association. *Maximizing the Role of Nutrition in Diabetes Management*. Alexandria, Va.: American Diabetes Association; 1994.

20. *Being Healthy Rocks!* Minneapolis, Minn: International Diabetes Center; 2002.

21. National Diabetes Education Program. Tips for kids with type 2 diabetes: eat healthy foods. Available at: http://ndep.nih.gov/diabetes/pubs/Youth_Tips_Eat.pdf. Accessed October 21, 2004.

22. National Diabetes Education Program. Tips for kids with type 2 diabetes: stay at a healthy weight. Available at: http://ndep.nih.gov/diabetes/pubs/Youth_Tips_Weight.pdf. Accessed October 21, 2004.

23. National Diabetes Education Program. Tips for kids with type 2 diabetes: what is diabetes? Available at: http://ndep.nih.gov/diabetes/pubs/Youth_Tips_Diabetes.pdf. Accessed October 21, 2004.

24. Betschart Roemer J, McGee T. Type 1 diabetes in youth. In: *A Core Curriculum for Diabetes Education: Diabetes in the Life Cycle and Research*. 5th ed. Chicago, Ill: American Association of Diabetes Educators; 2003:33–62.

25. Drash A. Management of the child with diabetes mellitus: clinical course, therapeutic strategies, and monitoring techniques. In: Lifshitz F, ed. *Pediatric Endocrinology: A Clinical Guide*. 2nd ed. New York, NY: Marcel Dekker; 1990:681–700.

26. Campbell RK, White JR. *Medications for Treatment of Diabetes*. Chicago, Ill: American Dietetic Association; 2000:14–15.

27. Skyler JS, ed. *Medical Management of Type 1 Diabetes*. 3rd ed. Alexandria, Va: American Diabetes Association, 1998.

28. Tamborlane WV, Gatcomb PM, Savoye M, Ahern J. Type 1 diabetes in children. In: Lebovitz HE, ed. *Therapy for Diabetes Mellitus and Related Disorders*. 3rd ed. Alexandria, Va: American Diabetes Association; 1998:61–69.

29. Campbell RK, White JR. *Medications for the Treatment of Diabetes*. Alexandria, Va: American Diabetes Association; 2000:14–16.

30. Ahern JA, Boland EA, Doane R, Ahern JJ, Rose P, Vincent M, Tamborlane WV: Insulin pump therapy in pediatrics: a therapeutic alternative to safely lower HbA1C levels across all age-groups. *Pediatr Diabetes*. 2002;3:10–15.

31. Weissberg-Benchell J, Antisdel-Lomaglio J, Seshadri R: Insulin pump therapy: a meta-analysis. *Diabetes Care*. 2003;26:1079–1087.

32. Franz M. Diabetes and exercise: guidelines for safe and enjoyable activity. *Diabetes Care*. 1994;17:924–937.

33. Sothern MS, von Almen TK, Schumacher H. *Trim Kids*. New York, NY: HarperResource; 2001.

34. Sothern MS, Schumacher H, von Almen TK, Carlisle LK, Udall JN. Committed to kids: an integrated, 4-level team approach to weight management in adolescents. *J Am Diet Assoc*. 2002;102(3 Suppl):S81–S85.

35. American Diabetes Association. Position statement: management of dyslipidemia in children and adolescents with diabetes. *Diabetes Care*. 2003;26:2194–2197.

36. Berenson G, Srinivasan S, Bao W, Newman W, Tracy R, Wattigney W, for the Bogalusa Heart Study. Association between multiple cardiovascular risk factors and atherosclerosis in children and young adults. *N Engl J Med*. 1998;338:1650–1656.

37. Newman W, Freedman D, Voors A, Gard P, Srinivasan S, Cresanta J, Williamson GD, Webber L, Berenson G. Relation of serum lipoprotein levels and systolic blood pressure to early atherosclerosis. *N Engl J Med*. 1986;314:138–144.

38. Strong J, Malcolm G, McMahan CA, Tracy R, Newman W, Herderick E, Cornhill JF, for the Pathobiological Determinants of Atherosclerosis in Youth Research Group (PDAY). Prevalence and extent of atherosclerosis in adolescents and young adults: implications for prevention from the Pathobiological Determinants of Atherosclerosis in Youth Study. *JAMA*. 1999;281:727–735.

39. Miller J, Silverstein J. Cardiovascular risk factors in children. *Practical Diabetology*. 2004;23(2):13–18.

40. US Department of Health and Human Services. Helping the student with diabetes succeed: a guide for school personnel. Available at: http://www.ndep.nih.gov/diabetes/pubs/Youth_NDEPSchoolGuide.pdf. Accessed October 25, 2004.

ADDITIONAL RESOURCES

American Diabetes Association Youth Zone Web site. Available at: http://www.diabetes.org/youthzone/youth-zone.jsp. Accessed October 27, 2004.

Betschart-Roemer J. *Diabetes Care for Babies, Toddlers, and Preschoolers: A Reassuring Guide*. New York, NY: John Wiley & Sons; 1998.

Betschart-Roemer J. *A Magic Ride in Foozbah-Land: An Inside Look at Diabetes*. New York: John Wiley & Sons; 1998.

Betschart-Roemer J, Thom S. *In Control: A Guide for Teens With Diabetes*. New York, NY: John Wiley & Sons; 1998.

Brackenridge BP, Rubin RR. *Sweet Kids: How to Balance Diabetes Control and Good Nutrition With Family Peace*. Alexandria, Va: American Diabetes Association; 2002.

Chase HP. *Understanding Insulin Dependent Diabetes*, 10th ed. Denver, Colo: Children's Diabetes Foundation; 2002.

Children With Diabetes Web site. Available at: http://www.childrenwithdiabetes.com/index_cwd.htm. Accessed October 27, 2004.

Digiwalker (pedometers). Available at: http://www.digiwalker.com. Accessed January 22, 2005.

Evert A. Nutrition FYI: tools and techniques for working with young people with diabetes. *Diabetes Spectrum*. 2004;17:8–13.

First Step (pedometers). Available at: http://www. firststepprogram.com. Accessed October 27, 2004.

Geil PB, Ross TA. *Cooking Up Fun for Kids With Diabetes.* Alexandria, Va: American Diabetes Association; 2003.

Juvenile Diabetes Research Foundation International Kids' Web Site. Available at: http://kids.jdrf.org. Accessed October 27, 2004.

KidsRPumping Web site. Available at: http://members.aol. com/CamelsRFun. Accessed October 27, 2004.

Learn About Diabetes Web site. Available at: http://www. KidsLearnAboutDiabetes.org. Accessed October 27, 2004.

New Lifestyles (pedometers). Available at: http://www. new-lifestyles.com. Accessed October 27, 2004.

Pump Girls Web site. Available at: http://www.pumpgirls. com. Accessed October 27, 2004.

Rubin R, Bierman H, Toohey B. *Psyching Out Diabetes: A Positive Approach to Your Negative Emotions.* 3rd ed. New York, NY: McGraw-Hill; 1999.

Siminerio LM, Betschart J. *Guide to Raising a Child With Diabetes.* New York, NY: McGraw-Hill; 1999.

USDA Team Nutrition Web site. Available at: http://www. fns.usda.gov/tn. Accessed October 27, 2004.

Weight-control Information Network (WIN) Web site. Available at: http://www.niddk.nih.gov/health/nutrit/win. htm. Accessed October 27, 2004.

Wysocki T. *The Ten Keys to Helping Your Child Grow Up With Diabetes.* 2nd ed. Alexandria, Va: American Diabetes Association; 2004.

16

Diabetes in Older Adults

Sue McLaughlin RD, CDE

CHAPTER OVERVIEW

- Life expectancy in the United States has increased since the beginning of the 20th century. By 2030, the number of adults age 65 years and older will likely more than double the number in 2000, to approximately 71.5 million (1).
- Older adults, defined here as those older than 65 years, are frequently challenged by at least one chronic health condition; many have multiple health conditions. Diabetes, particularly type 2, is a major health care problem for older Americans that is often underdiagnosed and undertreated.
- By 2030, nearly 40% of adults older than 65 years will have either impaired glucose tolerance or diabetes; minority groups will likely comprise a disproportionate segment of this population (2).
- Diabetes in older individuals presents personal and health care costs. In 1997, two-thirds of the costs attributable to diabetes inpatient care, outpatient services, and nursing home care were related to the care of elders with diabetes (3).
- Intervention strategies for managing diabetes in older adults include nutrition therapy, medication, physical activity, and self-monitoring of blood glucose. Because few older adults have had previous diabetes education, and many may have poor

nutritional status, a thorough assessment and individualized nutrition intervention are particularly important, to evaluate diabetes knowledge and misconceptions as well as current nutrition needs.

DIABETES PREVALENCE

The risk of developing diabetes increases with age. The prevalence of diabetes is higher among elderly African Americans, Hispanics, Pima Indians, Micronesians, Scandinavians, and male Japanese than among whites (4). The same diagnostic criteria are used for all adults (see Chapter 4).

Glucose intolerance is one of many factors that have contributed to the dramatically increased prevalence of type 2 diabetes among older adults. Although glucose intolerance is not inevitable, it has been noted to rise, particularly after 75 years of age, in the United States (5,6). Other factors for the development of type 2 diabetes include the following (7):

- Increasing age
- Genetics
- Sedentary lifestyle
- Body composition
- Coexisting medical conditions
- Multiple medications

BOX 16.1

Nutrition Therapy Considerations for Older Adults

- Energy needs are less for older adults than for younger adults.
- Physical activity for older adults should be encouraged.
- Undernutrition in older adults is common; adequate intake should be a goal.
- Weight loss should be recommended with caution because medications may require dose adjustments.
- Residents of long-term-care facilities do not require restriction of sweets. They should be served regular (unrestricted) menus, with consistency in the amount and timing of carbohydrate.
- There is no evidence to support use of "no concentrated sweets" diets.

Source: Data are from reference 9.

NUTRITION THERAPY GOALS

Nutrition recommendations for older adults with diabetes must be extrapolated from what is known for the general population, because there is virtually no research on changes in nutrition needs of aging individuals with diabetes. See Chapter 6 for the goals of nutrition therapy that apply to all individuals with diabetes. A goal specific to older adults is to provide for the nutrition and psychosocial needs of the aging individual (8). Box 16.1 presents key nutrition therapy considerations for the older adult population (9).

PSYCHOSOCIAL ASSESSMENT

Older adults face a number of biological changes and psychosocial issues, which affect their ability to manage diabetes well. Psychosocial issues that shape the quality of life and diabetes management in older adults include the following:

- Depression
- Stress and anxiety
- Support systems
- Abuse
- Safety issues
- Living conditions
- Transportation difficulties
- Financial concerns
- Alcohol and drug abuse
- Sexuality
- Cultural practices
- Health beliefs
- Cognition changes/dementia

NUTRITION ASSESSMENT AND INTERVENTIONS

Malnutrition

Malnutrition affects a large number of older adults, including those with diabetes. Nutrition screening programs in a variety of institutional and community settings have reported malnutrition risk rates ranging from 25% to 85% in the elderly population as a whole (10).

Malnutrition can be either overnutrition or undernutrition, and it can be caused by physiological changes of aging, poor dentition, poor glycemic control, food insecurity, physical disabilities, medications, alcohol use, social isolation, boredom, depression, or other psychosocial issues. Many older adults are at risk for food insecurity, or rather the inability to afford or obtain food (11). In a study by Nelson et al (12), food insecurity was present in 25% of subjects with diabetes. Of the individuals who reported having hypoglycemia in the past year, half attributed this to the inability to afford food.

Long-term-care residents and hospitalized individuals are at increased risk for malnutrition. Underweight is more problematic than overweight, particularly in long-term care, and is associated with increased morbidity and mortality (8).

Appropriate interventions include the following:

- Screening regularly for signs of malnutrition
- Referring to social worker, state agencies, or senior congregate meal sites, if appropriate
- Implementing liberalized meal plans, including a consistent carbohydrate approach (see Chapter 18)
- Maintaining weight and preventing deterioration in overall health status as a goal for most long-term-care residents
- Anticipating financial costs associated with any dietary changes and providing alternative low-cost strategies as needed

Weight change is likely the most reliable indicator of poor nutritional status in older adults (8). Generally, an unintentional gain or loss of more than 10 lb or 10% of body weight in less than 6 months indicates need for further investigation (8).

Decreased Energy Requirements

Although energy requirements for older adults decrease by 10% to 20%, other nutrient needs remain constant or increase (4). Interventions to consider include basing meal plans on the diet history; increasing physical activity, if possible; evaluating need for weight loss carefully; and evaluating need for multivitamin/mineral supplements, to prevent deficiencies.

Hyperglycemia and Nutrient Deficiencies

Chronic hyperglycemia heightens the risk for protein-energy malnutrition, as well as micronutrient deficiencies. Older adults are at risk for nutrient deficiencies. The most common deficiencies are calcium, zinc, magnesium, vitamins A and D, and water-soluble vitamins. If appropriate, dietetics professionals should recommend a multivitamin and mineral supplement and should refer the individual for further laboratory testing to identify nutrient status and deficiencies. Other interventions are providing counsel regarding food and beverage choices, to boost intake of deficient nutrients, and referring to a social worker regarding financial concerns impacting food/beverage intake.

Dehydration

In older adults, the risk for dehydration increases because of changes in thirst perception and access to fluids. Hospitalized individuals and residents of long-term-care facilities are at increased risk of dehydration. Appropriate interventions include encouraging and monitoring fluid intake, and improving glycemic control to prevent fluid losses through polyuria.

Increased Protein Needs

Protein needs can be increased, because of the aging process, wound healing, infection, and other stresses. Appropriate interventions include adjusting diet and considering nutrition supplements, such as protein powder and supplements specifically for individuals with diabetes.

Cardiovascular Disease and Decline in Renal Function

In an older adult population, cardiovascular disease and decline in renal function can be observed. Interventions to consider include evaluating risk for coronary heart disease or stroke versus malnutrition before prescribing a modified fat diet, and monitoring hydration for renal function.

Constipation

Constipation due to inadequate fiber intake may result from decreased intake of plant products because of dentition changes, gastrointestinal disorder, or financial limits. Dietetics professionals should watch for terminal reservoir syndrome. An intervention for constipation is a gradual increase in fiber, with accompanying fluid intake. Fiber supplements may be helpful.

Alcohol Abuse

Alcohol abuse affects 10% of community dwellers and 40% of those in long-term-care facilities (13) and may cause nutrient deficiencies. Dietetics professionals should address abuse issues, as with other adults.

Hypertension

Adults who are sensitive to sodium are at increased risk of hypertension with high sodium intake. Individuals with a systolic blood pressure of 130 to 139 mm Hg or a diastolic blood pressure of 80 to 89 mm Hg should receive lifestyle and behavioral therapy alone for a maximum of 3 months. If targets are not achieved, then they should also be treated with a pharmacologic agent (14). Individuals with systolic blood pressure above 140 mm Hg or diastolic blood pressure above 90 mm Hg should receive drug therapy in addition to lifestyle and behavior therapy (14). In elderly hypertensive individuals, blood pressure should be lowered gradually to avoid complications (14). Nutrition interventions should focus on sodium reduction (particularly in individuals who are sensitive to sodium), reduced alcohol consumption, the Dietary Approaches to Stop Hypertension (DASH) eating plan (see Chapter 22), and regular aerobic physical activity.

THE VALUE OF A THOROUGH ASSESSMENT

Recognition of the biological changes, psychosocial issues, and nutritional concerns through a thorough assessment helps to ensure that the treatment plan meets the older adult's needs and promotes an improved quality of life. Because many older adults may not have had previous diabetes education, an assessment can also evaluate their level of knowledge about diabetes, in order to provide updated information and to clarify any misconceptions. See Table 16.1 (4,9,14,15) for assessment data and considerations.

TABLE 16.1 Assessment Data and Considerations for Older Adults

Areas to Assess	Special Concerns and Considerations
Relevant medical history	• Multiple coexisting medical conditions and chronic complications may be present; related stressors affect glycemic control. • Many physiologic changes of aging resemble signs and symptoms of diabetes. • Older women with diabetes are at increased risk for urinary incontinence.
Medications	• Polypharmacy is common. • Multiple medications and multiple daily dose schedules lessen likelihood of adherence and increase risk of drug-drug and food-drug interactions.
Clinical data (laboratory values, height, weight)	• Age-related declines in organ function may cause elevated laboratory values, which require dietary modifications and preclude use of some diabetes medications. • Increased risk for malnutrition (overnutrition or undernutrition).
Usual food intake	• Food groups may be omitted because of financial constraints, digestive disturbances, dentition problems, and unawareness of new food products. • Lifelong habits are often hard to change.
Physical activity	• Decrease in physical activity is often due to decline in physical condition, safety level, or environment; individuals are at greater risk for injurious falls. • Increased chance for injury without proper conditioning; medical clearance is necessary.
Blood glucose monitoring skills	• Older adults can be comparable to younger counterparts in ability to perform blood glucose monitoring. • The meter should be matched to the individual with attention to visual acuity, manual dexterity, complexity of operation, and ability to obtain adequate sample.
Individual's goals and priorities	• Older adults exhibit typical adult learner characteristics. • Seemingly simple goals may require manipulation of many factors. • Goals/priorities are based on lifelong experiences and perspectives.
Knowledge, skill level, attitude, and motivation	• Knowledge, skills, attitudes, and motivation vary widely in older adults, as in younger individuals. • Disproportionate numbers of older adults have no past diabetes self-management education and skills training. • Many older adults have outdated or inaccurate information. • Motivation may be influenced by chronic complications and remaining years of life anticipated.
Self-efficacy	• An individual's history of perceived success or failure throughout a lifetime of challenges influences his or her beliefs regarding whether positive behavior change is realistic and achievable. • Maintaining independence is a priority for older adults.
Support systems/presence of caregivers	• Support and care are often lacking, because of the death of spouse or friends and poor proximity to other family members. • There is a strong correlation between high level of support from adult children and successful diabetes management.
Readiness to learn and change behaviors	• Readiness is affected by health status and multiple psychosocial issues, especially losses. • Cognitive and physical changes (such as memory, vision, or auditory losses) prevent reception or retention of information. • Prior life experiences may hinder learning.
Psychosocial and economic issues	• With age, there is increased incidence of cognitive changes, anxiety disorders, depression, social isolation, transportation difficulties, elder abuse, poverty, alcoholism, and drug abuse. • Older adults may experience a decline in their level of safety and social support. • Minority group elders are at greatest risk for problems.
Cultural influences	• Cultural beliefs may conflict with recommended diabetes treatment.

Source: Data are from references 4, 9, 14, and 15.

MANAGEMENT OF TYPE 1 AND TYPE 2 DIABETES

Clinical Goals

Older adults should understand what their individual target goals are for blood glucose, blood pressure, lipids, and other indexes, as well as the value in reaching the targets to promote improved health and quality of life. Targets should be individualized, recognizing that they may need adjustment, as the health condition of the older adult changes over time. Clinical goals should not be relaxed simply because of advanced age.

When setting and prioritizing individualized treatment goals, the concerns and considerations in Table 16.1 must be taken into account, particularly the priorities and quality of life of older adults. Treatment plans that are complicated, uncomfortable, or costly may result in harmful side effects, reduction in adherence to the plan, and a decrease in overall well-being.

Individuals who can be expected to live long enough to reap the benefits of long-term intensive diabetes management and who are cognitively intact, physically active, and willing to undertake the responsibility of self-management are encouraged to pursue intensive management (14). Older adults who have developed microvascular complications but are otherwise in good health are likely to benefit the most from intensive glycemic control (15).

Teaching Strategies

To teach older adults effectively, the following guidelines are recommended. First, dietetics professionals should perform a thorough assessment and prioritize needs. Similarly, dietetics professionals should screen for depression, anxiety, and decline in cognition, which interfere with learning.

Next, dietetics professionals are encouraged to allow the older adult to choose between one-on-one and group education. With the individual's permission, family and/or caregivers may be included in education sessions. It is beneficial for the dietetics professional to address the individual's concerns first, listen actively, and build on information the individual already knows. Because hyperglycemia impairs learning and retention, instruction should be simple in format.

Like all learners, adult learners benefit from the presentation of material in a variety of teaching formats. Dietetics professionals should adapt teaching style and materials to the individual and beware of ageism. It can be helpful for individuals to bring food labels and other products to their counseling sessions for discussion. For the purpose of demonstration, needed skills should be practiced, and return demonstrations should be observed. Frequent practice opportunities and role-playing of real-life scenarios are beneficial. Meaningful, practical information should be provided, and medical jargon should be avoided.

Individuals learn better when time is set aside for questions and written information for key points is provided for later reference. Using cues, such as pill boxes, timers, and calendars, enhances memory, as does repeating key points and providing concrete familiar examples. As a general rule, learning should be evaluated often, especially when hyperglycemia or cognitive or sensory deficits are present.

When cognitive losses are present, it is appropriate to include family and/or caregivers in the teaching session. The teaching pace should be slowed, with sentences kept short and simple. When teaching tasks, it is productive to begin with the simplest and progress toward the complex. As a general rule, messages should be focused, and teaching sessions should be kept to no more than 45 minutes. As a reminder, important points should be summarized more frequently.

When hearing loss is present, teaching one-on-one may be preferable. Visual and auditory distractions in the room should be eliminated. Sentences should be kept short and delivered slowly with clear enunciation. The dietetics professional should speak toward the ear with the best hearing. Visual aids and tactile learning are encouraged whenever possible. Key points should be repeated, and drawn or written out. It is advisable to avoid changing topics abruptly.

When visual impairment is present, a well-lit room for teaching and low-vision aids, such as magnifiers, are needed. The dietetics professional should use much detail in verbal explanations and should involve other senses, whenever possible. Written handouts in a 14-point or larger simple font and dark ink, printed on white or pale yellow paper without glare, are recommended.

Nutrition Therapy

As discussed earlier in this chapter, factors that deserve special consideration when providing nutrition intervention to older adults include malnutrition, decreased energy requirements, hyperglycemia, nutrient deficiencies, dehydration, increased protein needs, cardiovascular disease, decline in renal function, constipation, alcohol abuse, and hypertension. The meal planning approaches reviewed in Chapter 18 may be implemented with older adults, adapting written materials and teaching methods, as needed.

If weight reduction is needed, the benefits and risks should be evaluated with any weight loss achieved gradually. Conversely, to promote weight maintenance or weight gain, the following should be considered (4):

- Preference and lifelong eating habits
- Palatability
- Food purchase and preparation
- Finances
- Cultural preferences/religious practices (see Chapter 20 for meal planning for ethnic populations)

Diabetes Medications

Older adults with diabetes can typically be treated with the same diabetes medications as younger adults, although extra attention is required when prescribing and monitoring the medications. See Table 16.2 (4,14) for potential contraindications associated with the various diabetes medications. For further information on diabetes medications, see Chapters 8 and 9.

When selecting a diabetes medication, the potential benefits should be weighed against the potential risks. Factors to consider include the following:

- Simplicity of plan/feasibility of dosing
- Cost
- Other drugs that may interfere with effectiveness
- Comorbidities that may create contraindications
- Side effects, including hypoglycemia risk
- Effect on weight and lipids

The medication of choice should always be initiated at the lowest dose and titrated upward gradually until target blood glucose is achieved or side effects develop (14). Dietetics professionals should note that second-generation sulfonylureas are frequently used initially, because of their safety profiles.

Insulin may be indicated if maximal doses of oral diabetes medications do not achieve blood glucose targets, especially when hyperglycemia puts older adults at risk of a hyperosmolar state. Rapid-acting insulin can be beneficial to reduce the likelihood of hypoglycemia in those with variable food intake or unpredictable digestion or absorption (4).

The dietetics professional should emphasize that type 2 diabetes is a progressive disease and that progression to insulin therapy does not indicate personal failure. In many cases, it may be preferable to make medication

TABLE 16.2 Diabetes Medications: Potential Contraindications for Use in Older Adults

Drug Class	Potential Contraindications for Use
Sulfonylureas	Hypoglycemia risk—glyburide metabolites can be cleared more slowly in the very old; glipizide has a shorter half-life and fewer hepatic metabolites
Meglitinides	Frequent dosing required
Biguanides	Renal insufficiency Hepatic insufficiency Heart failure
Thiazolidinediones	Congestive heart failure
Alpha-glucosidase inhibitors	Gastrointestinal disease
Insulin	Hypoglycemia risk Poor visual and motor skills of the older adult or caregiver Poor cognition

Source: Data are from references 4 and 14.

changes to control blood glucose rather than impose food restrictions (8).

Tips on Increasing Medication Adherence

To increase medication adherence, dietetics professionals should consider including family members involved in an older adult's care in the teaching process. Teaching aids are particularly useful—for example, pill-dosing dispensers for oral diabetes medications; adaptive aids, such as pill cutters or syringe magnifiers; timers to prompt dosing; and calendars to track doses. Additional tips to consider include the following:

- Incorporating the medication schedule into the daily routine
- Reviewing the dosing instructions and ensuring that the older adult understands them
- Supervising practice of insulin injections for those with visual or motor problems
- Checking injection technique on a regular basis

Hypoglycemia

Evidence suggests that frail older adults are at higher risk for severe hypoglycemia and hypoglycemic coma than healthier, more functional adults (15). The following conditions put older adults at higher hypoglycemia risk (4):

- Renal changes
- Slowed hormonal counterregulation
- Inadequate hydration
- Polypharmacy
- Inadequate or erratic food intake
- Slowed intestinal absorption

The first symptoms of hypoglycemia in an older adult may be lightheadedness, unsteadiness, poor concentration, sweating, or trembling—all of which are often inappropriately attributed to normal aging, comorbidities, drug side effects, or cardiac or cerebrovascular causes. As a result, the dietetics professional should advise avoidance of sole reliance on hypoglycemic symptoms to indicate hypoglycemia; symptoms may even be absent.

Oral diabetes medications without hypoglycemic effects should be used when possible. If a medication with hypoglycemia risk is selected, a bedtime snack can help prevent nocturnal hypoglycemia. Keeping glucose tablets or other appropriate treatment by the bed for

nocturnal hypoglycemia treatment can help prevent falls from unsteadiness while seeking treatment.

For individuals with a history of severe hypoglycemia, higher blood glucose targets may be indicated, along with a check-in system (where those who live alone check in with a family member at a preappointed time). Expert consensus suggests that self-monitoring of blood glucose may reduce the risk of severe hypoglycemia in older adults who use insulin or oral diabetes medications. For more information on hypoglycemia, see Chapter 12.

Physical Activity

Physical activity should be encouraged if the individual is functionally and cognitively able to participate. Exercise offers several benefits for the older adult with diabetes (8), including the following (4):

- Reduction of the decline in maximal aerobic capacity that occurs with aging
- Improvement of atherosclerotic risk factors
- Slowing the decline in age-related lean body mass
- Decrease in central adiposity
- Improvement of insulin sensitivity
- Reversal of some microvascular changes

The physical activity plan should be based on the individual's interests, activity preferences, functional ability, and the presence of coexisting conditions (such as cardiovascular, neurological, or ophthalmologic). A reasonable starting goal is 10 minutes three times daily at 50% to 60% of maximum heart rate, with gradual increase (4). Physical limitations may be accommodated through armchair exercises, swimming, water aerobics, and stationary cycling. For more information on exercise, see Chapter 7.

Self-Monitoring of Blood Glucose

Older adults can learn to monitor as accurately as younger adults. Concerns associated with blood glucose monitoring among the older adult population include manual dexterity, vision, and memory (of the procedure and technique).

Monitoring technique should be routinely reviewed. There is no identified optimal timing and frequency of blood glucose monitoring for older adults; timing and frequency should be dictated by the individual's needs, goals, ability/willingness, anticipated longevity, and blood glucose control/glycemic symptoms. Multidisciplinary interventions that provide education on medication use, blood glucose monitoring, and recognizing hypo- and hyperglycemia can significantly improve glycemic control (14).

Dementia, certain cognitive disorders, memory, energy level, and quality of life have been shown to improve with blood glucose control (4). For individuals with advanced diabetes complications, with life-limiting comorbid illness or life expectancy of less than 5 years, with cognitive/functional impairment, and in whom the risk of intensive glycemic control outweighs the benefits, it is reasonable to set less intensive target glycemic and A1C goals (such as 8%) (14,15). Dietetics professionals should note that A1C is affected by hemoglobinopathies, such as anemia, which may occur among older adults.

Although blood glucose control is important, a greater reduction in morbidity and mortality may result from control of cardiovascular risk factors than from tight glycemic control. For more information on monitoring, see Chapter 10.

ADDITIONAL CONSIDERATIONS

Hyperglycemic Hyperosmolar Syndrome

Hyperglycemic hyperosmolar syndrome (HHS) is often overlooked and confused with other illnesses or conditions. It is characterized by a blood glucose level greater than 600 mg/dL without the presence of ketones. HHS is most often seen among the elderly with untreated or undertreated type 2 diabetes, particularly those in long-term-care facilities. Mortality is highest in the oldest individuals.

Constructing the individual environment to support routine hydration and adequate monitoring is important in the prevention of HHS, especially when the individual lives alone or is in a long-term-care facility. See Chapter 12 for more information on causes, symptoms, treatment, and prevention of HHS.

Concerns for Hospitalized Older Adults and Residents of Long-Term-Care Facilities

A large segment of the older population lives in long-term-care or assisted-living facilities. Individuals residing in these facilities are at increased risk for malnutrition and dehydration due to lack of food choices, poor food quality, and unnecessary restrictions, followed by a downward trend in the overall health condition (16–18).

Priorities of Care

Care for older adults during hospitalization or for those residing in long-term-care facilities should be based on the older adult's personal priorities and the family's priorities (4). Additional priorities of care include the following:

- Promoting the best possible glycemic control and eliminating symptoms associated with hyperglycemia.
- Achieving or maintaining optimal daily functioning.
- Providing adequate nutrition, to improve or prevent further decline in the current level of health and quality of life.
- Making medication changes rather than food adjustments in many instances, to manage glycemia (17).
- Balancing treatment with overall prognosis.

Meal Service

The imposition of dietary restrictions is not warranted, because of the increased risk for dehydration and malnutrition. Experience shows that residents eat better when provided with less restrictive diets; improved intake, in turn, helps promote healing and prevent further decline.

Long-term-care residents should be served the regular unrestricted menus, with consistency in the timing and amount of carbohydrate (17). Severe calorie restrictions should not be imposed, in an effort to control blood glucose because of the risk of malnutrition. Fat restrictions also are not indicated for the majority, because of the risk of malnutrition (17).

Dietetics professionals should individualize meal plans as needed, using blood glucose monitoring to evaluate the effectiveness of the nutrition care plan (17). Diabetes medication should be matched to food intake rather than the reverse.

Diabetes Teaching

Initial, or survival level, diabetes teaching may be provided to hospitalized individuals or to long-term-care residents. Whether diabetes education is appropriate for the long-term-care resident depends on a number of factors, including the following:

- Previous diabetes education history
- Current cognitive function
- Likelihood of discharge
- Involvement of caregivers

In long-term care, education is often best provided to caregivers, so that they can assist in management when the resident goes on outings or when food is brought into the facility. After discharge, survival skills education can be reinforced and expanded on in an outpatient setting.

SUMMARY

As the incidence of impaired glucose tolerance and diabetes continues to rise, and as Americans live longer, dietetics professionals will find an increasingly greater percentage of their clientele to be 65 years or older.

Older adults with diabetes are faced with many challenges, in addition to those related to diabetes management. It is critical that the health care team work closely with community agencies, organizations, and family members/support systems, to improve care and the quality of life for people with diabetes as they age.

Dietetics professionals can help improve the lives of older adults with diabetes by listening carefully, performing a thorough assessment, individualizing treatment recommendations, and providing guidance in setting goals that reflect positive changes in lifestyle habits and that promote desired outcomes.

REFERENCES

1. Older Americans 2004: Key Indicators of Well-Being. Available at: http://www.agingstats.gov. Accessed December 30, 2004.

2. *National Diabetes Fact Sheet, 2002*. Atlanta, Ga: Centers for Disease Control and Prevention; 2002.

3. American Diabetes Association. Economic consequences of diabetes mellitus in the U.S. in 1997. *Diabetes Care*. 1998;21:296–309.

4. Nettles AT. Diabetes in older adults. In: *A Core Curriculum for Diabetes Education: Diabetes in the Life Cycle and Research*. 5th ed. Chicago, Ill: American Association of Diabetes Educators; 2003:179–201.

5. Kenny SJ, Aubert RE, Geiss LS. Prevalence and incidence of non-insulin-dependent diabetes. In: *National Diabetes Data Group. Diabetes in America*. 2nd ed. Bethesda, Md: National Institutes of Health; 1995:49–52. NIH publication 95-1468.

6. Samos LF, Roos BA. Diabetes mellitus in older persons. *Med Clin North Am*. 1998;82:791–803.

7. Halter JB. *Diabetes Update: Elderly Patients with Non-Insulin Dependent Diabetes Mellitus*. Kalamazoo, Mich: Upjohn Co; 1990.

8. American Diabetes Association. Position statement: evidence-based nutrition principles and recommendations for the treatment and prevention of diabetes and related complications. *J Am Diet Assoc*. 2002;102:109–118.

9. *American Dietetic Association Medical Nutrition Therapy Evidence-Based Guides for Practice: Nutrition Practice Guidelines for Type 1 and Type 2 Diabetes* [CD-ROM]. Chicago, Ill: 2001.

10. Peter D. *National Survey on Nutrition Screening and Treatment for the Elderly*. Washington, DC: Hart Research Associates; 1993.

11. Position of the American Dietetic Association: domestic food and nutrition security. *J Am Diet Assoc*. 2002;102:1840–1847.

12. Nelson K, Brown ME, Lurie N. Hunger in an adult patient population. *JAMA*. 1998;279:1211–1214.

13. Egbert AM. The older alcoholic: recognizing the subtle clinical clues. *Geriatrics*. 1993;48:63–69.

14. American Diabetes Association. Position Statement: Standards of medical care in diabetes. *Diabetes Care*. 2005;28(Suppl 1):S4–S36.

15. Brown AF, Mangione CM, Saliba D, Sarkisian CA; California Healthcare Foundation/American Geriatrics Society Panel on Improving Care for Elders with Diabetes. Guidelines for improving the care of the older person with diabetes mellitus. *J Am Geriatr Soc*. 2003;51(suppl): S265–S280.

16. Elderweb. *Average Length of Nursing Home Stay*. Available at: http://www.elderweb.com/default.php?PageID= 2770. Accessed March 13, 2004.

17. American Diabetes Association. Position statement: diabetes nutrition recommendations for health care institutions. *Diabetes Care*. 2004;27(Suppl 1):S55–S57.

18. Position of the American Dietetic Association: liberalized diets for older adults in long-term care. *J Am Diet Assoc*. 2002;102:1316–1323.

ADDITIONAL RESOURCES

Administration on Aging Web site. Available at: http://www. aoa.gov. Accessed September 20, 2004.

American Diabetes Association Web site. Available at: http://www. diabetes.org. Accessed January 20, 2005.

American Diabetes Association. Evidence-based nutrition principles and recommendations for the treatment and prevention of diabetes and related complications (position statement). *Diabetes Care*. 2003;26(Suppl 1):S51–S61.

Centers for Disease Control and Prevention Web site. Available at: http://www.cdc.gov. Accessed September 20, 2004.

Franz MJ, Bantle JP, Beebe CA, Brunzell JD, Chiasson JL, Garg A, Holzmeister LA, Hoogwerf B, Mayer-Davis E,

Mooradian AD, Purnell JQ, Wheeler M. Evidence-based nutrition principles and recommendations for the treatment and prevention of diabetes and related complications (technical review). *Diabetes Care.* 2002;25: 148–198.

McLaughlin S. Nutrition therapy for the older adult with diabetes. In: Franz M, Bantle J, eds. *American Diabetes Association Guide to Medical Nutrition Therapy for Diabetes.* Alexandria, Va: American Diabetes Association; 1999:249–273.

National Institute on Aging Web site. Available at: http://www.nia.nih.gov. Accessed September 20, 2004.

National Policy & Resource Center on Nutrition and Aging Web site. Available at: http://www.fiu.edu/~nutreldr. Accessed September 20, 2004.

Rose D, Oliveira V. Nutrient intakes of individuals from food insufficient households in the United States. *Am J Public Health.* 1997;87:1956–1961.

17

Diabetes in Pregnancy and Lactation

Diane Reader, RD, CDE

CHAPTER OVERVIEW

- Women with diabetes or gestational diabetes mellitus (GDM) can have healthy babies, but normal blood glucose control is needed for a successful outcome.
- Nutrition therapy provided by experienced registered dietitians (RDs) is a key component of both preconception counseling and the management of GDM and pregnancy complicated by preexisting diabetes.
- Nutrition therapy recommendations and self-management guidelines should be guided by the desired clinical outcomes and should follow research-based practice guidelines, such as those of the *Nutrition Practice Guidelines for Gestational Diabetes Mellitus* (1).

GESTATIONAL DIABETES MELLITUS

GDM is defined as "glucose intolerance of variable severity with onset or first recognition during pregnancy" (2). In the second and third trimesters of pregnancy, the placenta produces large amounts of hormones that cause insulin resistance. Most pregnant women are able to double or triple their insulin production to overcome this (3). Women who are not able to increase insulin secretion develop GDM.

In the United States about 2% to 5% of all pregnancies, or about 200,000 births per year, are complicated with GDM. The prevalence ranges from 1% to 14% and is in direct proportion to the prevalence of type 2 diabetes in a given population (4).

The risk of developing GDM is influenced by the following factors (2):

- High body weight
- Inactivity
- Older age
- History of GDM
- Previous large-for-gestational-age infant
- Family history of diabetes
- Member of high-risk ethnic group

SCREENING AND DIAGNOSIS OF GDM

GDM is usually without symptoms, so maternal screening during pregnancy is necessary for diagnosis and treatment. In the United States, a two-step process is used for screening and diagnosis of GDM: first, an initial 50-g oral glucose challenge is given any time of day (1 hour after the glucose challenge test [GCT], blood glucose should be < 140 mg/dL); second, if blood glucose is 140 mg/dL or higher, then the second step, a fasted 100-g oral glucose tolerance test (OGTT), is taken. Blood glucose levels are measured during fasting and at

1, 2, and 3 hours postprandial. The diagnosis of GDM is made if two or more of the OGTT values are equal to or greater than the following (2):

- Fasting: 95 mg/dL
- 1 hour postprandial: 180 mg/dL
- 2 hours postprandial: 155 mg/dL
- 3 hours postprandial: 140 mg/dL

It is recommended that a minimum of 150 g of carbohydrate (or about a 1,500-kcal diet) be consumed on the days before the test, but there is no need to prepare for the OGTT with a carbohydrate-loading diet. Current screening guidelines for GDM recommend determining the mother's risk of developing GDM at the first prenatal visit (2).

High-risk individuals should be tested as early as possible. In clinics that serve high-risk populations, the 50-g GCT is given at the first prenatal visit, to identify women who already have carbohydrate intolerance. For women with average risk of developing GDM, screening is recommended between the 24th and 28th weeks of gestation (2). Women at low risk for the development of GDM do not need to undergo screening by glucose challenge (2). This includes women who meet all the following criteria: younger than 25 years and of normal body weight, no family history of diabetes, no history of abnormal glucose tolerance or poor obstetric outcome, and not members of an ethnic group with increased rates of diabetes (2).

NUTRITION THERAPY FOR GESTATIONAL DIABETES

After diagnosis, the individual should be referred to an RD to receive nutrition therapy for GDM. Nutrition therapy includes assessment, diagnosis, intervention, and monitoring and evaluation of clinical outcomes. Box 17.1 (1) and Table 17.1 (1,5–7) outline key assessment parameters, nutrition recommendations, and meal planning tips for GDM.

GDM Nutrition Practice Guidelines

The American Dietetic Association has developed nutrition practice guidelines for GDM (1), which outline optimal nutrition therapy in GDM and desired clinical outcomes. Figure 17.1 (1) provides an overview of nutrition therapy for GDM.

BOX 17.1

Nutrition Assessment in Gestational Diabetes Mellitus

Collecting the following data during the nutrition assessment will assist the dietitian in designing a food plan appropriate for the woman's educational level and lifestyle and will facilitate achievement of clinical outcomes.

- Medical and obstetric history
- Anthropometric data: height, current weight, prepregnancy weight and body mass index, weight-gain goal for pregnancy
- Laboratory data: glucose challenge test, oral glucose tolerance test, hemoglobin, hematocrit, blood pressure, urine ketones, A1C
- Lifestyle factors: type of work and schedule, education level, family, cultural/ethnic/religious issues, financial concerns, food assistance use, substance use
- Gastrointestinal factors: appetite, eating disorders, discomforts, allergies, intolerances, cravings, aversions, pica
- Infant feeding plans
- Food recall: meal and snack times, food choices and portions; food preparation methods, food preferences, supplement use
- Exercise: typical exercise/activity pattern, restrictions

Source: Data are from reference 1.

Clinical Outcomes

Clinicians need to be aware of the clinical outcomes they are trying to achieve before they develop a nutrition plan. Clinical outcomes that the RD can affect and evaluate are blood glucose values, weight changes, ketone levels, and food selection (1). The individual will need to record daily food intake, blood glucose values, and fasting ketone tests, and will return for regular follow-up visits.

There are three clinical outcomes for GDM: (*a*) achieving and maintaining normoglycemia; (*b*) consumption of adequate energy to promote appropriate weight gain and to avoid maternal ketosis; and (*c*) consumption of food providing nutrients necessary for maternal and fetal health.

Achieving and Maintaining Normoglycemia

Blood glucose levels for the pregnant woman without diabetes are lower than in the nonpregnant state. Fasting

TABLE 17.1 Nutrition Recommendations for Gestational Diabetes Mellitus

Nutrient or Food Type	Recommendation	Meal-Planning Tips
Energy	Intake should be sufficient to promote adequate, but not excessive, weight gain and to avoid ketonuria.	• Include 3 small- to moderate-sized meals and 2–4 snacks. Space snacks and meals at least 2 h apart. • A bedtime snack (or even a snack in the middle of the night) is recommended, to diminish the number of hours fasting.
Carbohydrate	Recommendations are based on effect of intake on blood glucose levels. Intake should be distributed throughout the day. Frequent feedings, smaller portions, with intake sufficient to avoid ketonuria.	• Common carbohydrate guidelines: 2 carbohydrate choices (30 g) at breakfast, 3–4 choices (45–60 g) for lunch and evening meal, and 1–2 choices (15 to 30 g) for snacks. • Recommendations should be modified based on individual assessment and blood glucose self-monitoring test results.
High-sucrose/ high-energy foods	Inclusion should be based on individual's ability to maintain blood glucose goals, nutritional adequacy of diet, and contribution of these foods to total meal plan.	• Eliminate foods containing large amounts of carbohydrates, such as sweets and sweetened drinks.
Protein	RDA for adult women (0.8 g/kg DBW) + 25 g/day, or 1.1g/kg DBW.	• Protein foods do not raise postmeal blood glucose levels. • Add protein to meals and snacks, to help provide enough calories and to satisfy appetite.
Fat	Limit saturated fat.	• Fat intake may be increased because of increased protein intake; focus on leaner protein choices.
Sodium	Not routinely restricted.	
Fiber	For relief of constipation, increase intake.	• Use whole grains and raw fruits and vegetables. • Activity and fluids help relieve constipation.
Nonnutritive sweeteners	Generally safe in pregnancy. Use in moderation.	
Vitamins and minerals	Preconception folate. Assess for specific individual needs: multivitamin throughout pregnancy, iron at 12 weeks, and calcium especially in last trimester and while lactating.	
Caffeine	Limit to < 300 mg/day.	
Alcohol	Avoid.	

Abbreviations: DBW, desired body weight; RDA, recommended dietary allowance.
Source: Data are from references 1 and 5–7.

values average 74 to 88 mg/dL and postprandial values rarely exceed 130 mg/dL at 1 hour or 120 mg/dL at 2 hours (8).

Optimal blood glucose targets in GDM are still controversial, and each clinic/hospital team needs to agree on targets, such as consistently recommending testing at either 1 or 2 hours postmeal, to avoid giving conflicting information. Optimal blood glucose targets and testing plans have not been established. National organizations have recommended thresholds at which insulin therapy should be started; these numbers are thresholds, *not* blood glucose targets. See Table 17.2 (2,9).

Referral to Dietitian made within 48 hours of diagnosis for self-management

⇩

Initial visit within 1 week of referral:
Assessment
Nutrition Therapy
Exercise
Self-Management Education Tools:
   a. appropriate food plan for patient
   b. daily food records
   c. SMBG records
   d. ketone testing if needed
Insulin if needed
First follow-up within 1 week
*Documentation/Communication

Clinical Outcomes of MNT:

Blood glucose maintained at these levels:

	Whole Blood *mg/dL*	Plasma *mg/dL*
Fasting	≤95	≤105
1 hr PP	≤140	≤155
2 hr PP	≤120	≤130

- achieve and maintain normoglycemia
- consume adequate calories to promote appropriate gestational weight gain and avoid maternal ketosis
- consume food providing nutrients necessary for maternal and fetal health
- decrease nutrition related complications

*Documentation/Communication
- to referral source
- summarize assessment
- specify therapy plan and recommendations
- specify follow-up plan

⇩

Follow-up Visit
Evaluate patient outcomes

⇩

Is patient achieving clinical outcomes and is patient using self-management techniques correctly?

YES ⇩   ⇩ NO

Provide support, answer questions
a. Adjust food/exercise plan to individual needs
b. Continue/review self-management education
c. Adjust testing regimen if appropriate
*Documentation/Communication

— Evaluate cause(s) that prevent achieving clinical outcome
— Determine barriers that may prevent implementing therapy
— Provide intervention
   a. adjusted food/exercise plan
   b. continue/review self-management education
   c. determine need for insulin therapy/make referral
*Documentation/Communication

Determine Follow-up Plan

Birth

Postpartum visit

Follow-up Visit Schedule:
If patient needs insulin, make referral immediately
— Second visit within 1 week
— Third visit 1–3 weeks
— Subsequent follow-up 2–3 weeks until birth

FIGURE 17.1 Nutrition practice guidelines for gestational diabetes. Abbreviations: PP, postprandial; SMBG, self-monitoring of blood glucose. Adapted with permission from *American Dietetic Association Medical Nutrition Therapy Evidence-Based Guides for Practice: Nutrition Practice Guidelines for Gestational Diabetes Mellitus* [CD-ROM]. Chicago, Ill: American Dietetic Association; 2001.

TABLE 17.2 Initiation of Insulin Therapy in Gestational Diabetes

	Threshold, mg/dL*	
	American Diabetes Association	*American College of Obstetrics and Gynecology*
Fasting	≤ 105	< 95
1 hour postprandial	≤ 155	< 130
2 hour postprandial	≤ 130	< 120

* Initiate insulin therapy when blood glucose values exceed these levels.
Source: Data are from references 2 and 9.

Many centers recommend four tests per day: while fasting, after breakfast, after lunch, and after dinner. Many women with GDM will require insulin (or glyburide) to meet glucose targets.

Consumption of Adequate Energy to Promote Appropriate Weight Gain and to Avoid Maternal Ketosis

Maternal weight gain is the preferred measure to determine whether energy intake is adequate to support fetal growth. Weight-gain guidelines are based on the woman's prepregnant body mass index, as shown in Table 17.3 (1). Dietetics professionals should note the following:

- Thin women need to gain more weight than overweight women.

- There are no special weight-gain recommendations for women with diabetes. Guidelines for all pregnant women can be used.
- Because many women with gestational diabetes are obese, a minimum gain of 15 lb is recommended, not more or less.

Weight change should be monitored and recorded at each visit. The specific energy intake recommendation should be individualized, based on assessment, prepregnancy weight, physical activity level, and weight gain to date in pregnancy.

No agreement has been reached on a minimum energy requirement for women with GDM. One study concluded that euglycemia and appropriate weight gain and birth weights were achieved with 23 to 25 kcal/kg of current body weight for obese women with GDM and 30 to 34

TABLE 17.3 Weight-Gain Recommendations for 2nd and 3rd Trimesters of Pregnancy

BMI Range	% DBW Range*	Recommended Weight Gain, lb (kg)
Underweight, < 19.8	< 90	28–40 (12.7–18.2)
Normal weight, 19.8–26.0	100–120	25–35 (11.3–15.9)
Overweight, > 26.0–29.0	> 120	15–25 (6.8–11.3)
Obese, > 29.0	> 135	15 (6.8)
Twins gestation		35–45 (15.9–20.5)

Abbreviations: BMI, body mass index; DBW, desired body weight.
*Based on pregravid weight status.
Source: Adapted with permission from *American Dietetic Association Medical Nutrition Therapy Evidence-Based Guides for Practice: Nutrition Practice Guidelines for Gestational Diabetes Mellitus* [CD-ROM]. Chicago, Ill: American Dietetic Association; 2001.

kcal/kg for women of normal weight (10). Other research indicates that a daily minimum of 1,700 to 1,800 kcal of carefully selected food choices prevents ketosis (11). Intakes below 1,700 to 1,800 kcal/day are generally not advised and often result in inadequate maternal weight gain, weight loss, and/or ketosis (4).

Ketones are formed when the body resorts to burning fat due to inadequate carbohydrate or energy supply. One study showed that elevated ketone levels affect neurologic development of the infant (12–14). By age 4 years, a decrease in intelligence quotient scores were shown in the children of mothers with ketonemia compared with children of nonketotic pregnant women. Ketone formation can be a special problem in pregnancy with diabetes, because blood glucose control is achieved with controlled food intake, and undereating is a common way to control postprandial glucose level.

There is no consensus or national standard regarding ketone testing in pregnancy. Some clinics ask women to test the first urine specimen of the day for ketones, and the goal is a negative result. Other centers institute ketone testing only when there is a concern that the woman's energy or carbohydrate intake is insufficient. Because of variations in the renal threshold during pregnancy, the urine test is not a very reliable test.

Consumption of Food Providing Nutrients Necessary for Maternal and Fetal Health

Achieving the balance of blood glucose control and appropriate weight gain can be a challenge. However, it is important to also instruct and encourage the woman to make excellent food choices and to not compromise good nutrition to achieve glucose control. The pregnant woman with GDM (or preexisting diabetes) does not have unique nutritional requirements, but she should get four or more servings of dairy, two or more servings of protein, three or more fruits, three or more vegetables, and adequate starches, to equal her energy needs.

Use of artificial sweeteners is acceptable during pregnancy. Saccharin does cross the placenta and remains in fetal tissue, so its use should be monitored during pregnancy (15). Alcohol intake should be avoided.

Self-Management Education Tools

Desired outcomes can only be achieved when individuals participate in the daily management of their diabetes. Dietetics professionals should make sure that the individuals know how and when to contact their health care provider with results, and should provide instruction and support on the following:

- *Food plan:* Using a food plan to keep blood glucose levels within target range.
- *Food records:* Keeping records of all food and beverages consumed and comparing records to blood glucose and urine ketone checks.
- *Self-monitoring of blood glucose:* Self-monitoring of fasting and postprandial blood glucose levels with use of a glucose meter. Recording and using results to make necessary changes.
- *Ketone testing:* Testing urine for ketones; recording and using results.
- *Insulin therapy:* Using insulin, if needed. Reviewing how to administer, record doses, treat hypoglycemia, manage sick days, dispose of sharps, etc.
- *Physical activity:* Planning activity to benefit blood glucose control.

When to Advance Therapy to Insulin

If an individual's blood glucose levels are outside target goals, the RD should contact the primary care provider for initiation of insulin. Insulin therapy should be started if, within a 1- to 2-week interval, on two or more occasions, capillary blood glucose is above the target goals selected by the institution.

In many cases, women with GDM follow their food plan carefully, but they are not able to achieve glucose control. In other situations, individuals are not able or willing to change their dietary intake to reach the level of glucose control compatible with a successful outcome. In these circumstances, blood glucose control may be acceptable but other clinical outcomes are not (eg, when a woman undereats to achieve glucose control or when a woman loses weight and spills ketones).

Insulin therapy may be initiated simultaneously with the initiation of nutrition therapy in cases with marked elevation of fasting blood glucose, because, in such cases, nutrition therapy alone is seldom sufficient to meet glycemic goals and prevent fetal complication. Glyburide is not currently approved for use in pregnancy. However, in one randomized clinical trial (16), it did not cross the placenta and was successful in management of women with GDM.

PREGNANCY AND PREEXISTING TYPE 1 OR TYPE 2 DIABETES

Research has shown that the risks of fetal anomaly are no greater in women with diabetes than in women without diabetes when blood glucose control is near normal during organogenesis, which occurs during the first trimester (17). Ideally, women with diabetes should achieve excellent glucose control, defined as an A1C value of up to 1% above normal, about 3 months before conceiving (18). Health care professionals need to review with all women and teenage girls of childbearing years the need for contraception, potential plans to conceive, and the importance of preconception glucose control. Women with diabetes will need to test blood glucose values at least four times per day, but more likely eight times per day. Multiple insulin injections or an insulin pump, balanced with a healthy food plan, are needed to achieve glucose control.

The Food and Drug Administration (FDA) has not approved any oral agents for use with pregnancy. Therefore, women with type 2 diabetes on oral-agent therapy probably need to switch to insulin therapy in the preconception phase. As noted earlier in this chapter, in one randomized clinical trial, glyburide did not cross the placenta and successfully managed women with GDM (16). Although the FDA has not approved the use of glyburide in pregnant women, some providers do use it off-label.

Metformin has also been used during pregnancy. Some women with polycystic ovary syndrome who are diagnosed with infertility are able to become pregnant when taking metformin (19). When the drug is discontinued, miscarriage occurs at a high rate. Therefore, continued use of metformin may help to prevent miscarriage in this population (20).

CLINICAL MANAGEMENT OF PREEXISTING DIABETES AND PREGNANCY

First Trimester

Ideally, a woman works with her diabetes team to achieve glucose control before becoming pregnant. If not, achieving good control becomes a top priority.

To achieve good glucose control and pregnancy outcomes, a woman with diabetes who becomes pregnant and has not been seeing her diabetes care team will need intensive education on a food plan, energy and nutrient needs, and monitoring. Conversely, a woman who has good glucose control before conception will need minor modifications to her food plan, with an emphasis on hypoglycemia prevention, alcohol restriction, and the addition of a multivitamin-mineral supplement.

Excellent glucose control usually requires use of an insulin pump or an intensified insulin plan of three or more injections per day. In recent years, the rapid-acting insulin analogs lispro (Humalog, Eli Lily & Co, Indi-

anapolis, IN 46285) and aspart (Novolog, Novo Nordisk, Princeton, NJ 08540) have commonly been used in intensified plans because they allow for more precise glucose control and better coordination of insulin with carbohydrate intake. The FDA has not approved these analogs for use in pregnancy; however, one study found no adverse effects with the use of lispro (21).

Hypoglycemia is more common in the first trimester, because insulin requirements decrease and morning sickness may cause food intake to be less consistent (22). The dietetics professional should review with the woman the physiologic changes that occur in pregnancy and insulin or food adjustments that may help to prevent serious hypoglycemia. After the first trimester, insulin needs increase and hypoglycemia is less common. Use of an insulin pump can facilitate improved overnight blood glucose control.

Energy needs do not increase in the first trimester, unless a woman is underweight. Most RDs prefer to base energy recommendations on a woman's actual intake rather than on formulas.

Second and Third Trimesters

During the second and third trimesters, insulin requirements increase weekly, so that by the end of the pregnancy, the insulin dose will double (23). This is a normal part of all pregnancies caused by the increase in placental hormones and the increased weight of the woman. For the second and third trimesters of pregnancy, the 2002 Dietary Reference Intake for energy equals the Estimated Energy Requirement (EER) plus 8 kcal/wk for increased total energy expenditure plus 180 kcal/day for energy deposition during pregnancy (24).

Regular bimonthly or monthly visits are needed to keep blood glucose levels in the target range. The food plan should be established by this time, and a focus should be on consistency. If insulin-to-carbohydrate ratios are used to determine mealtime insulin dosage, it must be adjusted weekly or monthly.

POSTPARTUM ISSUES FOR WOMEN WITH PREEXISTING DIABETES

Immediately after delivery, insulin requirements drop to prepregnancy levels, and insulin doses need to be decreased to those more similar to prepregnancy doses. There is no reason why a woman with diabetes should not breastfeed. If breastfeeding is planned, the woman should continue with the energy intake during pregnancy. Because some women experience hypoglycemia after breastfeeding their newborn, an additional snack in the middle of the night with breastfeeding is often needed. If not breastfeeding, the woman can return to her prepregnancy meal plan and energy requirements.

POSTPARTUM ISSUES FOR WOMEN WITH GESTATIONAL DIABETES

Although in most cases blood glucose levels will return to normal after delivery, women who have had GDM are at increased risk of developing GDM in subsequent pregnancies and diabetes later in life. The recurrence rate of GDM ranges from approximately 30% to 65% in subsequent pregnancies (2).

Forty to sixty percent of women with GDM will develop type 2 diabetes within 15 to 20 years of the pregnancy (25). Risk factors for developing diabetes in the years ahead include the degree of abnormality of the diagnostic glucose tolerance test, degree of obesity, family history of type 2 diabetes, and certain ethnicities. Intervention strategies to prevent or reduce the risk of diabetes in the future are important components in postpartum care. Strategies include counseling to promote healthy food and lifestyle habits, such as weight management and regular physical activity (see Chapter 5).

SUMMARY

Nutrition therapy for women with GDM includes assessment, diagnosis, intervention, and monitoring and evaluation of clinical outcomes. The three clinical outcomes for GDM are (*a*) achieving and maintaining normoglycemia; (*b*) consumption of adequate energy to promote appropriate weight gain and to avoid maternal ketosis; and (*c*) consumption of food providing nutrients necessary for maternal and fetal health. Blood glucose values, weight changes, ketone levels, and nutritious food selection are clinical outcomes that the dietitian can affect and evaluate.

REFERENCES

1. *American Dietetic Association Medical Nutrition Therapy Evidence-Based Guides for Practice: Nutrition Practice Guidelines for Gestational Diabetes Mellitus* [CD-ROM]. Chicago, Ill: American Dietetic Association; 2001.

2. American Diabetes Association. Position statement: gestational diabetes mellitus. *Diabetes Care.* 2004;27(Suppl 1):S88–S90.

3. Spellacy WN, Goetz FC. Plasma insulin in normal late pregnancy. *N Engl J Med.* 1963;268:988–991.

4. Coustan DR. Gestational diabetes. In: *Diabetes in America.* 2nd ed. Bethesda, Md: National Institutes of Diabetes and Digestive and Kidney Diseases; 1995:703–717. National Institutes of Health Publication No. 95-1468.

5. International Diabetes Center. *Gestational Diabetes: Caring for Yourself and Your Baby.* Minneapolis, Minn: International Diabetes Center, Park Nicollet Institute; 2001.

6. Peterson CM, Jovanovic-Peterson L. Percentages of carbohydrate and glycemic response to breakfast, lunch, and dinner in women with gestational diabetes. *Diabetes.* 1991;40:172–194.

7. Regenstein A, Coulston A, Flanagan G, Druzin M. Metabolic response to carbohydrate variations in gestational diabetes. *Diabetes.* 1996;45(Suppl 2):A1259.

8. Cousins L, Rigg L, Hollingsworth D, Brink G, Aurand J, Yen SS. The 24-hour excursion and diurnal rhythm of glucose, insulin and c-peptide in normal pregnancy. *Am J Obstet Gynecol.* 1980;136:483–488.

9. American College of Obstetricians and Gynecologists Committee on Practice Bulletins—Obstetrics. ACOG Practice Bulletin. Clinical management guidelines for obstetrician-gynecologists. Number 30, September 2001 (replaces Technical Bulletin Number 200, December 1994). Gestational diabetes. *Obstet Gynecol.* 2001;98:525–538.

10. Metzger B, Coustan DC. Summary and recommendations of the Fourth International Workshop-Conference on Gestational Diabetes Mellitus. *Diabetes Care.* 1998;21(Suppl 2):B161–B167.

11. Knopp RH, Magee MS, Raisys V, Benedetti T, Bonet B. Hypocaloric diets and ketogenesis in the management of obese gestational diabetic women. *J Am Coll Nutr.* 1991;10:649–667.

12. Rizzo T, Metzger B, Burns W, Burns K. Correlations between antepartum maternal metabolism and intelligence of offsprings. *N Engl J Med.* 1991;325:911–916.

13. Churchill J, Berendes H, Nemore J. Neuropsychological deficits in children of diabetic mothers. *Am J Obstet Gynecol.* 1969;105:257–268.

14. Naeye RL, Chez RA. Effects of maternal acetonuria and low pregnancy weight gain on children's psychomotor development. *Am J Obstet Gynecol.* 1981;139:189–193.

15. Position of the American Dietetic Association: use of nutritive and nonnutritive sweeteners. *J Am Diet Assoc.* 2004;104:255–275.

16. Langer O, Conway D, Berkus M, Xenakis E, Gonzalez OL. A comparison of glyburide and insulin in women with gestational diabetes mellitus. *N Engl J Med.* 2000; 343:1134–1138.

17. Kitzmiller JL, Gavin LA, Gin GD, Jovanovic-Peterson L, Main EK, Zigrang WD. Preconception care of diabetes:

glycemic control prevents congenital anomalies. *JAMA.* 1991;265:731–736.

18. American Diabetes Association. Position statement: preconception care of women with diabetes. *Diabetes Care.* 2004;27(Suppl 1):S76–S78.

19. Nestler JE, Jakubowicz DJ, Evans WS, Pasquali R. Effects of metformin on spontaneous and clomiphene-induced ovulation in polycystic ovary syndrome. *N Engl J Med.* 1998;338:1876–1880.

20. Glueck CJ, Wang P, Goldenberg N, Sieve-Smith L. Pregnancy outcomes among women with polycystic ovary syndrome treated with metformin. *Hum Reprod.* 2002;17: 2858–2864.

21. Jovanovic L, Ilic S, Pettitt DJ, Hugo K, Gutierrez M, Bowsher RR, Bastyr EJ. Metabolic and immunologic effects of insulin lispro in gestational diabetes. *Diabetes Care.* 1999;22:1422–1427.

22. Brown F, Hare J. *Diabetes Complicating Pregnancy: The Joslin Clinic Method.* New York, NY: Wiley-Liss, Inc; 1995.

23. Langer O, Anyaegbunam A, Brustman L, Guidetti D, Levy J, Mazze R. Pregestational diabetes: insulin requirements throughout pregnancy. *Am J Obstet Gynecol.* 1988: 159:616–621.

24. Institute of Medicine. *Dietary Reference Intakes: Energy, Carbohydrate, Fiber, Fat, Fatty Acids, Cholesterol, Protein, and Amino Acids (Macronutrients).* Washington, DC: National Academy Press; 2002. Available at: http://www. nap.edu. Accessed January 20, 2005.

25. O'Sullivan JB. Subsequent morbidity among gestational diabetic women. In: Sutherland HW, Stowers JM, eds. *Carbohydrate Metabolism in Pregnancy and the Newborn.* New York, NY: Churchill Livingstone; 1984:174–180.

Part 5

Nutrition Education: Meal Planning

18

Diabetes Meal-Planning Strategies

Joyce Green Pastors, MS, RD, CDE, Janelle Waslaski, RD, CDE, and Heidi Gunderson, MS, RD, CDE

CHAPTER OVERVIEW

- Diabetes nutrition therapy and self-management training should be based on a comprehensive nutrition assessment, which includes the individual's diabetes self-care treatment plan, health status, learning ability, readiness to change, and current lifestyle.
- When selecting a meal-planning approach, dietetics professionals need to take into account the long-term nature of diabetes education and the likelihood that a combination of different meal-planning approaches and resources may be needed.
- Every meal-planning approach and resource used to educate individuals with diabetes has advantages and disadvantages. The key is to tailor the meal-planning approach and resources to the current needs of each individual.

MEAL-PLANNING APPROACHES

There are many meal-planning approaches that can be used to teach individuals with diabetes how and what to eat. Some approaches offer the individual less structure, some offer more flexibility, and some are more structured and specific, requiring the individual to match more precisely insulin requirements with food choices. In this chapter, a variety of meal-planning approaches

are described, along with tools that can be used to supplement the educational process.

FOOD PYRAMIDS

Food pyramids have become increasingly popular tools for teaching basic diabetes meal planning. The shape is easy to remember, and most individuals are familiar with the concept that a person should eat more of foods that form the base of the pyramid and less of foods at the tip of the pyramid. *The First Step in Diabetes Meal Planning* brochure (1) is a simplified meal-planning tool for diabetes, which is based on the diabetes food pyramid. The diabetes food pyramid (2) is similar to the US Department of Agriculture Food Guide Pyramid (the version released in 1992) but is preferred for teaching individuals with diabetes because it emphasizes serving sizes and carbohydrate-containing foods to help improve blood glucose management.

Strategies for using the diabetes food pyramid include assessing eating habits by comparing usual intake with recommended number of servings shown for each food group on the pyramid. Dietetics professionals should discuss with individuals how their usual food intake compares with recommendations for number of servings and serving size. The dietetics professional and the individual should review sections of the pyramid and what counts as a serving in each section and should discuss the number of servings the individual may need each day to meet his or her energy requirements and blood glucose goals.

Dietetics professionals should help individuals review guidelines for healthful food choices—such as choosing whole fruits, unsweetened fruit juices, whole-grain foods, and low-fat meats and milk—in each section of the pyramid and should compare these options with the individual's usual food choices. The diabetes pyramid can also be used to review the common misconception that all carbohydrates or starches are bad for blood glucose control and diabetes management.

If the individual comprehends the basic nutrition concepts of the pyramid, the dietetics professional can introduce the following nutrient-specific information:

- The main food groups that contain carbohydrate (grains, beans and starchy vegetables section, fruit section, milk section)
- Effect of macronutrients (carbohydrate, protein, fat) on blood glucose level.
- Guideline of three to five carbohydrate servings at each meal and one to two carbohydrate servings at snacks (if needed).

HEALTHY FOOD CHOICES

Diabetes guidelines for healthful eating provide individuals with an understanding of the connection between nutrition and diabetes. They give direction in making appropriate food choices for managing diabetes. *Healthy Food Choices* (3)—a joint publication of the American Dietetic Association and the American Diabetes Association—is a pamphlet that promotes healthful eating practices.

Strategies for teaching diabetes guidelines for healthful eating should be broad in focus and yet allow for individualization of the nutrition message. In addition to providing information that explains the relationship between food and diabetes, the dietetics professional should help the individual set goals that will promote changes in eating behaviors.

The "Guidelines for Healthy Eating" section of *Healthy Food Choices* can help individuals identify habits that could be changed to improve general health and diabetes management. Dietetics professionals can use the menu and meal-plan section of the pamphlet to discuss meal timing and sample menu ideas. *Healthy Food Choices* can be used as part of a two-step approach with individuals who have just learned that they have diabetes

and who may become overwhelmed with more complex meal-planning concepts. This pamphlet can also be used to simplify nutrition messages for individuals who may have multiple health concerns and multiple nutrition recommendations.

If the individual comprehends the basic nutrition concepts, the dietetics professional can introduce the following nutrient-specific information:

- Review the main food groups that contain carbohydrate (grains, beans and starchy vegetables section, fruit section, milk section) and amounts
- Explain the effect of macronutrients (carbohydrate, protein, fat) on blood glucose
- Discuss the fat content of specific food groups
- Describe the use of food labels in meal planning

PLATE METHOD

The plate method for meal planning helps individuals easily select meals with acceptable food portions. Individuals estimate serving sizes without measuring, to promote consistent carbohydrate content in meals. Various groups have adapted this method for diabetes meal planning. It is particularly useful for initial or simplified diabetes meal planning, basic portion control, and weight management. The plate method is also appropriate for people with poor reading and math skills, cognitive limitations, or difficulty using more structured approaches, and for those who do not speak English.

Strategies for teaching the plate method include reviewing the food groups and using a copy of a plate to compare the individual's usual intake with the recommended portions. The standard meal pattern (see Box 18.1) should be reviewed. The sample plate format should be used to plan a day's meals and snacks. This meal plan provides about 45 to 75 g carbohydrate at each meal or 3 to 5 carbohydrate servings. Calories can vary based on food choices. Serving sizes for snacks are the same as for meals.

MENUS

The menu is the basis of all meal-planning approaches. It is the written description of what to eat. Written menus reflect individualized nutrition recommendations necessary to meet medical nutrition therapy goals. Ideally, dietetics professionals will incorporate some degree of menu planning into whatever nutrition education method is chosen.

BOX 18.1

Plate Method: Standard Meal Pattern*

Breakfast
- ¼ to ½ plate of bread or cereal
- 8-oz glass of milk
- A piece of fruit or ½ cup fruit juice or ¼ cup dried fruit
- Optional ¼ plate of meat or protein
- If individual does not, or should not, drink milk at all meals, a bread/cereal serving can be added in place of the milk.

Lunch or Dinner
- ¼ plate of bread, grain, or starchy food (bread, rolls, rice, crackers, cereal, starchy vegetables, including potatoes, corn, winter squash, and legumes)
- ¼ plate of meat, fish, or poultry
- ½ plate of nonstarchy vegetables, including broccoli, green beans, carrots, mushrooms, tomatoes, cauliflower, spinach, peppers, and salad greens
- 8-oz glass of milk
- A piece of fruit
- If individual does not, or should not, drink milk at all meals, a bread/cereal serving can be added in place of the milk.

*Based on 9-inch plate.

Dietetics professionals should have the individuals record what they usually eat and categorize food consumed into carbohydrate choices, exchange list servings, or food pyramid servings. A person's typical food intake should be used to create a meal plan and sample menu, making necessary changes for nutrition guidelines and diabetes therapy.

Individuals who have fairly routine eating habits and who eat at consistent times and places are likely to do better than people who have no routine. However, even individuals who have no regular routine can benefit because the menu encourages some structure. Menus are useful for

- initial or simplified diabetes meal planning.
- people who have little experience or little interest in meal planning.
- individuals with poor reading and math skills, cognitive limitations, and difficulty using more structured approaches.

EXCHANGE SYSTEM

Background

The concept of "exchange," or substitution, of different foods that are acceptable for use by people with diabetes was developed in 1950 by the American Dietetic Association, the American Diabetes Association, and the US Public Health Service. The goal was to develop an educational tool that would provide uniformity in meal planning and would allow a wider variety of foods to be included (4).

The exchange lists originally grouped foods into six lists: starch/bread, meat and meat substitutes, vegetables, fruit, milk, and fat (4). Each list was a group of measured foods of approximately the same nutritional value. To simplify teaching of carbohydrate-control concepts, in recent revisions the food groups have been reduced to three (4,5): carbohydrate, meat and meat substitutes, and fat (see Table 18.1) (6). In addition, the exchange lists identify foods that are good sources of dietary fiber; are high in sodium; and are combination foods, such as casseroles, pizza, and soups, which fit into more than one exchange group.

Nutrition Assessment

The food exchange method can be used effectively for both nutrition assessment and nutrition intervention. To convert an individual's nutrition history into exchange list values (Figure 18.1), dietetics professionals should do the following:

1. Categorize the individual's usual food intake into food exchange groups and servings according to his or her pattern of meals and snacks.
2. In a chart similar to the one shown in Figure 18.1, record grams of carbohydrate, protein, and fat allowed in the individual's total number of exchanges per day.
3. Calculate the number of grams of carbohydrate, protein, and fat and the number of calories consumed by an individual in a day. Determine the percentages of carbohydrate, protein, and fat in the person's diet.

Nutrition Intervention

After the nutrition assessment is completed and individualized goals are established with the individual, a nutrition intervention is initiated. The nutrition intervention may or may not include the use of exchange lists,

TABLE 18.1 Macronutrient Content of the Exchange Lists				
Groups/Lists	Carbohydrate (grams)	Protein (grams)	Fat (grams)	Calories
Carbohydrate group				
• Starch	15	3	0–1	80
• Fruit	15	0	0	60
• Milk				
∘ Fat-free, low-fat	12	8	0–3	90
∘ Reduced-fat	12	8	5	120
∘ Whole	12	8	8	150
• Other carbohydrates	15	varies	varies	varies
• Nonstarchy vegetables	5	2	0	25
Meat and meat substitutes group				
• Very lean	0	7	0–1	35
• Lean	0	7	3	55
• Medium-fat	0	7	5	75
• High-fat	0	7	8	100
Fat group	0	0	5	45

Source: Reprinted with permission from *Exchange Lists for Meal Planning*. Alexandria, Va, and Chicago, Ill: American Diabetes Association and American Dietetic Association; 2003:5.

depending on the needs, abilities, and interests of the individual.

Dietetics professionals should try to individualize the meal plan based on individuals' usual food intake and their input, so people can more easily implement the changes. Meals and snacks should be distributed according to the individual's lifestyle and activity patterns and diabetes medications.

With increasing use of more flexible insulin plans, it is usually not necessary to divide the meal plan, or carbohydrate, into various fractions throughout the day. If individuals are reasonably consistent in their carbohydrate intake day to day, insulin therapy can generally be adjusted to match their intake. Box 18.2 (4,7) includes some additional hints that may be helpful in calculation of meal plans using exchange lists.

CARBOHYDRATE COUNTING: OVERVIEW

Teaching carbohydrate counting is one of the most commonly used methods of diabetes meal planning. The use of carbohydrate counting is supported by research, which shows that carbohydrate is the primary nutrient affecting postprandial blood glucose level, and thus insulin requirements (8), and that all sources of carbohydrate (monosaccharides, disaccharides, or polysaccharides) affect blood glucose level similarly when eaten in the same gram amounts (7,9).

The Diabetes Control and Complications Trial (DCCT) reported that carbohydrate counting was the most successful meal-planning approach used by subjects with type 1 diabetes (10,11). The American Diabetes Association nutrition recommendations emphasize the importance of focusing on the total amount of carbohydrate eaten (7,9), because careful attention to both carbohydrate quantity and distribution can improve metabolic control. Focus on the source of carbohydrate (eg, using the glycemic index as a meal planning approach) may provide an additional benefit over that observed when total carbohydrate is considered alone (12). However, these types of approaches are more complex and less practical for people to learn (for Web sites with information on the glycemic index, see Appendix A).

Nutrition History

Breakfast
1 cup orange juice (2 fruit)
1 slice toast with margarine (1 starch, 1 fat)
1 cup dry cereal with 2 Tbsp raisins
 (1 starch, 1 fruit)
1 cup 2% milk (1 milk)
Coffee, black (free)

Lunch
Sandwich: 2 slices bread (2 starch),
 2 oz ham (2 meat), 1 oz cheese
 (1 meat, 1 fat), 1 Tbsp mayonnaise (3 fat)
1 small bag potato chips (1 starch, 2 fat)
1 diet cola (free)

Dinner
Spaghetti: 1 cup pasta (3 starch), ½ cup tomato sauce
 (1 vegetable), 4 oz grilled chicken breast, sliced (4 meat)
1 cup raw vegetables (1 vegetable)
2 Tbsp ranch dressing (2 fat)
2 slices garlic bread (2 starch, 2 fat)
1 cup 2% milk (1 milk)

Bedtime Snack

1 cup mint chocolate chip ice cream (2 starch, 2 fat)

Exchange List Values

| Food Group | Number of Servings | | | | | | | Macronutrients | | | |
	Meal	Snack	Meal	Snack	Meal	Snack	Total	Carbo-hydrate, g/d (g/serving)	Protein, g/d (g/serving)	Fat, g/d (g/serving)	Energy, kcal/d (kcal/serving)
Starch	2		3		5	2	12	180 (15)	36 (3)	6 (0.5)	960 (80)
Fruit	3		2				5	75 (15)	0 (0)	0 (0)	300 (60)
Milk (2%)	1				1		2	24 (12)	16 (8)	10 (5)	240 (120)
Vegetables					2		2	10 (5)	4 (2)	0 (0)	50 (25)
Meat & meat substitutes			3		4		7	0 (0)	49 (7)	35 (5)	525 (75)
Fat	1		6		4	4	15	0 (0)	0 (0)	75 (5)	675 (45)
							TOTAL GRAMS	289	105	126	
							TOTAL KCAL*	1156	420	1134	2710
							% of kcal	43	15	42	

*To calculate total kcal for carbohydrate or protein, multiply total grams by 4 (there are 4 kcal per gram of carbohydrate or protein). To calculate total kcal for fat, multiply total grams by 9 (there are 9 kcal per gram of fat).

FIGURE 18.1 Converting a nutrition history into exchange list values.

BOX 18.2

Helpful Hints for Calculating Exchange List Meal Plans

- Energy level estimates in calculated meal plans should be rounded to the nearest 50 or 100 kcal, because calculations of food intake based on the exchange system are not accurate enough to allow more precision. Because self-reports of food intake generally underestimate calories, values should be rounded up rather than down.
- Individuals may consume up to 50 or 60 kcal from free foods before they have to count them as exchanges.
- Foods from the starch, fruit, and milk lists all contain similar carbohydrate and energy content, and foods from one of these lists may be interchanged with foods from the other two. If fruits or starches are regularly substituted for milk, calcium intake may be decreased. Substitution of other food groups for milk can also decrease protein intake in children.
- Many foods from the "other carbohydrate" list in the carbohydrate food group, the combination foods list, and the fast foods list are also interchangeable with the starch, fruit, and milk lists. When making exchanges, use caution to ensure sufficient intake of calcium, fiber, and protein. Most of the dessert-type foods on the "other carbohydrate" list are higher in sugars and fat and need to be used within the context of a healthful meal plan. The dietetics professional needs to provide specific guidelines for interchanging foods.
- Vegetables are included in the carbohydrate group and should be a part of the meal plan. However, because three servings of nonstarchy vegetables are the equivalent of one carbohydrate choice, individuals wanting only one or two servings per meal need not count the calories or macronutrients, unless they are tightly controlling energy and/or carbohydrate intake. This guideline encourages consumption of vegetables and simplifies meal planning.
- The types of meat and meat substitutes typically consumed by the individual should be used to calculate the meal plan. Lean meats or medium-fat meats will probably be used most often. It is not recommended that individuals add or subtract fat exchanges when choosing meats that are different from meats ordinarily consumed.
- For calculating protein amounts for diabetes renal meal plans, use the average value of 2.3 g protein per starch exchange or the average grams of protein given for each subcategory on the starch list.

Source: Data are from references 4 and 7.

In its simplest form, carbohydrate counting can be used to help people with diabetes become more aware of carbohydrate in foods and focus on the consistency of their food consumption at meals and snacks. At a more advanced level, the focus is on adjustment of food, medication, and activity, based on patterns from daily food and blood glucose records (see Chapter 11 for additional information). To use the advanced level of carbohydrate counting, it is essential that the dietetics professional and the individual understand intensive insulin therapy (ie, how to make food and/or insulin adjustments based on blood glucose monitoring results).

BASIC CARBOHYDRATE COUNTING

To teach basic carbohydrate counting, dietetics professionals should emphasize the following topics:

- Elementary facts about carbohydrates
- Sources of food that contain carbohydrate

- Carbohydrate consistency (measuring portions)
- Label reading
- Calculating energy needs and amounts of carbohydrate to be consumed

Elementary Facts About Carbohydrates

Persons with diabetes need to understand (*a*) the function of carbohydrate; (*b*) the types of carbohydrate; and (*c*) the effect of carbohydrate on blood glucose. For example, dietetics professionals should review the importance of carbohydrate as an energy source, the brain's dependence on glucose, and storage of excess carbohydrate in the liver as glycogen for use as needed. The different forms of carbohydrate—starches (long chains of ten or more sugar molecules), sugars (short, simple chains of fewer than ten sugar molecules), and fiber (nondigestible carbohydrate)—should be explained. Dietetics professionals should also point out that the most common sugars in the foods people eat are sucrose (table sugar), fructose (sugar in fruits), and lactose (sugar in milk).

The major macronutrients in foods that contain calories (carbohydrate, protein, and fat) should be defined. Dietetics professionals should also explain that carbohydrate has the most pronounced effect on blood glucose and that most carbohydrates have a similar effect on blood glucose when eaten in similar quantities.

Sources of Carbohydrate

Dietetics professionals should explain to individuals the three major food groupings (carbohydrate, meat and meat substitutes/protein, and fat) and should identify the primary sources of carbohydrate:

- Breads, crackers, and cereals
- Pasta, rice, and grains
- Starchy vegetables, such as potatoes, corn, and peas
- Nonstarchy vegetables, such as broccoli, salad greens, and carrots
- Milk and yogurt
- Fruits and juices
- Sweets and desserts

The dietetics professional should explain that many sweets and desserts provide a significant amount of calories from fat and do not contribute vitamins and minerals. Nutrient density and quality of food choices should also be discussed with individuals with diabetes.

Carbohydrate Consistency (Measuring Portions)

When teaching basic carbohydrate counting, dietetics professionals should explain that carbohydrates can be measured in grams or carbohydrate servings and should teach the individual the relationship between the two measurements: one carbohydrate serving is a portion of food that contains 15 g carbohydrate. (One carbohydrate serving equals 15 g.)

Some people may find it easier to count the number of carbohydrate servings consumed than to track carbohydrate intake by grams. Box 18.3 (6) provides a brief list of portions of foods equal to one carbohydrate serving.

Dietetics professionals need to teach individuals with diabetes that one serving of nonstarchy vegetables equals 5 g carbohydrate. A single serving of nonstarchy vegetables is considered free (ie, it is not counted). If an indi-

---

BOX 18.3

Portion Sizes Equivalent to One Carbohydrate Serving (15 g Carbohydrate)

Grains, Breads, Cereals, Pasta
1 slice or 1 oz bread
¾ cup cold cereal
½ cup cooked cereal
⅓ cup cooked pasta or rice

Milk and Yogurt
1 cup milk
⅔ cup (6 oz) unsweetened or sugar-free yogurt

Fruits
1 small fresh fruit
½ cup canned fruit in own juice
1 cup melon or berries
¼ cup dried fruit
½ cup fruit juice

Vegetables
½ cup potato, peas, or corn
3 cups raw vegetables
1½ cups cooked vegetables
(Small portions of nonstarchy vegetables are free.)

Sweets and Snack Foods
½ cup or ¾ oz snack food (pretzels, chips, 4–6 crackers)
1 oz sweet snack (2 small cookies)
½ cup ice cream
1 Tbsp sugar

Source: Data are from reference 6.

---

vidual eats three or more servings in a meal, the individual counts them as one carbohydrate serving.

Dietetics professionals should help individuals practice estimating and measuring portions using various methods (food scale, measuring cups, measuring spoons). Box 18.4 provides tips for teaching people to calculate carbohydrate servings.

Label Reading

The Nutrition Facts panel on a food label is the best source of carbohydrate information for packaged foods. Food lists and reference books are also available (see Additional Resources at the end of the chapter).

BOX 18.4

Tips for Teaching Individuals to Calculate Carbohydrate Servings

- Encourage the individual to use a food scale, measuring cups, measuring spoons, and a calculator.
- Clarify that the serving size listed by weight in grams on a food label is not the same as the number of grams of total carbohydrate per serving.
- Emphasize that the serving size on the food label may not be the same as the portion a person will consume or the portion equal to one carbohydrate serving.
- Review foods to be measured by weight (ounces) vs volume (cups) and the difference between a level and a heaping measuring cup or tablespoon.
- Teach techniques to assess portion size skills. For example, have individuals "guesstimate" before they actually measure, and then compare their two answers; or conduct a "food lab" demonstration with hands-on practice.
- Begin teaching portion-size skills on combination foods, such as casseroles, pizza, and baked goods.

The following are steps for using food labels for counting carbohydrate:

1. Find the standard serving size on the label and the grams of total carbohydrate for one standard serving of food. Remind individuals that sugars are included in the total grams of carbohydrate.
2. Compare the standard serving size of food from the label to the portion being eaten. Remind individuals that many packages contain more than one serving of food. If the portion eaten is different from the standard serving listed on the label, then the number of grams of carbohydrate consumed is also different from the label amount.
3. Calculate the number of carbohydrate servings by dividing the total number of grams of carbohydrate in the portion of food being eaten by 15.
4. If a food has more than 5 g of fiber per serving, subtract the grams of fiber from the total grams of carbohydrate before calculating the number of carbohydrate servings.
5. If a food has more than 10 g of sugar alcohols (which have approximately half the caloric value of other carbohydrates and a smaller effect on blood

glucose) per serving, subtract half the amount of sugar alcohol before calculating carbohydrate choices.

Calculating Energy Needs and Amount of Carbohydrate

In the last component of teaching basic carbohydrate counting, the dietetics professional discusses with the individual the amount of carbohydrate to eat. Ideally, the amount of carbohydrate should be individualized and based on usual carbohydrate intake, nutrition goals set by the individual and dietetics professional, and the person's therapeutic plan.

Individuals should be provided with a meal plan with individualized carbohydrate goals. If a dietetics professional is not available to provide an individualized meal plan or if there is not adequate opportunity to complete a comprehensive assessment, a reasonable starting place is to use three to five carbohydrate servings at each of three meals and one to two carbohydrate choices at snacks if they are appropriate or desired.

ADVANCED CARBOHYDRATE COUNTING

Key topics to cover when teaching advanced carbohydrate counting include the following:

- Record keeping
- Pattern management
- Calculating insulin-to-carbohydrate ratios and premeal correction factors
- Calculating energy needs and amount of carbohydrate

Record Keeping

For advanced carbohydrate counting, individuals must keep and study several weeks of detailed records of food, medication, physical activity, and blood glucose results. Dietetics professionals should use fax and e-mail to review records and provide feedback, when possible.

Initially, the diabetes care team will make insulin adjustments, but over time individuals assume responsibility for making adjustments, with appropriate coaching. To learn the effects of carbohydrate intake on blood glucose, it is necessary for individuals to check blood glucose level before and 2 hours after the start of some meals, to see trends in their blood glucose level. The following information must be tracked for advanced carbohydrate counting and pattern management:

- Time of meal
- Amount and type of food eaten
- Estimated carbohydrate per food item
- Total amount of carbohydrate for each meal and snack
- Changes in insulin dosage
- Unusual circumstances (eg, illness, stress, menstrual cycle)

Pattern Management

The second component of advanced carbohydrate counting is pattern management (see Chapter 11). This is a systematic approach to identifying patterns in blood glucose readings, to determine whether changes are needed in medical management to improve blood glucose control.

The characteristics of pattern management, which is an anticipatory approach, include the following:

- It adjusts to insulin therapy based on blood glucose patterns over several days.
- It responds to causes of problems (eg, schedule, carbohydrate, activity, insulin dose).
- It is a problem-solving approach.
- Patterns reflect previous insulin dose.

In contrast, the characteristics of the commonly used sliding scale method, a compensatory approach, are as follows:

- It adjusts insulin to correct a single blood glucose level at a given moment.
- It does not consider lag time, time of day, or causes of problems.
- It is a quick-fix approach.
- It asks insulin to "work backward."
- It requires hyperglycemia or hypoglycemia before action.

Calculating Insulin-to-Carbohydrate Ratios and Correction Factors

The last component of advanced carbohydrate counting is figuring insulin-to-carbohydrate ratios and calculating a correction factor. An insulin-to-carbohydrate ratio tells a person how much rapid- or short-acting insulin is needed to "cover" the carbohydrate that is eaten at a meal or snack. Knowing how to match insulin doses with what the individual eats allows greater flexibility of lifestyle along with improved glucose control.

Food Record Method for Calculating Insulin-to-Carbohydrate Ratios

The preferred method for calculating an insulin-to-carbohydrate ratio uses several days of food records, blood glucose records, and total daily dose (TDD) of insulin. In general, about half the TDD is background (basal) insulin and half is mealtime (bolus) insulin.

This method involves four steps:

1. *Study food records.* The individual calculates average carbohydrate intake at each meal and snack for at least 3 days.
2. *Practice consistency.* The individual should practice eating consistent amounts of carbohydrate at consistent times, so that baseline insulin requirements can be established.
3. *Study glucose records.* Using pre- and postprandial testing, the effects of food type and amount on blood glucose are determined, and it is determined what and how much food is eaten when blood glucose is in target range.
4. *Calculate the insulin-to-carbohydrate ratio.* The number of grams of carbohydrate eaten at the meal is divided by the units of premeal insulin. For example, if the individual uses 5 units of premeal insulin and eats 75 g carbohydrate, the insulin-to-carbohydrate ratio is 15 (75 divided by 5), which equals 1 unit of insulin per 15 g carbohydrate, a 1:15 ratio. This calculation assumes that the premeal blood glucose is in target range. If the premeal blood glucose is above or below target range, an additional correction bolus is needed (see Chapter 11).

Insulin-to-carbohydrate ratios can vary from meal to meal, between active days and sedentary days, or because of illness or stress. Thus, it may be necessary to use a different insulin-to-carbohydrate ratio for different meals or from day to day, depending on activity level.

Other Methods

Two other methods used to calculate insulin-to-carbohydrate ratios are the 450–500 rule and the "weight method." These methods are not as accurate as food records, because they do not take into account individual amounts of carbohydrate eaten at meals.

TABLE 18.2   Calculating the Insulin-to-Carbohydrate Ratio

Weight, lb	Ratio
120–129	1:15
130–139	1:14
140–149	1:13
150–169	1:12
170–179	1:11
180–189	1:10
190–199	1:9
> 200	1:8

Source: Data are from reference 13.

The 450–500 rule uses the following formulas for calculating the insulin-to-carbohydrate ratios:

- For regular insulin: 450 divided by TDD
- For rapid-acting insulin (lispro [Humalog, Eli Lily & Co, Indianapolis, IN 46285] or aspart [Novolog, Novo Nordisk, Princeton, NJ 08540]): 500 divided by TDD.

For example, if the TDD is 50 units and the patient is using rapid-acting insulin, the insulin-to-carbohydrate ratio would be 10 (500/50).

The weight method uses the data shown in Table 18.2 (13) to calculate the insulin-to-carbohydrate ratio.

Calculating the Correction Factor

The last component of calculating an insulin-to-carbohydrate ratio is calculation of a correction factor. This factor is used to determine the adjusted insulin dosage needed to correct a high or low blood glucose level before a meal. A correction factor is added to, or subtracted from, the premeal bolus insulin dose. To calculate the correction factor, use the following formulas:

- For rapid-acting insulin: Divide 1,800 by TDD.
- For regular insulin: Divide 1,500 by TDD.

For example, if a person's TDD is 50 units of lispro used before meals, the correction factor would be 36 (1,800 divided by 50). This means that 1 additional unit of insulin lowers blood glucose approximately 36 mg/dL. If a person's blood glucose level is 169 mg/dL

before lunch, and the target blood glucose range is less than 130 mg/dL, the individual needs 1 additional unit of insulin to correct for the premeal high blood glucose (169 minus 130 equals 39). This extra unit of insulin would be added to the premeal bolus insulin dose calculated using the lunch insulin-to-carbohydrate ratio. If the insulin-to-carbohydrate ratio is 10, and the person plans to eat 60 g carbohydrate, he or she would take 6 units of rapid-acting insulin to cover the meal plus 1 additional unit of rapid-acting insulin to compensate for the initial high blood glucose, or 7 units total.

Additional Factors to Consider in Advanced Carbohydrate Counting

In addition to calculating insulin-to-carbohydrate ratios and correction factors, advanced carbohydrate counting takes into account other considerations in diabetes management.

Weight Management

There is a potential for weight gain with increased flexibility in food choices. With advanced carbohydrate counting, individuals may be less focused on fat and meat choices, feel more comfortable eating out, and increase their substitution of sweets. Weight management and improved glycemic control should therefore be discussed with individuals, so steps can be taken to minimize weight gain.

Hypoglycemia

People using intensive management need to understand the signs and symptoms of hypoglycemia and should be taught about the possibility of hypoglycemia unawareness (ie, the inability of the person to recognize signs and symptoms of hypoglycemia). Individuals must also learn about appropriate hypoglycemia treatment and should be cautioned that overtreatment can be a cause of weight gain. See Chapter 12 for more information on hypoglycemia.

CASE STUDIES

Using The First Step in Diabetes Meal Planning, Month of Meals, *and Menu Planning Materials*

Mary is age 52 years and was recently diagnosed with type 2 diabetes during a routine physical exam. She was somewhat surprised but told her doctor that she had been experiencing increased thirst and urination over the past several weeks. In addition, Mary has a family history of diabetes: both her mother and grandmother had type 2 diabetes later in their lives. Mary's physical exam yields the following data: height, 5 feet 3 inches; weight, 175 lb; blood pressure, 125/80 mm Hg. Laboratory values: total cholesterol, 202 mg/dL; high-density lipoprotein (HDL) cholesterol: 52 mg/dL; low-density lipoprotein (LDL) cholesterol, 108 mg/dL; triglycerides (TG), 211 mg/dL. Her fasting blood glucose is 147 mg/dL. She takes no medications.

Mary tells her physician that she has been under a lot of stress at work lately. She has not had time to exercise (in fact, she has not been physically active in many years), and she has paid little attention to her diet. She and her doctor agree that Mary will do the following: meet with a diabetes educator to learn how to self-monitor her blood glucose level, see a registered dietitian (RD) for healthful eating guidelines, increase her physical activity, and follow up with her physician in 1 to 2 months. No medications will be started until then, and only if necessary.

Mary meets with an RD the following week. She brings in a 3-day food record for the RD to review. Mary has several questions about what she can eat now that she has diabetes. Mary has not followed any type of diet in the past but states that she is interested in losing weight. She has started to walk for 30 minutes a day during her lunch hour. Her blood glucose record reveals that Mary is checking her blood glucose twice a day at various times, and most readings meet the goals that her doctor gave her. Mary wonders why some of the readings were elevated.

Mary's food records reveal she eats three meals a day, with an occasional snack. Mary's typical habits are to buy a sweet roll in the morning, eat lunch in the cafeteria at work or go out for fast food, and eat dinner at home, which is quite variable in content. She always feels "rushed" and admits that she spends little time planning her meals.

The RD senses that Mary is feeling somewhat overwhelmed with her recent diagnosis and the changes in her lifestyle that were recommended to her, although she is already in the "action" stage of change for activity and blood glucose monitoring. She is preparing to make changes in her food choices but needs more information on diabetes and healthful eating. The RD chooses to use *The First Step in Diabetes Meal Planning* (1) as a resource to explain basic information about how foods affect blood glucose levels, meal-planning guidelines, and portion sizes. Based on Mary's food choices from her food record, a sample menu is created. Mary is also encouraged to increase her intake from some food

groups that were low, such as fruit and milk. The RD helps Mary problem-solve why she still has some elevated blood glucose readings, and Mary concludes that a few might be related to large portion sizes that she had eaten.

Mary's goals from her initial nutrition appointment are to take her lunch and snacks to work (lunch and snack ideas are discussed) at least three times per week, plan several evening meals in advance of grocery shopping, and measure portion sizes of foods eaten at home for the next week. The RD recommends the American Diabetes Association's "Month of Meals" publications (see Additional Resources) for guidance in menu planning, and encourages Mary to continue with her exercise plans and to return to see the RD in 2 to 4 weeks.

Using Healthy Food Choices *and the Plate Method*

John is a 68-year-old man who has had type 2 diabetes for more than 10 years. He currently takes oral diabetes medications (metformin and glyburide) to manage his diabetes and takes lisinopril and atorvastatin for elevated blood pressure and cholesterol levels. John's wife died 6 months ago. He had been her primary caregiver while she was ill, and, because of this, he has not been to his doctor for more than a year. At this appointment, a random blood glucose reading is 205 mg/dL and blood pressure is 145/90 mm Hg. John is 5 feet, 9 inches tall and weighs 182 lb, having lost about 15 lb since his last clinic appointment. He cannot remember what his last A1C or cholesterol levels were or when they were measured, because his wife usually kept track of his medical information. The doctor asks how John is doing since his wife's death. He answers, "I'm struggling because she did all the cooking and took care of me and my diabetes. Since she died I've been cooking for myself and I'm not sure what I'm supposed to eat. I've been eating out a lot (mainly buffets) and not sure what meals are best for people with diabetes. So I'm eating whatever looks good."

The doctor suggests that John make an appointment to talk with an RD for basic meal planning for dining out and preparing easy meals at home. The RD is in the office that day and is able to briefly speak with John. She gives him the *Healthy Food Choices* brochure (3), to provide some survival education until he can be seen in the clinic. She also suggests that he complete a 3-day food diary before the appointment in the clinic.

Two weeks later, John goes to the clinic and meets with the RD. He brings his food diary and the *Healthy Food Choices* brochure. Using the tips page and food groups poster, the RD and John review 1 day of his food record, focusing on serving sizes and areas where his food choices differ significantly from guidelines. Together they identify that he has no consistency in meal times when he ate at home; instead, John is grazing throughout the day. The RD reinforces the importance of eating meals and snacks at regular times each day and monitoring serving sizes. John decides that it would be realistic for him to focus on regular meals and snacks while he is at home. They fill out the "menu ideas" section to help get him started.

John then asks, "What do I eat when I'm dining out at buffets?" Because there are only 5 minutes remaining of the 60-minute consultation, the RD draws a circle on a piece of paper and sections it into four. She advises that when going through the buffet line, John should try to fill half of the plate with vegetables, one-fourth of the plate with a starch, and one-fourth of the plate with meat, adding a piece of fruit for dessert and a glass of milk for a beverage. John thinks this is a great tool. Therefore, the RD suggests scheduling a follow-up appointment to discuss the plate method in more detail and to review laboratory results and blood glucose records using these meal planning methods.

Using Advanced Carbohydrate Counting

Jackie is a 23-year-old single woman who has type 1 diabetes and works as an accountant for a large firm. She is interested in improving her diabetes control while becoming more independent with her management. Her endocrinologist has referred her to an RD who specializes in diabetes, to fine-tune her diabetes control using carbohydrate counting and insulin-to-carbohydrate ratios.

Jackie is 5 feet 6 inches tall and weighs 132 lb. Her laboratory values are: A1C, 9.7%; HDL cholesterol, 57 mg/dL; LDL cholesterol, 98 mg/dL, TG, 85 mg/dL; albumin, normal; blood pressure, 115/68 mm Hg. Her blood glucose ranges are: fasting, 65–210 mg/dL; before lunch, 40–100 mg/dL; before lunch (weekends), 90–160 mg/dL; before dinner, 50–180 mg/dL; before bedtime, 150–200 mg/dL. Her insulin schedule is: 18 units NPH in the morning; 10 units NPH in the evening; regular insulin before meals (7 units at breakfast; 8 units at lunch; 9 units at dinner). Her insulin plan is being changed to 20 units glargine at bedtime and lispro before meals based on insulin-to-carbohydrate ratio and correction factor.

Jackie is currently physically active, using a treadmill and cross-trainer 2 nights per week after work and on Saturday morning. She is very interested in continuing this schedule of physical activity.

Jackie's new blood glucose targets are: premeal, 90–130 mg/dL; 2-hour postmeal, less than 180 mg/dL. Her A1C target level is less than 7%.

At the initial visit, the RD focuses on assessing Jackie's current diabetes self-management skills (testing, recording, and interpreting blood glucose results; experience and ability in adjusting insulin levels based on glucose results; and coordinating food intake and physical activity with insulin schedules). Jackie reports that she exercised twice after work during the past week and felt hypoglycemic each time. Her blood glucose level on these days before evening meals was between 40 and 50 mg/dL.

An assessment of Jackie's usual food intake and patterns of eating reveals the following:

- Breakfast (7:30–8:00 am): 2 slices of toast, 8 oz of orange juice, hot tea (four carbohydrate servings)
- Lunch (12:00–1:30 pm): 6 oz of yogurt, 5 crackers, and fresh fruit; or deli sandwich with chips, diet soda (three carbohydrate servings)
- Dinner (6:30–7:30 pm): chicken vegetable stir-fry, egg roll, 1 cup rice, tea (four carbohydrate servings)
- Evening snack (9:00–10:00 pm): 3–4 cookies (two carbohydrate servings)

Jackie's estimated energy intake is approximately 1,800 to 2,000 kcal. Her frequent low blood glucose levels before dinner on days she exercises indicate a need for food-insulin adjustment—ie, less insulin before the dinner meal and/or an additional afternoon carbohydrate snack before exercising.

The RD introduces the concept of establishing an insulin-to-carbohydrate ratio and explains how to calculate a correction factor before meals. She provides Jackie with the educational resource *Advanced Carbohydrate Counting* (13) and recommends that Jackie keep combined food, glucose, insulin, and exercise records and begin to count grams of carbohydrate, using the following pattern for meals and snacks:

- Breakfast: 60 g carbohydrate
- Lunch: 60 g carbohydrate
- Afternoon snack: 15 to 30 g carbohydrate
- Dinner: 60 g carbohydrate
- Evening snack: 15 to 30 g carbohydrate

The RD recommends that on exercise days Jackie eat half of her evening snack (15 g carbohydrate) before exercise and the other half at bedtime (15 g carbohydrate). Jackie is asked to return in 1 week.

At her next visit, Jackie's random blood glucose level (2 hours postprandial) is 132 mg/dL, and she reports that she had no problems with hypoglycemia after her exercise sessions when she included a snack before her exercise session. The RD assists Jackie in establishing an insulin-to-carbohydrate ratio using the formula 500 divided by TDD. Jackie's current dose of insulin is 20 units glargine at bedtime, 5 units lispro before breakfast, 4 units lispro before lunch, and 5 units lispro before dinner, for a TDD of 34 units. Because 500 divided by 34 equals 15, the insulin-to-carbohydrate ratio is 1:15 (1 unit of insulin covers 15 g carbohydrate).

In addition, the RD teaches Jackie how to calculate a correction factor to correct for a high or low blood glucose level before meals. Using the formula 1,800 (standard rule for rapid-acting insulin) divided by 34 (Jackie's TDD), the correction factor is 53, which means that adding or subtracting 1 unit of insulin increases or decreases Jackie's blood glucose by 53 mg/dL.

The RD provides Jackie with a copy of *Eat Out, Eat Right!* (14), to obtain carbohydrate values of foods in popular fast-food and ethnic restaurants. In addition, the RD gives Jackie a reference, *Basic Carbohydrate Counting,* for looking up carbohydrate, fat, and energy values of foods (15).

The RD asks Jackie to continue to keep daily diabetes self-care records over the next few weeks, recording carbohydrate intake at each meal, insulin dosage, physical activity, and blood glucose results before each meal, snack, bedtime, and exercise session. Jackie will begin adjusting rapid-acting insulin based on her insulin-to-carbohydrate ratio and correction factor before each meal and will fax self-care records to the RD for follow-up by phone. Jackie's RD will update her endocrinologist and communicate progress. The RD will also see Jackie, as needed, to review food and blood glucose records and to assist in making insulin and meal-plan adjustments as needed.

SUMMARY

There are many educational approaches and resources available to dietetics professionals who work with people who have diabetes. There is no one ideal educational approach or teaching tool. Optimal nutrition therapy and diabetes outcomes can be achieved when the nutrition assessment, desired clinical goals, and preferred lifestyle of the person with diabetes are used to guide creative diabetes meal planning. A review of the meal-planning approaches discussed in this chapter can be found in Table 18.3.

TABLE 18.3 Meal Planning Tools

Meal-Planning Tool	Key Messages	Appropriate Population	Strengths	Weaknesses
Healthful eating guidelines				
The First Step in Diabetes Meal Planning (1)	• Food pyramid concept • Serving sizes • General guidelines for servings per day • Healthful food choices	• Individuals newly diagnosed with diabetes • Individuals with fixed medication/insulin plans • Individuals who need basic concepts or prefer visual approach to learning • Individuals following a low-fat meal plan • Individuals with poor math skills • Individuals who are unable or unwilling to	• Easy-to-follow format, simple concept • Can be used to assess nutritional adequacy and quality of individual's usual eating pattern • Basic healthful lifestyle tips • Tips for choosing healthful, low-fat foods • General guidelines for servings per day (could be given to patients before their first RD visit)	• Limited number of foods listed • No space for sample menu • Does not specifically discuss carbohydrate control • Does not review carbohydrate label reading • Does not cover combination and fast foods

(continued)

TABLE 18.3 (*Continued*)

Meal-Planning Tool	Key Messages	Appropriate Population	Strengths	Weaknesses
		use a more complex meal planning system	• Space for individualized meal plan and personal goals • Food-group nutrient composition provided (allows teaching of introductory carbohydrate concepts) • Available in Spanish	
Healthy Food Choices (3)	• Healthful lifestyle including physical activity • Food groups • Portion control • Healthful food choices • Basic carbohydrate concepts	• Individuals newly diagnosed with diabetes • Individuals with pre-diabetes (piece does not say diabetes in text) • Individuals with fixed medication/insulin plans • Individuals following a low-fat meal plan • Individuals who are not ready or do not require detailed carbohydrate counting information	• Can be used to assess nutritional adequacy and quality of individual's usual eating pattern • Detailed healthful lifestyle tips: exercise, variety, low fat, fiber, weight, alcohol • Space for individualized meal plan and sample menu • General guidelines for servings per day and nutrient composition • Information on combination foods and fast foods • Basic carbohydrate and meal timing concepts • Goal setting tips and space for personal goals • Available in Spanish	• Less intuitive format • Does not specifically discuss carbohydrate counting • Does not review carbohydrate label reading

Plate method

Meal-Planning Tool	Key Messages	Appropriate Population	Strengths	Weaknesses
Box 18.1	• General portion control • Consistency • Basic food categories	• Individuals newly diagnosed with diabetes • Individuals in long-term care • Individuals with poor reading or math skills • Individuals with fixed medication/insulin regimens • Individuals who are unable or unwilling to use more complex meal planning systems • Individuals who do not require detailed carbohydrate information	• Simple and intuitive • Does not require measurement of foods • Easy to use and teach • Useful when counseling non-English speaking individuals • Good tool for visual learners	• Broad portion control method • Portions may vary • Need to adapt for people who do not drink milk • May not emphasize healthful foods • May not cover carbohydrate concepts • Does not review label reading

(*continued*)

TABLE 18.3 (*Continued*)

Meal-Planning Tool	Key Messages	Appropriate Population	Strengths	Weaknesses
Menus				
Individualized menus	• Portion control • Meal spacing	• Individuals who have routine eating habits and eat at consistent places • Individuals with fixed medication/insulin regimens • Individuals who are unable or do not wish to use a meal planning system • Individuals with multiple nutrition restrictions and limited ability to integrate the various guidelines	• Easy to use and teach • Does not require meal planning skills • Can model healthful eating and variety • Can be individualized to individual's needs for fat, protein, sodium intake, meal pattern, and carbohydrate intake	• Highly structured • Does not teach guidelines for selecting healthful foods • Does not cover carbohydrate concepts
Exchange system				
Eating Healthy with Diabetes: An Easy Read Guide (16)	• Exchange system food groups • Portions • Low-fat, low-sugar food choices • Combination foods	• Individuals with fixed medication/insulin regimens • Individuals who need basic concepts • Individuals with poor math skills • Individuals who are unable or unwilling to use more complex meal planning systems	• Many pictures of foods, food groups, and combination foods • Simplified exchange system • Pictures showing how to count combination foods • Space for personal meal plan by meal	• High degree of structure • Limited food lists • Does not cover carbohydrate concepts or label reading • Does not review healthful lifestyle • Does not show meal plan for day on one page
Exchange Lists for Meal Planning (6)	• Exchange system • Macronutrient information and calories • Portion sizes • Healthful food choices and tips	• Individuals with good reading and math skills • Individuals with fixed medication/insulin regimens • Individuals who are willing to measure foods • Individuals with a desire to have increased flexibility in food choices • Individuals who need to limit total fat, saturated fat, or calories • Individuals who are already familiar with exchange-based meal planning	• Can be used for nutrition assessment • Can be used for calculation of macronutrient content and calorie level of meal plan or recipes • Detailed food lists (including combination and fast foods) and nutrient information • Space for individual meal plan and detailed menu ideas • Detailed information for people limiting fat and calorie intake • Allows more flexibility in food choices	• High degree of structure • Requires multiple visits for instruction • Information too detailed or complex for some people • Requires good reading and math skills • Does not specifically discuss carbohydrate counting

(*continued*)

TABLE 18.3 (*Continued*)

Meal-Planning Tool	Key Messages	Appropriate Population	Strengths	Weaknesses
			• Basic carbohydrate concepts • High-sodium foods identified • Reviews label reading • Basic meal timing information • Available in Spanish	

Carbohydrate counting

Meal-Planning Tool	Key Messages	Appropriate Population	Strengths	Weaknesses
Basic Carbohydrate Counting (15)	• Basic carbohydrate concepts • Basic blood glucose management concepts • Consistent carbohydrate intake • Portion control	• Individuals with moderate reading and math skills • Individuals who need a focused education message • Individuals who do little medication and insulin adjustment • Individuals with a desire to have increased flexibility in food choices • Individuals who eat out or use foods with labels frequently	• Space for individualized meal plan • Information on combination foods and fast foods • Single nutrient, focused education topic • Consistent carbohydrate and meal spacing concepts • Limited space for setting personal goals	• No general guidelines for servings per day for food groups • Little space for menu ideas • Limited information on healthful food choices
Advanced Carbohydrate Counting (13)	• Advanced carbohydrate counting concepts • Advanced blood glucose and pattern management • Record keeping • Portion control	• Individuals with good reading and math skills • Individuals who are willing and able to monitor blood glucose levels frequently, keep detailed records, and measure or weigh foods • Individuals who use flexible insulin plans, understand insulin action profiles, and feel confident with insulin dose adjustment • Individuals with variable meal times or food intake • Individuals who want maximal flexibility in food choices • Individuals who eat out or use foods with labels frequently • Individuals who already understand basic carbohydrate counting and label reading	• Single nutrient-focused education topic • Detailed review of record keeping • Basic review of blood glucose monitoring and postprandial blood glucose • Reviews how to calculate insulin-to-carbohydrate ratios, insulin sensitivity factors, and pattern management with practice exercises • Basic troubleshooting for weight gain and hypoglycemia • Insulin adjustment for fiber and fat	• Requires multiple visits for instruction • Concepts too complex for many people • Requires good reading and math skills • Does not include any food lists, so must be used with another resource that provides nutrient composition of foods • Does not cover label reading • Does not review insulin action • Limited information on healthful food choices

REFERENCES

1. *The First Step in Diabetes Meal Planning.* Alexandria, Va, and Chicago, Ill: American Diabetes Association and American Dietetic Association; 2003.

2. American Diabetes Association. Diabetes food pyramid. Available at: http://www.diabetes.org/nutrition-and-recipes/nutrition/foodpyramid.jsp. Accessed January 10, 2005.

3. *Healthy Food Choices.* Alexandria, Va, and Chicago, Ill: American Diabetes Association and American Dietetic Association; 2003.

4. Exchanges. In: Holler HJ, Green Pastors J, eds. *Diabetes Medical Nutrition Therapy: A Professional Guide to Management and Nutrition Education Resource.* Chicago, Ill: American Dietetic Association; 1997:167–178.

5. Franz MJ. Exchange lists for meal planning: what you should know about the 1995 version. *On the Cutting Edge.* 1996;17(2):12–15.

6. *Exchange Lists for Meal Planning.* Alexandria, Va, and Chicago, Ill: American Diabetes Association and American Dietetic Association; 2003.

7. American Diabetes Association. Technical review: evidence-based nutrition principles and recommendation for the treatment and prevention of diabetes and related complications. *Diabetes Care.* 2002;25:148–198.

8. Nuttall FQ. Carbohydrate and dietary management of clients with insulin-requiring diabetes. *Diabetes Care.* 1993;16:1039–1042.

9. American Diabetes Association. Nutrition recommendations and principles for people with diabetes mellitus. *Diabetes Care.* 1994;17:519–522.

10. Diabetes Control and Complications Trial Research Group. The effect of intensive treatment of diabetes on the development and progression of long-term complications in insulin-dependent diabetes mellitus. *N Engl J Med.* 1993;329:977–986.

11. Anderson EJ, Richardson M, Castle G, Cercone S, Delahanty L, Lyon R, Mueller D, Snetselaar L; Diabetes Control and Complications Trial Research Group. Nutrition interventions for intensive therapy in the Diabetes Control and Complications Trial. *J Am Diet Assoc.* 1993;93:766–772.

12. American Diabetes Association. Standards of medical care in diabetes. *Diabetes Care.* 2005;28(Suppl 1):S4–S36.

13. *Advanced Carbohydrate Counting.* Alexandria, Va, and Chicago, Ill: American Diabetes Association and American Dietetic Association; 2003.

14. Warshaw HS. *Eat Out, Eat Right!* Chicago, Ill: Surrey Books; 2003.

15. *Basic Carbohydrate Counting.* Alexandria, Va, and Chicago, Ill: American Diabetes Association and American Dietetic Association; 2003.

16. *Eating Healthy with Diabetes: An Easy Read Guide.* Alexandria, Va, and Chicago, Ill: American Diabetes Association and American Dietetic Association; 2003.

ADDITIONAL RESOURCES

Carbohydrate Counting. Minneapolis, Minn: International Diabetes Center; 2002.

Idaho Plate Method Web site. Available at: http://www.platemethod.com. Accessed January 11, 2005. Offers nutrition materials based on the Idaho Plate Method.

The Month of Meals series. Alexandria, Va: American Diabetes Association. Five books that teach the menu-planning approach. Each book contains 28 days of complete menus written for a basic meal plan of 1,500 kcal/day, including three meals plus two 60-kcal snacks or one 125-kcal snack. Instructions are provided for how to adjust the calorie level upward or downward with sample patterns for 1,200 kcal, 1,800 kcal, and 2,100 kcal included. Menus provide 45% to 50% of energy from carbohydrate, 20% from protein, and about 30% from fat. Some recipes are included.

My Food Plan. Minneapolis, Minn: International Diabetes Center; 2004. An easy-to-read booklet that teaches the basics of carbohydrate counting and label reading.

My Food Plan Made Easy. Minneapolis, Minn: International Diabetes Center; 2004. A simplified, large-print version of *My Food Plan* for individuals who have difficulty with carbohydrate counting. Useful with the elderly, hospitalized patients, and the "math challenged."

Tabletop Nutrition Web site. Available at: http://www.tabletopnutrition.com. Accessed January 11, 2005. Offers diabetes and nutrition placemats based on the plate method.

Warshaw H, Bolderman K. *Practical Carbohydrate Counting: A How-to-Teach Guide for Health Professionals.* Alexandria, Va: American Diabetes Association; 2000.

Warshaw H, Kulkarni K. *Complete Guide to Carb Counting.* Alexandria, Va: American Diabetes Association; 2000.

19

Advanced Topics in Diabetes Nutrition Management

Hope S. Warshaw, MMSc, RD, BC-ADM, CDE

CHAPTER OVERVIEW

- Topics covered in this chapter may be considered advanced. However, some individuals with diabetes may need this information at their first visit with a dietetics professional. (See Appendixes B and C for other advanced topics.)
- Assessment of the person's wants, needs, lifestyle, medication plan, and diabetes goals helps determine the content to cover and when to cover it.
- People gain the most understanding of content when they actually need to use it. Thus, focus should be on teaching the content that the individual with diabetes needs at that moment. To help individuals make decisions, it is better to strengthen their problem-solving and decision-making skills, and to teach use of blood glucose monitoring results, instead of providing absolute information or guidelines.
- Because today's more flexible diabetes treatment plans present few absolute guidelines for many aspects of diabetes nutrition management, a "whatever works" approach can be used with many individuals. Dietetics professionals should take an active role and work with the individual's other health care providers to help the individual find a plan that fits his or her lifestyle.

SNACKING

Because there are a variety of medication and insulin plans available to manage diabetes, an individual's preferred food and lifestyle schedule should be the first consideration in assessing whether he or she snacks. Inclusion of snacks should be a matter of want, not need.

Assessment

To assess an individual's snacking habits, the dietetics professional should ask him or her the following questions:

1. Do you currently include snacks in your daily eating plan?
2. If yes, why? If no, why not?
3. If yes, how many snacks and when?
4. If yes, what do you eat?
5. Do you feel that eating snacks helps you control your appetite and/or blood glucose levels or not?
6. Do you want to continue to include snacks? If so, which ones? If no, why not?
7. For children: What is the snack schedule in school? For other individuals (if relevant): Do you snack differently in different environments? For example, do you snack during coffee breaks at work?

The dietetics professional should consider the individual's medication schedule and whether it requires planned snacks to prevent hypoglycemia. However, if the individual does not want to snack, then the dietetics professional should assist in having the medication schedule changed. In the past, many diabetes meal plans automatically included a snack before bed and between meals. Dietetics professionals should educate individuals who erroneously believe they must eat this way because they have diabetes.

Individuals with diabetes may also erroneously believe that snacks, particularly before bed, must contain sources of carbohydrate and protein. In fact, although protein can be converted to glucose, this glucose does not enter the bloodstream when the insulin supply is adequate. Therefore, the carbohydrate content of snacks is most important, and small amounts of protein do not prevent hypoglycemia several hours after food is consumed or during the night. Inclusion of protein in snacks should be determined based on personal preference and the individual's energy and nutrient requirements (1,2).

The dietetics professional should determine whether the individual's medication schedule is well coordinated with his or her preferred food and lifestyle schedule. If it is not, the counselor should recommend a more suitable medication plan to the individual and his or her health care provider.

Snacking and Type 2 Diabetes (No Diabetes Medications)

Controlling energy intake to promote weight loss or maintenance is a priority in type 2 diabetes. Dietetics professionals should help individualize snacking guidelines. Some people find eating more than three times a day helps them to control their hunger and to limit overall energy intake. Others find that they consistently overeat when they snack, so eating less frequently works better for them.

Frequent snacking between meals may not allow sufficient time for blood glucose to return to normal. However, for individuals who can control energy intake more successfully with five or six small meals a day, blood glucose excursions may be diminished each time they eat.

A delayed and/or diminished first-phase insulin release is an early defect in type 2 diabetes. Therefore, it can take 4 to 5 hours after food intake for blood glucose to normalize, unless oral diabetes medications or insulin are used.

Snacking and Type 1 Diabetes or Insulin-Requiring Type 2 Diabetes

New rapid- and long-acting insulin analogs have affected snacking requirements for individuals with diabetes who use these types of insulin. With these insulin plans, snacking is not necessary unless (*a*) it is physiologically necessary for growth (as for infants and small children), or (*b*) it is a part of a person's desired eating pattern and/or lifestyle.

People who use rapid-acting insulin analogs may need to take additional bolus insulin with snacks that contain more than 10 to 15 g carbohydrate. Snacks may be necessary to provide adequate nutrition in children with type 1 diabetes and should be a part of their usual daily schedule. A regular source of carbohydrate can help prevent hypoglycemia in young children with sporadic activity levels.

IRREGULAR MEALTIMES

Eating meals on time can be a challenge for individuals with fast-paced lifestyles. People using insulin or oral diabetes medications that can cause hypoglycemia need to be aware that delayed meals and snacks can lead to hypoglycemia. Dietetics professionals should review individuals' lifestyles, eating patterns, and medications, to determine whether changing their medication plans would increase flexibility and/or decrease problems, such as hypoglycemia, that may be caused by irregular mealtimes.

Assessment

The dietetics professional should ask individuals with diabetes the following questions about delayed meals:

1. How often do you find that you are not able to eat your meals at regular times?
2. Which meals do you have the most problem with?
3. What are the variables in your life that cause irregular mealtimes?
4. What problems do you encounter when you do not eat on time?
5. What solutions have you tried? How well do they work?
6. Do you think that a more flexible medication plan would be helpful? (Many people may not know enough to answer this question.)
7. Do you know the symptoms of hypoglycemia and the appropriate treatment?

If irregular mealtimes are common, individuals should be encouraged to carry snacks or consider a more flexible medication plan. If individuals are interested, dietetics professionals should help them advocate for therapy changes with their health care providers.

Teaching Points

When discussing irregular mealtimes with individuals with diabetes, dietetics professionals should describe the symptoms, treatment, and prevention of hypoglycemia (see Chapter 12), and review and individualize the guidelines for delayed meals presented in Table 19.1 (3).

TRAVELING

Some individuals with diabetes need detailed information about managing their diabetes while traveling, but others may never need any education in this subject because they do not travel or travel infrequently. When teaching concepts related to diabetes management and traveling, the dietetics professionals should use role-playing and the individual's past experiences to make the advice concrete and practical.

Assessment

Dietetics professionals should ask individuals the following questions about traveling:

1. How often do you travel?
2. Do you travel for work, pleasure, or other reasons?
3. How do you travel (for example, by car, plane, or train)?
4. How far do you travel? Do you cross time zones?
5. What is the average length of time you are away?
6. How do you prepare for travel?

Teaching Points

Dietetics professionals should encourage individuals with diabetes to keep as close to their usual food and medication schedule as possible when traveling. Travelers with diabetes should carry enough portable, easy-to-eat foods and a quick source of glucose to manage delays or emergencies that may occur.

Individuals with diabetes should also carry enough supplies (eg, insulin, strips, pump supplies, extra pump batteries, ketone strips) to last the length of the trip plus an additional few days (in case there are unexpected

TABLE 19.1 Guidelines for Responding to Delayed Meals

Insulin Plan	Delay < 30 min, Blood Glucose Level > 150 mg/dL	Delay ≤ 1 h, Blood Glucose Level 90–130 mg/dL*	Delay > 1 h, Blood Glucose Level 90–130 mg/dL*
Oral diabetes medication	No additional carbohydrate needed.	Take 15 g carbohydrate and eat a smaller amount of carbohydrate at the next meal (3).	• Take ≥ 15 g carbohydrate.†
Rapid-acting insulin	No additional carbohydrate needed.	Take ≤ 15 g carbohydrate‡ and take needed bolus with meal.	• Take background insulin at scheduled time; take bolus insulin at time of the meal.
Fixed insulin	No additional carbohydrate needed.	Take 15 g carbohydrate and take usual insulin dose with meal.	• Persons who mix own insulin should take background insulin at scheduled time; take bolus insulin at time of the meal. • Persons taking premixed fixed insulin should take insulin at regular time with additional carbohydrate; consider switching usual meal with a later snack.

*Level should be near premeal target.
†Amount will vary with activity level, medication plan, and length of delay.
‡For individuals who need minimal carbohydrate to raise their blood glucose more than 50 mg/dL, less than 15 g carbohydrate may be appropriate. Suggest they start with 8–10 g carbohydrate.

delays). When flying, medications, insulin, and a blood glucose meter should be placed in carry-on luggage to avoid loss or damage. Dietetics professionals should remind individuals that insulin and meters need to remain close to room temperature and should not be packed in suitcases that will be transported in the cargo area of an airplane, which is subject to extreme temperature changes. For extended travel, individuals with diabetes should bring prescriptions for usual supplies and medications as well as over-the-counter and prescription medications to manage unexpected illnesses.

During all times of travel, individuals with diabetes should wear their diabetes medical identification and should carry the emergency contact phone numbers of their diabetes educator, primary care provider, and pharmacy. If individuals are traveling by plane or crossing borders, they should also carry several copies of a letter of medical necessity for supplies, such as syringes, meter, insulin, and glucagon.

To pass airport security, insulin and glucagon need to be in their original boxes with their prescription labels, and meters must show the manufacturers' names directly on them. Travel guidelines vary by airline and are subject to change. Individuals should contact the airline the day before travel. Concerns or problems with airport security should be reported by contacting the Transportation Security Administration (866/289–9673).

The timing and amount of diabetes medication that individuals take may need to be adjusted if they cross time zones. The dietetics professional should individualize time-zone advice to suit the individual's medication routine and trip schedule. See Table 19.2 (4) for general guidelines.

The dietetics professional should also suggest ways to eat healthfully and maintain weight when traveling. Tips outlined in the following section can be used.

EATING AWAY FROM HOME

Dietetics professionals should approach the topic of eating in restaurants and other places away from home in a practical, hands-on manner, using examples of foods that their clients eat and restaurants that they frequent.

Assessment

To determine the number of times the individual with diabetes eats away from home and to learn about his or her food choices, the dietetics professional should ask the following questions:

1. How often do you eat away from home? Daily, weekly, monthly?
2. Which meals or snacks do you most frequently eat away from home?
3. Which restaurants or other food outlets do you visit?
4. What are you most likely to order at each of these restaurants?
5. Do you ever order take-out or to-go foods? If yes, what foods do you select? Include full meals and parts of meals.
6. Could you change what you order when eating away from home? If yes, what changes are you willing to make?

Teaching Points

When discussing eating away from home, dietetics professionals should help individuals understand the potential pitfalls of foods and meals purchased or eaten away from home, such as large portion size, high calorie and fat content, large servings of protein, and high sodium content (3). To demonstrate areas of concern, dietetics professionals should choose meals that individuals typically eat to serve as examples.

Educators can help individuals assess whether the number of meals they are eating out can be curtailed. Dietetics professionals also can help individuals develop skills to eat healthfully when eating away from home, such as choosing foods with less fat, saturated fat, and cholesterol; choosing restaurants wisely; practicing portion control; and using the menu creatively. When teaching these skills, the dietetics professional should consider the individual's nutrition priorities.

When demonstrating how to estimate food portions properly, dietetics professionals should make the point that the more the individual weighs and measures foods at home, the better he or she will be able to estimate portions in restaurants (5). Dietetics professionals should teach individuals with diabetes how to use consumer resources to find the carbohydrate content and other nutrients in foods (see Additional Resources at the end of this chapter).

Dietetics professionals may use nutrition information and menus from local restaurants to help individuals identify healthful alternatives to less healthful foods. Taking a group of people to a restaurant for a hands-on experience can be another way to teach eating-out skills.

TABLE 19.2 General Guidelines for Adjusting Insulin When Crossing Time Zones

Note: These guidelines are *not* applicable in all cases. Individualized guidelines should be created for specific persons based on their particular sensitivities to insulin and time change.

Time Zone Change in Hours (Direction of Travel)	Insulin Plan	Insulin Adjustments
< 3 (Any direction)	Any	• On day of travel, take insulin based on home time. • Begin using local time in morning of first full day at destination.
> 3 (East)*	1 insulin injection/day	• On day of travel, take insulin as usual or decrease dosage 10%–20%. • On first full day at destination, take usual dose based on local time schedule. Continue taking insulin at the same time each day using local time.
	≥ 2 insulin injections/day	• On day of travel, decrease final daily dose of intermediate- or long-acting insulin by 20%. • On first full day at destination, take usual doses of insulin based on local time schedule. Continue taking insulin based on local time.
> 3 (West)†	1 insulin injection/day	• On day of travel, follow usual insulin plan. • Because travel day may be > 24 hours, a second injection of insulin in early evening may be needed. • If an extra meal is eaten, an injection of rapid-acting insulin may be needed to cover carbohydrate content of meal.
	Intermediate-acting insulin	• If only intermediate-acting insulin is taken at breakfast, a second injection of same insulin may be needed before dinner. Injection time should be based on home time, not destination time. Dosage should be equal to ⅓ of morning dosage.
	Intermediate-acting insulin and short- or rapid-acting insulin	• If morning injection is a combination injection, use same combination for second injection. • Second injection should be given before dinnertime at home, not at destination. Dosage should be equal to ⅓ of morning dosage.
	Insulin mix of 70/30, 75/25, or 50/50	• Take the morning injection based on home time. • Second injection should be equal to ⅓ of dosage of breakfast injection and taken at dinnertime at home.
	≥ 2 insulin injections/day	**DAY OF TRAVEL:** • *Breakfast insulin:* Take as usual based on home time schedule. • *Lunchtime insulin:* If insulin is taken at lunchtime, take usual dose based on home time schedule. • *Dinnertime insulin:* Take usual dinnertime rapid- or regular-acting insulin. If final daily injection of intermediate-or long-acting insulin is usually at dinnertime, delay injection 3 hours and decrease the dosage by 20%. • *Bedtime insulin:* If final daily injection of intermediate- or long-acting insulin is usually taken at 9–10 pm, take injection at same time based on home time, and decrease dosage by 10%. **OTHER DAYS IN NEW TIME ZONE:** • Awaken on destination time and take insulin doses based on destination time schedule.
Any change (Any direction)	Insulin pump	• Until destination is reached, do not change time on pump. • At destination, change time on pump to local time. (Keep in mind that pump delivers basal insulin at the rate set for the time set on the pump.) • If individual is as active as usual, the temporary basal feature can be used for a number of hours on long travel days to increase the amount of insulin delivered. Check blood glucose levels frequently. Glucose levels are the best information on which to base dosage changes.

*Travel day shortened.
†Travel day lengthened.
Source: Data are from reference 4.

HOLIDAYS AND SPECIAL OCCASIONS

Dietetics professionals should encourage individuals with diabetes to enjoy holidays and special occasions and should provide practical information about managing their diabetes during these times.

Assessment

To learn more about special occasions and how they affect the individual's ability to manage his or her diabetes, the dietetics professional should ask the following questions:

1. Which holidays and special occasions do you celebrate?
2. How does what you eat change at these times? Do you fast, avoid certain foods, or eat certain special foods during these holidays and special occasions?
3. Do the times of your meals or snacks change during these holidays and special occasions?
4. Do you have any holidays and special occasions coming up soon? Can we problem-solve possible solutions?

Teaching Points

People have varying education needs with regard to holidays and special occasions. Some individuals may be interested in finding more healthful versions of favorite family recipes. Others may need problem-solving skills to help prevent overeating or may want advice about how to manage their diabetes when meals are delayed. A person's answers to the assessment questions can help the dietetics professional identify the skills and knowledge that the particular individual needs. Many of the concerns related to holidays and special occasions (irregular meal times, eating away from home, alcohol) are covered elsewhere in this chapter. For discussion of adjusting insulin and medications, managing hypoglycemia, and fitting sweets into the meal plan, see Chapters 8 and 9, 12, and 18, respectively.

MANAGING ILLNESSES THAT AFFECT FOOD INTAKE AND TIMING

When illness occurs, the person with diabetes must be prepared to handle the situation properly and know when and how to contact the appropriate health care providers. Dietetics professionals should help individuals review guidelines or provide written information for managing illness.

Assessment

The dietetics professional should ask the individual with diabetes the following questions about managing illnesses:

1. How often are you so sick that you are unable to eat regularly?
2. Do you know how to handle an illness that disrupts your usual way of eating (eg, vomiting, diarrhea, or flu)?
3. Do you keep foods and supplies at home to help you manage sick days?
4. What are you most likely to consume if you cannot eat regularly?
5. Have you ever been in diabetic ketoacidosis (DKA) or a hyperglycemic hyperosmolar nonketotic state?
6. Do you know how and when to test for ketones? Do you have ketone testing equipment?
7. Do you know when to contact your health care providers if you are ill?

Teaching Points

When teaching individuals to manage diabetes during times of illness, dietetics professionals should encourage them to notify health care providers, if possible, in advance of surgery, dental work, or other situations that may require a change in their medication routine or food intake.

Symptoms and treatment of hypoglycemia should be reviewed, and the importance of taking insulin and diabetes medications as close to the regular schedule as possible should be stressed. Similarly, dietetics professionals should review the effects of illness, infection, and stress on blood glucose levels (ie, the potential for levels to increase) and the potential need for increased insulin or medication. More frequent monitoring of glucose levels (every 2 to 4 hours) should also be encouraged during times when the person with diabetes is not able to eat as usual. Dietetics professionals should use the individual's blood glucose results to guide care and actions. Individuals with diabetes who experience illness should be advised to test for urine ketones when blood glucose levels are above 250 mg/dL, and repeat the ketone test every 4 to 6 hours if blood glucose levels remain elevated. Because ketone strips are not used very often, individuals should be encouraged to purchase individually wrapped ketone strips. They have the longest shelf life.

Individuals with diabetes should keep soft, mild, easily eaten foods and fluids on hand for occasions when they cannot consume the foods they usually eat. Dietetics professionals should encourage individuals to stock both carbohydrate-containing and carbohydrate-free selections that have a long shelf life.

Adequate hydration is necessary when an individual with diabetes experiences vomiting or diarrhea, to help restore and maintain the depleted vascular volume and the kidney's ability to excrete excess glucose, which lessens hyperglycemia (3). Dietetics professionals should encourage individuals to keep both caloric and noncaloric beverages on hand for managing illness.

Dietetics professionals should review with individuals when and how they should contact their health care provider, and what information to provide when they call. Important information includes symptoms, temperature, blood glucose readings, medication doses, and food intake. Most health care providers request that individuals with diabetes call if they have blood glucose readings consistently above 240 mg/dL, have the presence of moderate to large ketones, or are unable to keep down liquids for 12 to 24 hours.

ALCOHOL AND DIABETES MANAGEMENT

Before prioritizing what to teach and when to teach this topic, the dietetics professional should assess the individual's usual alcohol intake and the degree of guidance he or she wants or needs. It is also important for the dietetics professional to know which diabetes medications individuals use, their blood glucose control, and their triglyceride and lipid levels. All of these factors influence what individuals need to learn about alcohol and diabetes.

Alcohol is rapidly absorbed, and blood concentrations peak within 30 to 90 minutes (3,6). Alcohol intake affects many biochemical pathways and can lead to hypoglycemia, hyperglycemia, hyperlipidemia, or lactic acidemia in people with diabetes (6).

Metabolism of alcohol occurs in the liver and can impair the ability of the liver to convert glycerol, lactic acid, and amino acids to glucose, potentially leading to hypoglycemia in people who use oral hypoglycemics or insulin. Due to peripheral insulin resistance and increased liver glycogen breakdown, alcohol can cause hyperglycemia in the fed state. The metabolism of alcohol produces carbon dioxide, water, and acetyl-CoA, which can be converted to fatty acids.

Under normal circumstances, when diabetes is well controlled, blood glucose levels are not significantly affected by the moderate use of alcohol (no more than two drinks per day for men and no more than one drink per day for women) (7). See Table 19.3 (8) for the portion size and nutrient composition of alcoholic beverages.

Individuals who take insulin may have an increased risk of late-onset hypoglycemia with alcohol intake. For this reason, people using insulin should consume alcohol only with food. They should not decrease food or carbohydrate intake to compensate for energy intake from alcohol (7).

Excess alcohol can elevate triglyceride levels, and regular alcohol intake should be avoided by individuals with diabetes who also have elevated triglycerides. Some people with type 2 diabetes can limit the amount of fat in

TABLE 19.3 Nutritional Content of Alcoholic Beverages

Beverage	Serving Size, oz	Carbohydrate, g	Alcohol, g	Energy, kcal
Beer, regular	12	11	12.8	146
Beer, light	12	4.6	11.3	99
Wine, red table	5	2.5	13.5	106
Wine, white table	5	1.1	13.5	100
Distilled liquor (gin, rum, vodka, whiskey), 80 proof	1.5*	0	14	97

*1 shot.
Source: Data are from reference 8.

their meal plan to compensate for the energy intake from alcohol, but this sort of adjustment is not practical for most individuals. Therefore, dietetics professionals should advise individuals with diabetes who consume alcohol to consume it in addition to regular food intake, but individuals should also be cautioned about the extra energy intake from the alcohol (6).

Assessment

To assess an individual's alcohol intake, the dietetics professional should ask the following questions:

1. Do you drink alcohol?
2. How often do you drink alcohol (daily, weekly, monthly, yearly)?
3. What alcoholic beverages do you drink?
4. When you drink, how much do you drink?
5. Have you experienced any problems with your diabetes related to your alcohol intake? If yes, what problems?
6. Do you change your insulin and medication plan or what you eat when you use alcohol? If yes, what changes do you make?

Teaching Points

Dietetics professionals should promote the safe use of alcohol and caution people to drink only if their diabetes is well controlled (3). Dietetics professionals should reinforce precautions that are encouraged for everyone, such as moderate drinking and not drinking and driving. Nonalcoholic drinks (eg, club soda, diet tonic water, unsweetened or artificially sweetened tea, diet soda, or water) should be recommended as alternatives to alcohol consumption in social situations.

When individuals with diabetes drink alcohol, they should test blood glucose more frequently than usual. For example, an individual with diabetes should test his or her blood glucose before drinking. If the glucose level is low, the individual should eat a carbohydrate snack to raise it. Similarly, the individual should test his or her blood glucose before driving and eat a source of carbohydrate if the glucose level is low. The blood glucose test should be repeated to ensure that glucose level is normal before the individual drives, or someone else should be designated to drive.

An individual treated with a diabetes medication who drinks alcohol in the evening should test his or her blood glucose before going to bed. In people who use insulin

or oral diabetes medications that have the potential to cause hypoglycemia, evening alcohol consumption can lead to hypoglycemia overnight. Individuals should be encouraged to eat their usual evening snack (if they consume one), or to eat a snack with some carbohydrate, if their blood glucose level is less than 100 mg/dL.

Dietetics professionals should teach individuals that the symptoms of hypoglycemia and alcohol intoxication are similar. Individuals with diabetes should wear diabetes medical identification and should discuss the similarity of symptoms with companions, so that a hypoglycemic reaction is not mistaken for drunkenness. People taking metformin should discuss alcohol intake with their health care providers. Binge drinking may lead to lactic acidosis.

Women who are pregnant or are attempting to become pregnant should abstain from alcohol use. Other people who should abstain include those with frequent hypoglycemia or hypoglycemia unawareness, individuals with elevated triglyceride levels, and people with pancreatitis or neuropathy.

SUMMARY

There is a vast amount of material available for the nutrition management of diabetes, and dietetics professionals generally have a limited amount of time for counseling individuals. Therefore, educators must carefully evaluate the content they choose to cover in teaching sessions. The individual's specific needs and learning priorities should guide the professional in deciding what to teach and when.

REFERENCES

1. Warshaw H, Kulkarni K. Is snacking still a must? *Diabetes Self-Management.* Jan/Feb 2000;80–84.
2. Franz MJ. Protein: New research, new recommendations. *Diabetes Self-Management.* Nov/Dec 2001;85–87.
3. Kulkarni K. Adjusting nutrition therapy for special situations. In: Powers MA, ed. *Handbook of Diabetes Medical Nutrition Therapy.* Gaithersburg, Md: Aspen Publishers; 1996:437–457.
4. Kruger DF. *The Diabetes Travel Guide.* Alexandria, Va: American Diabetes Association; 2000.
5. Warshaw HS. *Guide to Healthy Restaurant Eating.* 2nd ed. Alexandria, Va: American Diabetes Association; 2002.
6. Franz MJ. Alcohol and diabetes. In: Franz MJ, Bantle JP, eds. *American Diabetes Association Guide to Medical Nutrition Therapy for Diabetes.* Alexandria, Va: American Diabetes Association; 1999:192–208.

7. American Diabetes Association. Evidence-based nutrition principles and recommendations for the treatment and prevention of diabetes and related complications (position statement). *J Am Diet Assoc.* 2002;102:109–118.

8. US Department of Agriculture, Agricultural Research Service. 2004. USDA Nutrient Database for Standard Reference, Release 17. Nutrient Data Laboratory Home Page. Available at: http://www.nal.usda.gov/fnic/foodcomp. Accessed September 20, 2004.

ADDITIONAL RESOURCES

Borushek A. *The Doctor's Pocket Calorie, Fat and Carbohydrates Counter.* Costa Mesa, Calif: Family Health Publications; 2000.

CalorieKing.com. Available at: http://www.calorieking.com. Accessed January 2, 2005.

Nutrition in the Fast Lane: The Fast Food Dining Guide. Indianapolis, Ind: Franklin Publishing; updated annually.

National Restaurant Association. Available at: http://www.restaurant.org. Accessed January 17, 2005.

Restaurant Web sites. Many chain restaurants provide nutrition information on company Web sites.

Warshaw HS. Fast food and restaurant fare column. *Diabetes Forecast.* June 2001–May 2003. Each column reviews one national restaurant chain and provides tips, sample meals at three calorie levels, and nutrition information.

20

Ethnic Populations

Tammy L. Brown, MPH, RD, BC-ADM, CDE

CHAPTER OVERVIEW

- Minority groups throughout the Unites States bear a disproportionate burden of type 2 diabetes.
- All people use food in culturally defined ways, and its meaning far exceeds that of simply providing sustenance.
- Cultural food patterns are defined by what foods are eaten, when they are eaten, how they are eaten, and with whom they are eaten.
- Diabetes medical nutrition therapy (MNT) is more successful when tailored to fit cultural practices, such as the use of traditional foods, social and religious traditions, and family and community customs, as well as beliefs about traditional medicines (1).
- Nutrition counseling considerations for Cajun and Creole, Chinese American, Filipino American, Hmong American, Indian and Pakistani, Mexican American, Northern Plains Indians, and soul and traditional Southern groups are reviewed in this chapter. General strategies outlined in this chapter can be applied to other population groups.

PREVALENCE OF TYPE 2 DIABETES IN US MINORITY GROUPS

With the steady increase in ethnic diversification, demographics in the US population have changed dramatically in the past 2 decades. With the rapid growth of ethnic minor-

ity groups, it is projected that by the year 2050, non-Hispanic whites will no longer be the "majority" group (2).

Minority groups throughout the United States suffer a disproportionate burden of type 2 diabetes. The rates of type 2 diabetes among American Indians and Alaska Natives, African Americans, and Hispanic Americans are two to six times greater than the rate in the non-Hispanic white population. These groups not only experience higher rates of type 2 diabetes, but its onset usually occurs at much earlier ages and the complications are more severe. The reasons for these ethnic differences are not well understood, although it is speculated that they may lie in the interaction of genetic susceptibility and modifiable environmental risk factors, such as poor diet and physical inactivity (3).

GENERAL CONSIDERATIONS WITH MULTICULTURAL NUTRITION COUNSELING

Multicultural nutrition counseling competencies can be developed using published models (4). The following sections outline basic skills required for an effective approach to nutrition counseling in any community.

Assessing Cultural Beliefs and Food Practices

To properly assess an individual's cultural beliefs and food practices, the dietetics professional should consider the person's ethnicity and his or her degree of affiliation with the ethnic group. For example, the individual's level of acculturation, religious practices, and patterns of decision making within the family should be examined.

The dietetics professional should ask the individual why he or she is seeking care. It is also useful to ask individuals with diabetes what they believe about diabetes. The individual's treatment choices and goals for care should be identified, as well as potential barriers to learning and behavior change, such as socioeconomic status, education level, and literacy skills.

The individual's previous or anticipated treatment should be explored, as well as his or her current and preferred diet. A proper assessment of cultural beliefs and food practices also depends on gleaning information about the meaning of food in the individual's life, food preparation methods, timing and frequency of meals, and food portions.

Adapting Communication and Interaction Patterns

To establish respect and trust and to maintain the individual's dignity, dietetics professionals should keep a nonjudgmental attitude and accept cultural differences. Dietetics professionals are more credible when they have knowledge of their clients' food habits and health beliefs. Dietetics professionals should also be sensitive to verbal and nonverbal styles of communication (eg, knowing the appropriate level of eye contact).

The dietetics professional must determine the primary language, written and verbal, used in the individual's home, and, when necessary, work with trained interpreters who understand medical terminology and the concepts being taught. The dietetics professional should also establish whether the individual prefers direct or indirect communication. For example, some people may be more comfortable with indirect communication, such as information presented in the third person ("Someone who has been asked to eat less fat, might do this") or diabetes nutrition concepts explained through the use of stories.

Information that is most pertinent to the individual (ie, need to know, rather than nice to know) should be provided. Experienced dietetics professionals find that positive messages are often most effective, such as focusing on prevention of complications, living well, and balance. When possible, consistency in the messages communicated should be maintained.

Additional strategies for adapting communication and interaction with individuals include working in partner-

ship with community leaders and social institutions (eg, churches, barber shops, and ethnic markets); training and collaborating with lay health workers as an essential cultural link to the ethnic community; and disseminating information through established channels (eg, ethnic radio, television, and newspapers).

Adapting Diabetes Education Approaches and Materials

Successful MNT requires adaptation of learning approaches and materials to the individual. Dietetics professionals should first determine the individual's preferred learning style (visual, auditory, experiential approaches) and then use an appropriate teaching method (one-on-one, didactic, peer educators, talking circles, storytelling, spiritual and gospel songs).

Dietetics professionals should consider incorporating rituals into nutrition interventions (eg, initiating a session with a prayer). During dietary recalls, specific questions should be asked. When initiating a course of MNT, the dietetics professional should assess the individual's reading level and consider using a single-concept approach to nutrition counseling.

Appropriate educational literature that is culturally sensitive should be used. The dietetics professional must evaluate the literature for complexity, font size, graphics, and reading level. When possible, dietetics professionals should consider creating culturally specific materials.

The following are additional counseling considerations (1,5–13):

- Include the individual in problem solving and developing strategies for behavior change.
- Build on health beliefs, preferred learning style, lifestyle preferences, and practices.
- Include family members involved in food preparation.
- Use familiar foods in meal planning as much as possible.
- Encourage incremental changes in food practices when medically feasible.
- Address myths and misconceptions about the role of foods in disease treatment and prevention.
- Explore the individual's use of folk remedies.
- Emphasize portion control.

When pointing out needed nutrition modifications, dietetics professionals should take care to not make individuals feel that they have made a mistake, because this may cause a loss of self-respect. Dietetics professionals should continually assess their personal cultural competency and take action to address deficiencies.

NUTRITION COUNSELING CONSIDERATIONS FOR SPECIFIC CULTURAL OR ETHNIC GROUPS

Traditional foods are defined as those consumed regularly—daily, seasonally, or ceremonially—before introduction of acculturation. The following sections review nutrition counseling considerations for Cajun and Creole populations, Chinese Americans, Filipino Americans, Hmong Americans, Indians and Pakistanis, Mexican Americans, Northern Plains Indians, and soul and traditional southern groups.

CAJUN AND CREOLE AMERICANS

Traditional Food Practices, Beliefs, and Customs

Food has played a central role in Cajun and Creole cultures, with French, African, Native American, and Spanish culinary influences (6). In Cajun and Creole cultures, there is a high standard of food preparation, with foods that are rich and well seasoned. As a general rule, recipes have been passed down through generations, with geographic location dictating the variety of foods available.

Both men and women participate in food preparation, with women generally preparing daily meals and men cooking during special events. On Fridays, meals are often meatless, in religious observance.

Some foods, such as rice, are considered too heavy (or to result in indigestion and disturbed sleep) to be eaten in the evening. Others, like fish and milk, are not eaten together, and oysters are not eaten during months with an "R" in their names (6).

Common beliefs are that diabetes is caused by eating too much sugar, and that one's life and health rest in God's hands. Cajun folk medicine includes belief in faith healers and herbal remedies. Many Louisianans value a healthful lifestyle but do not necessarily connect diet with illness risk factors. Some believe that a "normal" weight is unattractive and indicates poor health (6).

Current Food Practices

Traditional food practices are still common, with the meal pattern based on three meals per day. The heaviest meal typically occurs in the evening, although it can be midday. Specific types of meals may be eaten on specific days of the week (6).

A complete meal for Cajuns always includes "rice and gravy"; however, this is not necessarily true for Creoles. Popular beverages include sweet iced tea, fruit-flavored drinks, soft drinks, beer, and dark roast coffee with sugar and creamer. Family gardens are common, although vegetables are typically prepared with added fat. In addition to typical American snacks, other favorites in the Cajun region include *boudin* (pork sausage with French bread or crackers) and *gratons* (pork skin cracklings). Pica is observed in these groups (6).

Holidays, Celebrations, and Fasting

Year-round festivals honor the foods and heritage of southern Louisiana. Common holiday foods include gumbo, pork roast, wild duck or goose, turkey, ham, or a meat-based dish with rice or cornbread dressing. Standard New Year's fare is greens and black-eyed peas, and turtle soup is a common Easter dish among Creoles. Traditional Mardi Gras foods are chicken *filé* gumbo and New Orleans Mardi Gras king cake. Both Cajuns and Creoles adhere to Lenten fasting, in which no beef, pork, or poultry is eaten on Fridays and Ash Wednesday; many also abstain from meat on Holy Thursday (6).

Key Implications for Nutrition Counseling

When appropriate, dietetics professionals should encourage using smaller portions of lean meat in addition to using low-fat cooking methods. Cooking spray and mono- and polyunsaturated fats should be used in place of bacon grease or lard. Note that consumption of organ meats, tongue, sausage, chitterlings, boudin, and marbled, high-fat meats should be limited (6).

Nonfat or low-fat milk as a beverage and in coffee should be encouraged. Additionally, dietetics professionals should recommend consumption of brown rice instead of white, and use of dried beans and peas (6).

CHINESE AMERICANS

Traditional Food Practices, Beliefs, and Customs

The traditional Chinese diet includes predominately grains and legumes with soybean curd (tofu) and vegetables, and to a lesser extent, meat, fowl, seafood, fruits, and fats (7). Edible parts of plants, as well as vegetables preserved by salting, pickling, and drying, are also included.

Key protein sources include pork, poultry, and eggs, with regional consumption of lamb and fish. As a general rule, no part of the animal is wasted. Fats used include peanut and corn oil, and to a lesser extent, sesame oil, lard, and chicken fat (7). Rice, noodles, and dumplings or steamed buns are staples, depending on the ancestral region of China. Typically, 2 to 3 cups of rice are consumed at a meal (7).

Lactose intolerance is common in the adult population (14). Dairy products are not part of the traditional diet. The preferred beverage is clear hot tea, and the preferred dessert is fruit.

Common cooking methods include steaming, stir frying, deep frying, braising, roasting, smoking, and making soups (7). Many condiments are high in sodium.

The traditional meal pattern includes three meals, with foods served family-style. A typical meal includes soup, rice, and two or three mixed dishes.

Certain foods are classified as "neutral"; others are classified "yin" ("cold" foods) or "yang" ("hot" foods) (15). In classic Chinese medicine, a balance between these opposing forces results in harmony and good health, whereas imbalance results in sickness. How each food is classified is generally passed down within a family. Diabetes is considered a "hot" disease that should be treated with "cold" remedies, including use of steamed and boiled foods instead of fried and spicy foods (15).

Some Chinese Americans equate excess body weight with prosperity, and many believe that diabetes results from eating too much sugar. There is also the belief that foods play a central role in the prevention and treatment of disease. Self-diagnosis and self-treatment are common (16,17), and herbal home remedies are frequently used, including for treatment for diabetes. Eating animal pancreas is often believed to improve insulin production.

Current Food Practices

Adoption of the American diet varies and is based on length of time in the United States, degree of acculturation, and access to traditional foods (18–20). There is increased consumption of dairy products and high-fat meats and desserts.

Holidays, Celebrations, and Fasting

Special foods play an integral role in birthdays, weddings, the lunar new year celebration, dragon boat festival (on the fifth day of the fifth month), and mooncake festival (on the 15th day of the 8th month). Many of the foods are high in fat and sugar. At family feasts, foods are served in courses and include a variety of meat and vegetable dishes chosen to symbolize peace, prosperity, and good fortune. Overconsumption at these feasts can occur.

Key Implications for Nutrition Counseling

One of the primary challenges for dietetics professionals is to dispel myths and misconceptions. One of the ways to do so is to teach about foods according to their functions rather than their nutritional properties (eg, instead of teaching that foods are high in fat and cholesterol, the dietetics professional should teach that some foods can hurt the heart and arteries). Consumption of traditional foods should be encouraged as appropriate (7). For instance, tofu may be suggested as a calcium source.

As much as possible, the dietetics professional should involve the person who cooks—it could be the client, a spouse, a parent, or a grandparent. Dietetics professionals should recommend low-fat cooking methods, lean meats, and reducing fat used in cooking. Portion control, in the context of the traditional Chinese communal meal service, should be discussed, including the quantities of rice to be used at mealtimes. High-sodium seasonings should be discouraged, and the use of highly salted preserved foods should be minimized. A trained interpreter may be beneficial, to ensure that the message is communicated accurately (7).

FILIPINO AMERICANS

Traditional Food Practices, Beliefs, and Customs

Filipino culture is influenced somewhat by immigrants to the Philippines; Spain and the United States have exerted the strongest influence (8). Traditional food practices, the selection of foods available, and preparation methods vary depending on the geographic location, weather, indigenous foods, contact with non-Filipino cultures, urbanization, industry and commerce, and religious influences. Coconut is one of the country's main crops (8).

Current Food Practices

Although many Filipino immigrants to the United States prefer to maintain their traditional diet and ways of food preparation, they have adapted to the American way of eating in their consumption of high-fat sausages, canned fruit and juices, and other sweetened beverages and desserts (21). One-pot meals using all edible parts of the animal and plant products are common Filipino fare (8). High-sodium condiments are used generously during cooking and at the table. Snacking on high-carbohydrate, high-calorie snacks is prevalent. Dairy product consumption is not common, but canned evaporated milk may be used in food preparation or hot beverages. Babies and young children are often given reconstituted powdered milk.

Food is given as gifts for special occasions and to express appreciation, love, and gratitude (8). Certain foods carry special symbolic meaning. In particular, sweets play an important role in social life and are served to visitors as a gesture of hospitality; it is considered impolite to refuse these.

Filipino culture includes the following food and health beliefs related to diabetes (8):

- Honey is a cure for diabetes.
- Garlic provides a stabilizing agent for high blood pressure and diabetes.
- Herbs, such as thyme and marjoram, and tree blossoms, such as chamomile flowers, can treat diabetes.

One widely held belief is that "hot" and "cold" foods maintain good health and cure illness by balancing energy in the body. Although many Filipino immigrants prefer to maintain more traditional diet and food preparation methods, they have likely incorporated some American foods into their diets, including a variety of high-fat sausages, juices and canned fruits in the absence of traditional fruits, and sweet beverages and snacks.

Holidays, Celebrations, and Fasting

Most Filipinos are Catholic; other religious influences include Protestantism, Islam, and Buddhism, which have a strong effect on dietary practices (8). A wide variety of food is served at social occasions, including business lunches, lavish dinners, fiestas to celebrate the local patron saint, family reunions, weddings, baptisms, birthdays, and other parties. A buffet table may be laden with traditional and cosmopolitan dishes, including roast pig, caraboa (black-skinned cattle or water buffalo), goat, chicken entrees, fish and seafood, noodle dishes, and at least two rice dishes. Another table displays an assortment of desserts, candies, and fruits. Dietetics professionals should note that dining out is a popular way to strengthen bonds and resolve disputes.

Key Implications for Nutrition Counseling

As the typical Filipino diet is high in fat and sweets, gradual steps toward improving food choices may be indicated. Dietetics professionals should address snacking and encourage lower-calorie snack options. More lean meats, less use of organs, and more low-fat cooking methods should be encouraged. Similarly, salt and high-sodium condiments should be reduced. Dietetics professionals should consider that nutrition counseling may be viewed as a loss of culture, with subsequent resistance to adherence.

HMONG AMERICANS

Traditional Food Practices, Beliefs, and Customs

The Hmong belong to clans (groups), with every child at birth being assigned to the father's clan (9). Households include both nuclear and extended family.

Illness is attributed to a combination of natural, physical, and spiritual origins. There is heavy reliance on herbs, herbalists, and healers (22).

The traditional lifestyle is physically active. Hmong typically consume two to three meals per day, depending on income, without snacks (23). Women generally prepare the food. The Hmong diet is high in carbohydrates, with a typical meal consisting of rice; vegetables; and chicken, pork, beef, or homemade tofu. Meals are served family-style. Rice is the staple of the Hmong diet and is served at every meal. Noodles may also be eaten. Commonly consumed fruits include jackfruit, mango, papaya, coconut, guava, and pineapple.

Common food preparation methods include boiling, grilling, steaming, and stir-frying with pork lard, or, less frequently, vegetable oil. Soups and stews are also popular. Vegetable broth and water are common beverages. Dairy products are not used. Hmong dishes are prepared with a variety of sauces (many high in sodium), spices, herbs, and salt (10).

Current Food Practices

Staple foods in the Hmong-American diet include rice, mustard greens, and pork (23). Traditional fruits are generally unavailable or too expensive. Consumption of protein and refined carbohydrates has increased.

Hmong immigrants enjoy coffee with condensed milk and sugar or plain tea. Soft drinks are cost prohibitive and are typically reserved for guests. Men consume alcohol only on special occasions. Dairy products have been introduced to a limited extent (milk, cheese, and ice cream), with some complaints of lactose intolerance.

The Hmong-American lifestyle is much more sedentary than in their homeland, with subsequent weight gain. Many adult Hmong immigrants have a limited formal education.

Holidays, Celebrations, and Fasting

The new year is the one major holiday. It is celebrated each December or January when the community gathers together for several days, and men and boys do most of the food preparation (9).

Key Implications for Nutrition Counseling

To increase the likelihood that Hmong will seek care from US health care providers, health care professionals should present Western medical procedures as complementary to traditional methods. In many families, a male head of household makes the final decision on all aspects of family life. Therefore, it may be helpful to include this individual in the counseling session, although the privacy of the client should also be respected.

During nutrition counseling, dietetics professionals should consider the following:

- Encouraging traditional foods and recommending lower-sodium seasonings
- Encouraging decreased consumption of protein and low-nutrient-density, refined carbohydrates
- Reinforcing stir-frying and steaming as healthful ways to prepare foods and encouraging replacement of lard with vegetable oil
- Suggesting moderate portions of rice at meals

Most Hmong do not understand that high-fat foods contribute to overweight or that foods contain energy and nutrients (23). Therefore, the use of American foods with low-nutrient density should be discouraged. Because the role of physical activity in weight management is not well understood by many Hmong Americans, dietetics professionals should promote daily lifestyle activity.

INDIAN AND PAKISTANI AMERICANS

Traditional Food Practices, Beliefs, and Customs

Vast differences in religious practices among Indian and Pakistani Americans result in a wide range of eating prac-

tices. Most Indian immigrants to the United States are Hindu, but they may be Muslim, Christian, Sikh, Buddhist, or of another religion. Most Pakistani immigrants are Muslim; a small percentage are Christian, Parsi, or Hindu (10).

Hindu beliefs and food practices categorize foods depending on how they are perceived to affect the mind, mood, and physiology (24,25). Muslim beliefs promote the concept of eat to live, not live to eat. Forbidden foods include alcohol, pork, and the flesh of clawed animals.

Fasting is common in Indian and Pakistani cultures. A fast can last one meal per day, part of a day, or a few days, or it may involve eating sparsely or avoiding a particular food group. Ayurveda is an Indian practice of medicine that involves the use of foods and is based on the belief that certain substances within foods interact with the body to either maintain homeostasis or cause imbalance. Ayurvedic remedies are used to treat a variety of illnesses.

Eating is an integral component of socialization. There are a wide variety of desserts and snacks. Many of the traditional snacks are high in fat, sugar, and salt (10). It is considered impolite not to offer foods to guests and for guests to refuse the offering of food.

Obesity is disfavored. Laws of food consumption dictate the types of foods that can be eaten and the order in which they are to be consumed (25).

Vegetarianism is widely practiced in India and is derived from religious beliefs. Lacto-vegetarian diets are the most prevalent, followed by lacto-ovo vegetarian and vegan diets. During religious occasions, even nonvegetarians eat vegetarian meals.

Foods are classified into "hot" or "cold" groups. In India, depending on the region, wheat or rice is the staple; in Pakistan, wheat, rice, and corn are the staples. Protein sources include whole milk and dairy products, legumes, and, in some areas, goat, fish, poultry, and eggs in small amounts.

Most meals include one or more of the following, in varied forms: homemade bread; rice; dhal-legumes (also known as curry); meat, poultry, fish, and eggs for non-vegetarians; fried wafers; chutney; pickle salad; salt placed in one corner of a dish for optional use; desserts; spiced tea or coffee; and mouth fresheners, such as betel leaves or fennel seeds. Mixed entrees are common, such as vegetables cooked with grains, legumes, and other vegetables; milk or milk products with vegetables or fruits; and grains with meat, poultry, and seafood. A wide variety of spices and condiments flavor Indian and Pakistani cuisines; many of these are also used for medicinal purposes. Ghee (clarified butter), butter, mustard, and peanut, sesame, and vegetable oils are used in food preparation.

Tea or coffee is the beverage of choice, depending on the region. These beverages are often sweetened and served with milk. Dairy and soda consumption are limited because of cost, and alcoholic beverages are traditionally unacceptable.

Current Food Practices

Indians

As in many westernized cultures, consumption of alcoholic beverages and smoking are on the rise among Indian Americans. An increase in acculturation is observed, with an increase in the westernization of food practices (26). For example, the use of butter and ghee is decreasing, whereas the use of margarine is increasing. Indian Americans continue to consume rice, chapati (a homemade bread), yogurt, legumes, and curried vegetables, although consumptions levels are decreasing.

Pakistanis

Among Pakistani Americans, traditional ingredients are being replaced with readily available American ingredients, with traditional foods consumed at the main dinner meal and American or other ethnic food at other times of the day (27). Because of Islamic food codes, meat is not generally eaten in restaurants.

Holidays, Celebrations, and Fasting

In Muslim custom, a full month of fasting, known as Ramadan, is observed each year in the ninth month of the lunar calendar. Ramadan requires complete fasting between dawn and sunset. After sunset and before dawn, foods and beverages are consumed freely (28). Women in the midst of menarche are exempt, as are pregnant or lactating women.

Key Implications for Nutrition Counseling

Traditional Indian and Pakistani plant-based diets are high in carbohydrate and fiber, moderate in protein, and low in fat. With acculturation and westernization of the diet, there is increased consumption of fast foods and convenience foods, resulting in increased saturated fat and animal protein intake and decreased fiber intake.

The use of traditional cereal-lentil dishes as a vegetable protein source and the use of lean meat, fish, and poultry

should be encouraged. Dietetics professionals should suggest using monounsaturated fats and spices and condiments to bring out flavor while reducing use of oil and ghee. Artificial sweeteners could be used in the concentrated desserts of these cuisines. When sodium restriction is necessary, the use of spices and lemon juice should be encouraged to replace salt and to enhance taste (10).

MEXICAN AMERICANS

Traditional Food Practices, Beliefs, and Customs

The traditional Mexican diet has influences from Spanish, French, and American Indian cultures (29). Regional differences result in great diversity in Mexican-American cuisine. Widely available ingredients include chilies, tomatoes, tomatillos, and beans.

A typical traditional breakfast is tortillas with fried beans and eggs, or cereal, and a beverage. Lunch and dinner include beans and rice, bread or tortillas, and meat, often in a one-pot stew, and a beverage. Vegetables include squash, corn, lettuce, and tomatoes. Desserts are few; however, pastries and added sugar are popular.

Mexican culture includes a traditional belief in the benefits of "hot" and "cold" foods in the treatment of illness (30,31). Hot or cold foods may be used depending on the nature of the illness. Folk remedies may still be used to treat diabetes (32).

Current Food Practices

For many Mexican Americans, food practices resemble a typical American diet more than traditional Mexican food consumption patterns (33). Food patterns vary according to level of income, degree of acculturation, and availability of traditional foods (34).

Traditional staples that have remained a part of the diet are beans, tortillas, and salsa. Eggs are also often included because they are an inexpensive protein source. Mixed dishes of meat, starch, and vegetables are typical. Tomatoes, squash, onions, cabbage, iceberg lettuce, corn, peas, and potatoes are the vegetables most frequently used. Popular fruits, if income is adequate, include oranges, bananas, apples, papaya, pineapple, mango, and guava. Starchy foods include rice, macaroni, spaghetti, oatmeal, cold cereal, and bread. In addition to traditional Mexican desserts, other sugary foods, such as ice cream, cakes, and candy, have become popular.

Milk consumption is limited because many Mexican Americans have lactose intolerance. If milk is used, whole milk is generally preferred. Cheese is frequently added in cooking. Soft drinks are frequently consumed with meals.

Holidays, Celebration, and Fasting

Mixed dishes that are time consuming and expensive to prepare, such as tamales, enchiladas, and chicken or pork mole, are often served on Sundays, holidays, and other celebrations. Accompaniments may include tortillas or *bolillos* (yeast rolls). Traditional Mexican and contemporary desserts may also be served. Meals are generally served in late afternoon or early evening.

Key Implications for Nutrition Counseling

Dietetics professionals should emphasize positive food practices related to the traditional Mexican diet, which is low in fat and saturated fat and high in fiber, and emphasizes a variety of nutrient-dense fruits and vegetables (34). Meals are generally made from scratch, simply prepared, and nutritionally balanced. Additional nutrition therapy strategies include reviewing low-fat cooking methods and encouraging the consumption of lean meats and a reduction in the use of oil or lard in cooking (29). The dietetics professionals should inquire about whether the individual observes hot and cold food practices.

NORTHERN PLAINS INDIANS

Traditional Food Practices, Beliefs, and Customs

Northern Plains Indians traditionally have believed that people are interrelated with all other living things on earth. Animals were highly respected for their contributions of food, clothing, shelter, and medicines. Certain food taboos were observed by some Northern Plains people; for example, the Blackfeet Confederacy tribes did not eat spirit animals from underwater or animals with only one stomach (12).

The traditional Northern Plains diet was high in protein, moderate in carbohydrate, low in fat, and prepared with few seasonings. Animal protein, primarily buffalo and other wild game, was the predominant protein source (35). Carbohydrate sources included wild rice, wild onions, potatoes, turnips and other roots, wild greens, rose hips, herbs, milkweed, bitterroot, lamb's quarter, prickly pear, Jerusalem artichoke, and mushrooms (36). Many types of berries were collected and dried (35). Seeds and nuts were also gathered.

Many traditional food practices were forced to change during the colonization period, beginning in the 1880s. Subsistence hunting and gathering practices were restricted. Because tribes faced starvation, they came to rely on the rations provided by the US Army, which included wheat flour, sugar, beef, salt pork, coffee, and pilot bread. Baking and frying were introduced as new cooking methods. It was believed that eating too much sugar caused diabetes.

Current Food Practices

Many traditional foods remain an important part of the Northern Plains Indian diet. These include buffalo, elk, deer, antelope, wild turnips and plums, fry bread, dry-corn soup, pemmican (dried meat mixed with tallow, dried wild berries, and occasionally peppermint), wojapi (boiled, sweetened fruit thickened with cornstarch or flour), chokecherry pudding, and berry soup. The current diet is typically moderate to high in carbohydrate, low in fiber, moderate to high in protein, and high in fat and calories.

Awareness of diabetes has increased, and many Northern Plains Indians are trying to reduce fat, sugar, and calorie intake and eat more fruit and vegetables. Many Native American families living on reservations rely on Federal Food Assistance programs.

A typical meal plan often includes two main meals with a snack in between. Some people snack throughout the day and eat one evening meal. When breakfast is eaten, it is a large meal, including typical American breakfast foods. The noon meal may include leftovers from the previous evening meal, or a sandwich and/or homemade, canned, or packaged noodle soup with crackers. The evening meal is typically the largest meal of the day and may include soup, a meat or meat-based dish, starch (such as potato or macaroni), canned vegetables, fruit, bread, and a beverage. Few fresh vegetables are eaten.

Beverages include coffee or tea with evaporated milk, cream, or whole milk, and sugar; soft drinks and other sweetened beverages; and fruit juices from the Commodity Food Program. Milk is not a part of the traditional diet, and many individuals avoid it because they dislike the taste or are lactose intolerant.

Snack items are frequently high in fat and include foods such as fried vegetables, chips and dips, crackers and cheese, nuts or seeds, desserts, candy, soft drinks, or leftovers from a previous meal. Large servings of high-fat meats (hamburgers, cold cuts, frankfurters, sausages, and organ meats) are preferred, with frying being the favored method of food preparation. Fish is rarely eaten.

Commonly used fats are bacon fat, shortening, lard, butter, margarine, and mayonnaise. Convenience and fast foods have become increasingly popular, particularly among younger people.

Holidays, Celebrations, and Fasting

Hospitality and sharing food are highly valued in the American Indian culture. Food plays a significant role in social events and religious ceremonies. Foods that may be served during or after social or religious events frequently include soup, bannock bread, crackers, store-bought bread, pemmican, fry bread, boiled or dried meat, fried chicken, potato salad, gelatin and fruit salads, wojapi, and a wide variety of desserts, sweetened drinks, coffee, tea, and water. The Crow sun dance ceremony involves 3 to 4 days of fasting, prayer, and dancing by the participants, often followed by a feast at the end of the ceremony.

Key Implications for Nutrition Counseling

Whenever possible, dietetics professionals should encourage consumption of fewer high-calorie main-dish items and recommend smaller protein portions. Lean cuts of meat should be identified, and low-fat cooking methods should be discussed in addition to tips for reducing fat intake. Use of whole grains and more fruits and vegetables with skins on should be encouraged.

SOUL AND TRADITIONAL SOUTHERN CULTURES

Traditional Food Practices, Beliefs, and Customs

The origins of soul food practices lie in Europe and Africa (37). Soul food plays an integral role in the African-American culture. Traditional soul food cuisine is high in fat, cholesterol, and sodium, but also rich in vitamins, minerals, carbohydrate, and fiber. Pork is a main protein source, with the high-fat cuts, such as fatback and ham hocks, used to flavor dishes. Vegetables often used are corn, cabbage, collard and turnip greens, onions, peas, sweet potatoes, and squash. One-pot meals are common and contain high-fat meat and seasoned vegetables in a broth called pot liquor (13). The pot liquor is soaked up with corn pone (cornbread).

Common folk beliefs include the ideas that peppermint candy will prevent hypoglycemia; yellow root tea cures illnesses and lowers blood sugar; and "stringent" foods, such as vinegar, pickled foods, and garlic, lower high blood pressure. Some individuals also avoid fresh pork because they believe that this helps control hypertension. Overweight and obesity may be viewed as a sign of prosperity.

Current Food Practices

Typically, three meals per day are eaten, with noon being the largest meal in agricultural families. Meats typical of soul food cuisine include beef, pork, poultry, and fish. Packaged and canned sausages, frankfurters, and cold cuts are frequently consumed. Game meats are also available in some areas.

Staple vegetables are greens, spinach, pokeweed, corn, green tomatoes, squash, onion, pickle cucumbers, okra, and eggplant. Other popular vegetables are cabbage, beets, broccoli, string and pole beans, peppers, turnip roots, and rutabagas. Certain side dishes, often referred to as "vegetable dishes," include macaroni and cheese, coleslaw, potato salad, potatoes, and stuffing. Southerners also enjoy a variety of fresh, frozen, and canned fruits.

Staple starches include sweet potatoes, dried beans and peas, rice, grits, corn, cornbread/cornpone, hush puppies, biscuits, muffins, cereals, and macaroni. White and wheat breads are eaten less often. Popular accompaniments to meals are homemade pickles and relishes.

Boiling, stewing, pressure-cooking, and frying are common cooking methods. Meats are generally breaded and fried, but are also baked, broiled, pickled, grilled, and smoked. Fats added to foods for flavoring include bacon/bacon grease, pigtails, lard, ham hock, fatback, butter, margarine, and oil. Gravies are served with some foods.

Whole milk and buttermilk are commonly consumed, but lower-fat milks are growing in popularity. Other popular beverages include sweetened tea, lemonade, powdered drink mixes, and soft drinks.

Desserts are often consumed daily. Popular snacks include boiled peanuts, peanut butter with bread or graham crackers, Vienna sausages with saltines, and a variety of other cookies and chips. Among the economically disadvantaged, pica is fairly common (38).

Holidays, Celebrations, and Fasting

Religion and spirituality are central in the African American life. Sunday is typically a time to gather to worship, share food, and stories. There are many religious influences, such as Muslim, Rastafarian, and Christian. Each religious belief has its specific dietary practices (39). For example, the Muslim dietary laws require fasting on Mondays and Thursdays of each week, 3 days during each Islamic month, the month of Ramadan, and 6 days after Ramadan. There are also prohibited foods, such as swine.

From December 26 through January 1, many African Americans take part in the holiday of Kwanzaa, a Swahili word meaning "first fruit of the harvest." It is a family celebration of the rich African heritage, culture, and traditions. African-inspired dishes are served during this 7-day event. Juneteenth Day is a community event to celebrate the emancipation of the slaves. Typical southern African American foods are eaten on this occasion.

Key Implications for Nutrition Counseling

Dietetics professionals should suggest limiting high-fat meats, such as chicken wings, fried meat, sausage, bologna, and fried foods. Similarly, dietetics professionals should recommend using skinless smoked turkey necks, smoke flavoring, fat-free broths, and limited amounts of reduced-calorie margarine and vegetable oil for seasoning in place of lard, fatback, ham hocks, and bacon grease. Consumption of the traditional starches—dried beans and peas, rice, white and sweet potatoes, and corn—should be encouraged.

SUMMARY

Food practices, beliefs, and customs vary greatly among ethnic populations. Dietetics professionals should routinely assess personal cultural competency and take action to address deficiencies. To provide effective MNT to ethnic populations, the dietetics professional must assess cultural beliefs and food practices, then adapt communication and interaction, as well as diabetes education approaches and materials, to the individual.

REFERENCES

1. Tripp-Reimer T, Choi E, Kelly LS, Enslein JC. Cultural barriers to care: inverting the problem. *Diabetes Spectrum*. 2001;14(1):13–22.

2. Sucher KP, Kittler PG. Cultural considerations in diabetes nutrition therapy. In: Powers MA, ed. *Handbook of Diabetes Medical Nutrition Therapy*. Gaithersburg, Md: Aspen Publishers;1996:284–299.

3. Hosey G, Gordon S, Levine A. Type 2 diabetes in people of color. *Nurse Pract Forum*. 1998;9:108–114.

4. Harris-Davis E, Haughton B. Model of multicultural nutrition counseling competencies. *J Am Diet Assoc*. 2000;100:1178–1185.

5. Gehling E. The next step: stage-matching your patient education materials. *Diabetes Care and Education Newsflash*. 2002;23(5):24–26.

6. American Dietetic Association. *Ethnic and Regional Food Practices: Cajun & Creole Food Practices, Customs, and Holidays*. Chicago, Ill: American Dietetic Association; 1996.

7. American Dietetic Association. *Ethnic and Regional Food Practices: Chinese American Food Practices, Customs, and Holidays*. Chicago, Ill: American Dietetic Association; 1998.

8. American Dietetic Association. *Ethnic and Regional Food Practices: Filipino American Food Practices, Customs, and Holidays*. Chicago, Ill: American Dietetic Association; 1994.

9. American Dietetic Association. *Ethnic and Regional Food Practices: Hmong American Food Practices, Customs, and Holidays*. Chicago, Ill: American Dietetic Association; 1999.

10. American Dietetic Association. *Ethnic and Regional Food Practices: Indian & Pakistani Food Practices, Customs, and Holidays*. Chicago, Ill: American Dietetic Association; 2000.

11. American Dietetic Association. *Ethnic and Regional Food Practices: Mexican American Food Practices, Customs, and Holidays*. Chicago, Ill: American Dietetic Association; 1998.

12. American Dietetic Association. *Ethnic and Regional Food Practices: Northern Plains Indian Food Practices, Customs, and Holidays*. Chicago, Ill: American Dietetic Association; 1999.

13. American Dietetic Association. *Ethnic and Regional Food Practices: Soul and Traditional Southern Food Practices, Customs, and Holidays*. Chicago, Ill: American Dietetic Association; 1995.

14. Wang YG, Yan YS, Xu JJ, Du RF, Flatz SD, Kuhnau W, Flatz G. Prevalence of primary adult lactose malabsorption in three populations of northern China. *Hum Genet*. 1984;67:103–106.

15. The Asian/Pacific Islander Task Force on High Blood Pressure Education and Control Cultural Aspects Manual Committee. *Social and Cultural Considerations in the Treatment of Hypertensives in Selected Asian/Pacific Islander Populations*. Sacramento, Calif: Health Promotion Section, California State Department of Health Services; 1984.

16. Ludman EK, Newman JM, Lynn LL. Blood-building foods in contemporary Chinese populations. *J Am Diet Assoc.* 1989;89:1122–1124.

17. Ludman EK, Newman JM. Yin and yang in the health-related food practices of three Chinese groups. *J Nutr Ed.* 1984;16:3–5.

18. Lv N, Cason KL. Dietary pattern change and acculturation of Chinese Americans in Pennsylvania. *J Am Diet Assoc.* 2004;104:771–778.

19. Satia JA, Patterson RE, Taylor VM, Cheney CL, Shiu-Thornton S, Chitnarong K, Kristal AR. Use of qualitative methods to study diet, acculturation, and health in Chinese-American women. *J Am Diet Assoc.* 2000;100:934–940.

20. Satia JA, Patterson RE, Kristal AR, Hislop TG, Yasui Y, Taylor VM. Development of scales to measure dietary acculturation among Chinese-Americans and Chinese-Canadians. *J Am Diet Assoc.* 2001;101:548–553.

21. Claudio VA: Practical dietary issues in counseling the Filipino client with diabetes. *On the Cutting Edge.* 1991;12(6):13–14.

22. Hmong cultural and medical traditions. Available at: http://xpedio02.childrenshc.org/stellent/groups/public@xcp/@web@clinicsanddepts/documents/policyreferenceprocedure/web025019.asp. Accessed January 1, 2005.

23. Ikeda JP, Ceja D, Glass R, Harwood JO, Lucke K, Sutherlin J. Food habits of the Hmong in Central California. *J Nutr Educ.* 1991;23:168–174.

24. Hindu Americans. Available at: http://www.unix.oit.umass.edu/ efhayes/hindu.htm. Accessed January 1, 2005.

25. Religious food practices. Available at: http://asiarecipe.com/religion/html. Accessed January 1, 2005.

26. Karim N, Bloch DS, Falciglia G, Murthy L. Modifications of food consumption patterns reported by people from India living in Cincinnati, Ohio. *Ecol Food Nutr.* 1986;19:11–18.

27. Siddiqui M, Cross AT. *A Comparative Study to Assess the Impact of Immigration on Prevalence, Attitudes and Awareness of Obesity Among Native and Immigrant Pakistani Women* [master's thesis]. New York, NY: Columbia University; 1990.

28. Eliasi JR, Dwyer JT. Kosher and halal: religious observances affecting dietary intake. *J Am Diet Assoc.* 2002;102:911–913.

29. Warrix M. Cultural Diversity: Eating in America Fact Sheet—Mexican American. Ohio State University Extension. Available at: http://ohioline.osu.edu/hyg-fact/5000/5255.html. Accessed September 20, 2004.

30. Harwood A. The hot-cold theory of disease. *JAMA.* 1971;216:1153–1158.

31. Smith LK. Mexican-American views of Anglo medical and dietetic practices. *J Am Diet Assoc.* 1979;74:463–464.

32. Frati-Munari AC, Fernandez-Harp JA, de la Riva H, Ariza-Andraca R, del Carmen Torres M. Effects of nopal (Opuntia sp.) on serum lipids, glycemia and body weight. *Arch Invest Med* (Mex). 1983;14:117–125.

33. Dewey KG, Metallinos ES, Strode MA, All EM, Fitch YR, Holguin M, Kraus JA, McNicholas LJ. Combining nutrition research and nutrition education for dietary change among Mexican American families. *J Nutr Ed.* 1984;16:5–7.

34. Neuhouser ML, Thompson B, Coronado GD, Solomon CC. Higher fat intake and lower fruit and vegetables intakes are associated with greater acculturation among Mexicans living in Washington State. *J Am Diet Assoc.* 2004;104:51–57.

35. MSN Encarta. Native Americans of North America. Available at: http://encarta.msn.com/encyclopedia_7615570777_13/Native_Americans_of_North_America.html. Accessed September 17, 2004.

36. Kopper P. *The Smithsonian Book of North American Indians.* Washington, DC: Smithsonian Books; 1986.

37. O'Brien R. *The Encyclopedia of the South.* New York, NY: Facts on File Publishers; 1985.

38. Tayie F. Pica: motivating factors and health issues. African Journal of Food, Agriculture, Nutrition, and Development. 2004;4(1). Available at: http://www.ajfand.net/Issue-VI-files/IssueVI-Student%20section%20-%20Tayie.htm. Accessed January 1, 2005.

39. University of Minnesota: Ethnic Foodways in Minnesota. Available at: http://www.agricola.umn.edu/foodways. Accessed July 27, 2004.

ADDITIONAL RESOURCES

American Association of Diabetes Educators. Cultural sensitivity: definition, application, and recommendations for diabetes educators (position statement). *Diabetes Educ.* 2002;28:922–927.

American Dietetic Association's Diversity Resource List. Available at: http://www.eatright.org/public/7782_10928.cfm. Accessed January 1, 2005.

Curry KR. Multicultural competence in dietetics and nutrition. *J Am Diet Assoc.* 2000;100:1142–1143.

Curry KR, Jaffe A. *Nutrition Counseling and Communication Skills.* Philadelphia, Pa: WB Saunders Company; 1998.

Food and Nutrition Information Center. Cultural and ethnic food and nutrition education material: a resource list for educators. Available at: http://www.nal.usda.gov/fnic/pubs/bibs/gen/ethnic.html. Accessed January 1, 2005.

Health Disparities Collaboratives Web site. Available at: http://www.healthdisparities.net. Accessed September 20, 2004.

Kittler PG, Sucher KP. *Cultural Foods: Traditions and Trends.* Belmont, Calif: Wadsworth Publishing; 2000.

Kittler PG, Sucher KP. *Food and Culture* 4th ed. Belmont, Calif: Wadsworth Publishing; 2004.

Medline Plus. Population group topics. Available at: http://www.nlm.nih.gov/medlineplus/populationgroups.html. Accessed January 17, 2005.

Office of Minority Health Web site. Available at: http://www.omhrc.gov. Accessed January 17, 2005.

Robins LS. Cultural competence in diabetes care and education. In: Franz MJ, ed. *A Core Curriculum for Diabetes Education: Diabetes Education and Program Management.* 5th ed. Chicago, Ill: American Association of Diabetes Educators; 2003:99–120.

Part 6

Nutrition Education for Diabetes Comorbidities

21

Overweight and Obesity

Jackie L. Boucher, MS, RD, BC-ADM, CDE,
Jeffrey J. VanWormer, MS, and Gretchen A. Gates, RD

CHAPTER OVERVIEW

- The prevalence of overweight and obesity in the United States is becoming epidemic (1). More than two thirds of adults are considered overweight (body mass index [BMI] 25.0–29.9) or obese (BMI ≥ 30). Of those with type 2 diabetes, 80% to 90% are overweight (2).
- For some individuals with diabetes, weight loss can improve glycemic control (3). Intentional weight loss has also been associated with reduced mortality and improved lipid profiles, blood pressure, and quality of life (4,5).
- Dietetics professionals working with individuals with diabetes should familiarize themselves with effective weight-loss and weight-maintenance strategies (eg, behavioral changes, lifestyle changes, medication, and surgery), to help individuals with diabetes develop a treatment plan that integrates and prioritizes both health and body weight goals (see Chapter 5 for information on weight and preventing diabetes).

DIABETES AND WEIGHT

A modest weight reduction of 5% to 10% can improve glycemic control and many of the comorbidities associated with diabetes (eg, high blood pressure, dyslipidemia)

(5). Weight loss is most likely to improve glycemic control in persons with type 2 diabetes who are primarily insulin resistant; in individuals who are insulin deficient, it usually does not improve glycemic control (3,6–8). When working with individuals with type 2 diabetes, dietetics professionals should keep in mind the following points regarding weight management:

- *Weight loss may improve glycemic control early in the disease process.* Most individuals newly diagnosed with type 2 diabetes respond to a 5- to 7-kg (11- to 15.4-lb) weight loss (3).
- *Energy restriction is at least as important as, if not more important than, weight loss for improving glycemic control.* During the nutrition run-in period of the United Kingdom Prospective Diabetes Study (UKPDS), individuals with diabetes lost an average of 3.5 kg (8 lb). Individuals had a large decrease in fasting plasma glucose (FPG) during the first month and a slower decrease during the next 2 months, although they continued to lose weight from months 1 to 3 (3,9). The data suggest that reduction of energy intake is as important as losing weight and maintaining the weight loss if lowered FPG levels are to be maintained (3,7,9).
- *To achieve therapeutic targets, diabetes medications should be used in conjunction with weight-loss strategies.* Weight loss most often is not enough to

improve glycemic control. The greater the FPG, the greater the weight loss required to return FPG to a normal range (3). For example, if the FPG is greater than 252 mg/dL, a significant, and most likely unrealistic, weight loss would be required to achieve a normal FPG level.

- *Medications can increase or decrease weight.* Therapeutic options to improve glycemic control (oral diabetes medications and insulin) can often hinder weight management efforts by causing weight gain. Type 2 diabetes is a progressive disorder, and, as a result, therapy needs to be intensified over time (3). Thiazolidinediones, insulin secretagogues, and insulin can increase weight, whereas biguanides and alpha-glucosidase inhibitors can cause weight loss (10) (see Chapters 8 and 9 for more information on medications).

Dietetics professionals should educate individuals with diabetes on the following: (*a*) use of diabetes medications to improve glycemic control and how medications may increase or decrease weight; (*b*) the potential impact weight loss may have on blood glucose control, depending on whether the individual is insulin resistant or insulin deficient; (*c*) the importance of portion control (ie, energy restriction) in lowering blood glucose level and managing weight; and (*d*) providing assistance in prioritizing weight loss goals within the context of the individual's medical treatment plan.

WEIGHT-LOSS STRATEGIES

Behavioral weight-loss programs that focus on energy balancing, using a combination of decreased energy intake and increased physical activity, are the most effective approaches (5). People participating in programs that include diet or diet plus exercise can expect a weight loss of approximately 11 kg in 15 weeks (11). In addition to strategies on eating and activity, many successful programs offer education and guidelines on behavioral techniques. In the following sections, lifestyle strategies that promote weight loss are reviewed, along with more-intensive interventions, such as pharmacotherapy and bariatric surgery.

DIETS

The past 50 years have seen a proliferation of diets. These have ranged from total fasting to consuming 300 to 400 kcal/day of liquid supplements to eating 1,200 to 2,100 kcal with varying macronutrient distributions (5%–60% carbohydrate, 2%–70% fat, and at least 20% protein) (12).

Energy Restriction and Weight Loss

Recent reviews concluded that weight loss was associated with caloric intake (ie, energy deficit) and diet duration (5,13,14). In most weight-management programs, energy goals range from 1,200 to 1,500 kcal/day and are designed to produce an energy deficit of 500 to 1,000 kcal/day. The dietetics professional should determine an energy goal the individual can maintain. For the individual with diabetes, the focus should be on lowering energy intake while achieving blood glucose goals.

Macronutrient Composition and Weight Loss

Two different systematic reviews concluded that weight loss was associated with energy intake (ie, energy deficit) and diet duration, but not with nutrient composition (13,14). Most evidence in these reviews supported low-fat, lower calorie diets. However, since these reviews were published, several randomized controlled trials have compared low-carbohydrate diets with standard low-fat, hypocaloric diets. In three different studies, the low-carbohydrate diet groups lost significantly more weight at 6 months (5.8 to 8.5 kg) than subjects following more conventional diets (1.9 to 3.9 kg) (15–17). Studies with 1-year outcomes, however, do not find statistically significant differences in weight loss between conventional diets and low-carbohydrate diets (17,18). Additionally, study participants on the low-carbohydrate diet had a higher dropout rate and poor dietary adherence (18). Given the limited evidence in support of low-carbohydrate diets, the American Diabetes Association does not recommend low-carbohydrate diets (< 130 g/day) for management of diabetes (19). Dietetics professionals should work with individuals with diabetes to determine an eating plan that is realistic for the long term and that helps them achieve their metabolic goals (ie, glucose, lipid, and blood pressure).

Nutritional Adequacy of Diets

Current evidence suggests that low-fat diets are more nutritionally adequate than high-protein, high-fat, low-carbohydrate diets (14,20). Dietetics professionals working with individuals with diabetes should support them in their desired nutrition preferences; however, balanced eating plans that include a variety of foods should be encouraged, to support current nutrition recommendations for health and diabetes management.

Very-Low-Calorie Diets and Meal Replacements

Given that energy restriction is the key to weight loss, several different strategies for energy restriction have been evaluated. Two strategies that dietetics professionals may be familiar with are the use of very-low-calorie or low-calorie diets and meal replacements.

Very-low-calorie diets (VLCD) (400 to 500 kcal/day) and low-calorie diets (LCD) (1,000 to 1,500 kcal/day) have been demonstrated to reduce weight (5). LCDs can reduce total body weight by an average of 8% in 3 to 12 months. VLCDs produce greater initial weight loss than LCDs; however, the long-term (more than 1 year) weight loss is not different from that of the LCD, and weight gain for either diet is common (5). These options are currently available as part of a medically supervised program.

Meal replacements are an option of convenience for individuals trying to lose weight. A meal replacement is any food that provides a defined amount of energy (ie, food is in controlled portions). Meal replacements are typically a formulated product, such as formula shakes or bars or prepackaged meals. Most often, these formulated products are used to replace up to two meals and one snack per day, to achieve weight loss (21). Research suggests that meal replacements are an effective weight-loss strategy (22,23). In one study, at 1-year, individuals using meal replacements had a mean weight loss of 5.8 ± 6.8 kg compared with a mean weight loss of 1.7 ± 6.5 kg for the usual care diet. A separate analysis of individuals with diabetes in this study had similar positive findings at 1 year—a mean weight loss of 3.0 ± 5.4 kg for meal replacements compared with 1.0 ± 3.8 kg for usual care (23). Meal replacements may help individuals lose weight, because they are simple to use, reduce food choices, and control portions, thereby improving compliance.

PHYSICAL ACTIVITY

Physical activity is defined as any bodily movement that results in energy expenditure (24). A physically active lifestyle for individuals with diabetes is associated with numerous health benefits, including reduced blood glucose level and improved insulin sensitivity (25) (see Chapter 7 for more information on physical activity). Physical activity can be especially helpful in the context of weight management because it burns calories, thereby tipping the energy balance toward a deficit (5).

By itself, physical activity does not typically result in substantial weight loss (11). The combination of diet and exercise, however, provides the most favorable results for lifestyle interventions. This is not to undermine the importance of physical fitness, however, because many health benefits (eg, improved body composition or reduced cardiovascular risk factors) are often observed among individuals with diabetes who exercise, even in the absence of weight loss (26,27). Perhaps physical activity is best regarded as a key component of a comprehensive weight-management program that enhances the rate of weight loss and greatly improves the prospects for long-term weight maintenance (28).

The American College of Sports Medicine recommends at least 200 minutes per week of moderate physical activity for weight loss (29). Similarly, the Institute of Medicine recommends at least 60 minutes of moderate activity on most days of the week (ie, 240 min/wk) for weight management (30) (see Figure 21.1). Individuals with diabetes who are interested in weight management are advised to expend at least 1,000 kcal/wk via aerobic exercise (26). Some researchers have suggested that even more-intense programs are needed, perhaps daily participation in moderate physical activities for 60 cumulative minutes. Indirect evidence for this advice comes from a meta-analysis on exercise interventions for individuals with diabetes (27). Across the 14 studies included in the meta-analysis, participants exercised, on average, 3.3 days per week for 53 minutes per session for 18 weeks. Results did not show a significant reduction in BMI, indicating the need for further study on more vigorous physical activity programs.

The key physical activity message to impart to individuals with diabetes is "more activity is better than some, and some is better than none." For individuals who desire weight loss, about 1 hour of moderately intense activity every day (in combination with modest energy restrictions) may be the ideal mark. Although intense levels of exercise are difficult for overweight individuals to sustain, physical activity does not need to be formal or done all at once to be beneficial (24). Walking is one of the most accessible, beneficial, and advocated forms of activity (5,24) and may be a good place to start. Energy can also be expended in a number of other ways, ranging from simple household chores to formal participation in sports. For completely inactive individuals, physical activity can be initiated slowly and shaped over time with a gradual increase in intensity.

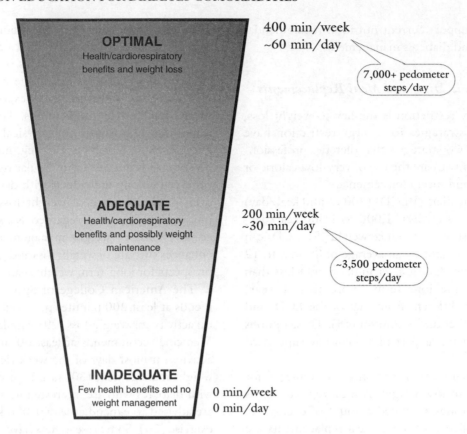

FIGURE 21.1 Physical activity recommendations for weight management. Reprinted with permission. Copyright © 2004 Health Partners, Center for Health Promotion, Minneapolis, Minn. All rights reserved.

BEHAVIOR THERAPY

Successful lifestyle approaches to weight management for individuals with diabetes primarily involve diet and exercise (31,32). Such lifestyle behavior changes are ineffective, however, if an individual fails to engage in them consistently. Knowing does not necessarily equate with doing, and some form of ongoing support is typically needed to help individuals with diabetes sustain their weight-management practices (33).

Behavior therapy is a broad term that encompasses a plethora of techniques designed to prompt and reward behavior change, as well as to overcome barriers (34). It is composed of both self-management skills and practitioner-led counseling techniques that support desirable weight management activities and extinguish undesirable ones (see Chapter 3). There are no firm recommendations on which behavior therapy activities work best for facilitating weight management, but techniques most common to successful behavioral weight-loss programs

include goal setting, self-monitoring, reinforcement, stimulus control, and problem solving (5).

Goal Setting

Setting a goal involves deciding on a target weight, key target behaviors, and a time frame in which to accomplish things. Goals should be specific, measurable, and achievable. Success breeds success. If the goal will be particularly difficult, a more gradual, shaping approach can be used. Also, it is important to keep in mind that goals for lifestyle behavior change are as important as goals for weight, and writing goals down in a contract for others to view can make them more effective.

Self-monitoring

Many overweight individuals will benefit from recording their weight and lifestyle activities. Behaviors can be recorded as events (eg, fruit/vegetable servings per day) or duration (eg, minutes walked). An easy and discrete recording method, such as a small diary to tally events or a wristwatch to record duration, should be used.

Reinforcement

Behavior that results in a favorable outcome will be repeated; behavior that results in an unfavorable outcome will be discontinued. Dietetics professionals should use praise frequently for improvements in target behaviors (or weight). Overweight individuals should also be encouraged to gain reinforcement by themselves via positive self-statements, encouraging thoughts, and social support (eg, recruiting a "buddy" or joining a local group or club).

Stimulus Control

Many cues in an overweight individual's environment are not set up in a manner that supports their desired change. For behaviors to be reduced (eg, eating high-fat foods), individuals should restrict the conditions where the target behavior occurs. For behaviors to be increased (eg, exercise), individuals need to confront themselves with conditions that cue the behavior to occur. Some examples of stimulus control strategies include shopping from a list, keeping high-fat foods out of sight, and limiting the time and place for meals.

Problem Solving

Overweight individuals must be able to problem-solve around barriers (eg, holidays, work demands, stress), in order to maintain a healthy lifestyle. The idea is to proactively try out different strategies until something is found that will modify or eliminate the barrier(s). There are five specific steps in problem solving: (*a*) list all the barriers, (*b*) brainstorm as many solutions as possible without any initial criticism, (*c*) choose the best solution(s), (*d*) put the solution(s) into action, and (*e*) review progress and make adjustments.

Behavior therapy is an integral part of a combined lifestyle approach to weight management (33). Directly applying the counseling techniques and teaching individuals how to use behavioral self-management skills requires a bit more time than standard education. Dietetics professionals do not have to be licensed therapists, however, to effectively deliver this aspect of care. If time is a limiting factor, a referral to other, more convenient

sources of behavior therapy assistance (eg, community program) should be considered. Other factors, such as maladaptive beliefs, negative attitudes, and a difficult history related to weight loss will likely affect discussions about weight management (5). Practitioners can add credibility to such discussions by exhibiting nonjudgmental attitudes and keeping expectations realistic.

PHARMACOTHERAPY

There are two medications currently approved for the long-term treatment of obesity: orlistat and sibutramine. Orlistat blocks the digestion and absorption of dietary fat by inhibiting gastrointestinal lipases. Sibutramine works by suppressing appetite. An additional medication approved for short-term treatment of obesity (ie, a few weeks) is phentermine. It is an amphetamine derivative that acts centrally as an anorectic drug.

Antiobesity medications result in modest weight loss in obese adults when used for 6 months to 1 year (5). In a meta-analysis (35) reviewing the efficacy of pharmacotherapy for weight loss in adults with type 2 diabetes, orlistat and sibutramine had a 2.6-kg and a 4.5-kg weight loss, respectively, at up to 26 weeks. This weight loss is lower than weight loss in nondiabetes populations, where weight loss ranges from 2 kg to 10 kg after treatment (36). Individuals with diabetes using antiobesity medications had only modest reductions in A1C: 0.4% reduction using orlistat and 0.7% reduction using sibutramine (35).

Currently, weight-loss drugs are recommended only as part of a comprehensive treatment plan involving lifestyle therapies. They are primarily recommended for individuals with a BMI of 30 or higher, or with a BMI of 27 or higher with concomitant obesity-related risk factors or diseases (5). Other medical conditions and medications should be evaluated to determine if there are any contraindications to pharmacotherapy for obesity. Additionally, individuals considering medication for obesity should also have realistic expectations about weight loss achievable through this form of therapy.

BARIATRIC SURGERY

Gastric restrictive procedures date back to the 1950s, and since that time they have evolved into a definitive treatment strategy for individuals with severe obesity. Although weight loss surgery (bariatric surgery) is highly effective, it is generally performed after obese individuals have failed to lose weight using lifestyle strategies. Surgery provides medically significant sustained weight loss for more than 5 years in most individuals and is recognized as the most effective approach for achieving long-term weight loss (37).

Bariatric surgery differs from other types of surgery because the outcome is directly related to behavioral change. Selection of surgical candidates is critical to the outcome of the surgery (38). Therefore, weight-loss surgery should be limited to "well-informed, highly motivated" individuals who meet one of the following criteria (37): (*a*) class III obesity (BMI > 40), or (*b*) class II obesity (BMI > 35) with diabetes and/or comorbidities related to obesity, including hypertension, heart failure, or sleep apnea.

Evaluation should be performed by a multidisciplinary team, with medical, surgical, psychiatric, and nutritional expertise to identify contraindications for surgery (38). The dietetics professional has an important role screening the individual who is a potential surgical candidate, to assist in selection of the optimal procedure for that individual. During the screening process, weight history, past efforts to lose weight, food preferences, and food-related behaviors (eg, binge eating) should be evaluated (39).

Types of Bariatric Surgeries

Bariatric surgery can be classified into two general categories: (*a*) restrictive procedures, which restrict the volume and rate of food intake; and (*b*) restrictive/malabsorptive procedures, which restrict the volume and rate of food intake but also produce varying degrees of malabsorption. Restrictive procedures include adjustable gastric banding (AGB) and vertical banded gastroplasty (VBG). Restrictive/malabsorptive procedures include Roux-en-Y gastric bypass (RYGB) and biliopancreatic diversion (BPD). This chapter focuses on the two procedures endorsed by the National Institutes of Health (NIH), VBG and RYGB.

Vertical Banded Gastroplasty

VBG, or "stomach stapling" (see Section A of Figure 21.2 [40]), involves creating a small pouch in the upper portion of the stomach, formed by applying a double row of staples parallel to the lesser curvature of the stomach. The outlet of the pouch is usually 1-cm in diameter and is reinforced by a gastric band. The pouch fills quickly and empties slowly, resulting in early satiety.

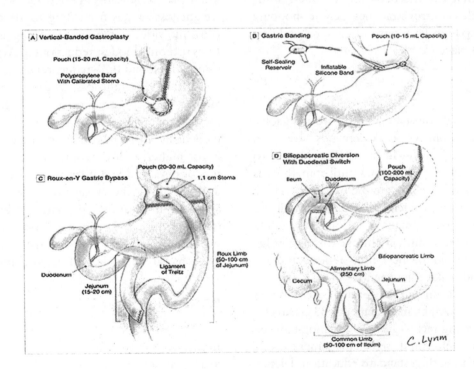

FIGURE 21.2 Surgical procedures for weight loss. Reprinted with permission from Brolin RE. Bariatric surgery and long-term control of morbid obesity. *JAMA*. 2002;288:2793–276. Copyrighted © 2002, American Medical Association. All Rights Reserved.

Roux-en-Y Gastric Bypass

RYGB is known as the "gold standard" for surgically treating obesity. This procedure is characterized by a reduced stomach capacity, usually 10 to 30 mL in size, bypassed duodenum, and varying length of the proximal jejunum. For an illustration of this procedure, see Section C of Figure 21.2 (40). The jejunum is then reconnected with the newly created stomach pouch, where a 1-cm diameter anastomotic gastrointestinal stoma regulates the rate of food consumption. Although the gastric bypass is often categorized as simply a restrictive procedure, it causes some malabsorption as a result of the bypassed stomach, duodenum, and upper jejunum. These changes in the anatomy of the digestive system dramatically alter nutrition management.

The Role of Dietetics Professionals

Dietetics professionals play an integral role in providing nutrition therapy, both preoperatively and postoperatively. A presurgical consult with a dietetics professional can help the individual prepare for alterations in lifestyle. Individuals considering surgery must understand the nature of the surgery, including its impact on diabetes management, weight loss, and nutritional status. Bariatric surgery should be limited to individuals who demonstrate motivation to comply with nutrition guidelines. Other than staple line disruption, excessive energy intake has been found to be the main modifiable cause of poor weight loss after gastric restrictive operations (41).

The goal with both VBG and RYGB is to restrict the volume and rate of food intake. The benefit of the VBG is that it maintains the normal digestive process; therefore, nutritional deficiencies are not a common occurrence. However, if foods are not chewed thoroughly or eaten slowly, individuals may develop postprandial vomiting, which can lead to protein-energy malnutrition (42,43). Postsurgery, individuals should be advised to take a multivitamin and mineral supplement, to ensure that they are meeting the recommended daily allowances for nutrients.

In contrast, individuals who have undergone RYGB may experience macronutrient and micronutrient deficiencies secondary to a bypassed gastric fundus, body and antrum, duodenum and varying length of the proximal jejunum. The most common nutrient deficiencies after RYGB include vitamin B-12, iron, calcium, and folate (42–45). Vitamin B-12 and calcium should be supplemented separately, in addition to the multivitamin and mineral supplement (43). Individuals should take a sublingual dose of B-12 or receive an injection every 4 to 6 weeks (42,44,45). Calcium should be taken in the form of calcium citrate (because of decreased gastric acid) in divided doses of 1,200 to 1,500 mg/day (42). Individuals who have anemia or who are menstruating may also need iron supplementation.

A complete medical exam should be performed annually, to assess hemoglobin, plasma mineral concentrations (iron, calcium, and magnesium), folate, and vitamin B-12 (44). In addition, individuals on oral diabetes medications or insulin need to be monitored frequently. Stabilization of blood glucose level happens rather quickly, often before substantial weight loss, and adjustments in medications or discontinuance from medications may be necessary (46,47).

Complications

Dumping syndrome occurs in some individuals after gastric bypass surgery. It occurs when the lower end of the small intestine (jejunum) fills too quickly with boluses from the stomach pouch. Individuals may experience dumping syndrome if they eat large amounts of food or drink energy-dense liquids that have a high sugar content. Symptoms usually occur during or right after a meal and include nausea, bloating, diarrhea, cold sweats, and/or lightheadedness. Dumping syndrome serves as a negative reinforcement to consuming concentrated sweets, as individuals fear developing unpleasant symptoms, and has been used as reason to choose surgical treatment in "sweet eaters" (41,44).

Protein deficiency is a rare occurrence after either VBG or RYGB. However, counseling individuals on adequate protein intake is pertinent both before and after surgery. Many cannot tolerate high-protein foods, which may jeopardize their ability to take in proper amounts of protein. These intolerances may be long-term, particularly with red meat. Individuals should be instructed to include at least 60 to 80 g of protein per day (45). Because achieving this level may be difficult, supplements are often used until adequate protein intake through solid foods can be maintained, usually about 6 months after surgery (42,45,48).

Surgeons vary in how quickly or slowly they choose to advance the diet, and, ultimately, this depends on the individual's compliance and readiness to advance (42). The diet is typically progressed in phases after weight loss surgery (see Table 21.1) (44). Some surgeons choose to use all phases, whereas other surgeons progress directly from liquids to soft foods. Initially after surgery, individuals will only be able to eat 1 to 2 tablespoons of food, so

TABLE 21.1 Dietary Guidelines After Bariatric Surgery*

Phase	Diet	Notes
I	Clear, nonacidic liquids (≥ 48 oz/day)	Emphasis should be placed on preventing dehydration.
II	Full liquids	Choices may include nonfat or soy milk, light yogurt, sugar-free pudding, sugar-free protein drink.
III	Pureed foods	Individuals reintroducing foods into their diet should be taught how to puree foods. Most fruits and vegetables can be pureed, although seeds and skins should be discarded.
IV	Soft foods	Individuals should be advised to chew food thoroughly to prevent vomiting.
V	Normal foods	

*Widely accepted nutrition guidelines include the following:

- Drink liquids 30 minutes before meals or 30 minutes after meals, *not* during meals.
- Eat protein first.
- Avoid foods that are high in sugar or fat.
- Chew well and eat slowly.
- Stop eating when satisfied, not full.
- Drink at least 6 to 8 cups of noncalorie liquids per day. Drink between meals.

Source: Data are from references 42 and 44.

they must know how to maximize nutrition with a limited volume of food.

The goal with bariatric surgery is to reduce complications associated with obesity (43). Several studies have shown a direct correlation between bariatric surgery and improved diabetes management or complete resolution of diabetes. In one clinical study, 91% of individuals with either type 2 diabetes or impaired glucose tolerance before surgery were able to maintain normal values of fasting blood glucose and A1C up to 14 years after surgery (47). In another clinical study, there was a reduction in diabetes medications and insulin use by 87% and 79%, respectively, after RYGB (49). In those individuals who still required diabetes medications or insulin, the quantity needed to manage blood glucose level

decreased. Furthermore, in 47% to 80% of individuals who had a restrictive procedure (as with VBG), and in 80% to 98% of individuals who underwent RYGB, there was actually clinical resolution of diabetes, defined as independence from all diabetes medications (oral and/or insulin) (49). Interestingly, euglycemia appears to occur before significant weight loss (46,47). The mechanisms behind diabetes resolution still require further investigation; however, several mechanisms have been proposed, including weight loss, reduced energy intake, delayed transit time from stomach to the jejunum due to the small gastric outlet, and changes in gut hormone secretion due to bypass of the foregut (46,47,49).

To date, bariatric surgery has been shown to be the most effective long-term weight-loss strategy for severely obese individuals. Surgery should be considered an option in individuals with both severe obesity and type 2 diabetes because surgery has shown a remarkable improvement in glycemic control and even resolution of the disease. However, surgery appears to have a greater impact on improving diabetes during the first 2 years after the disease is diagnosed (47); this is probably because individuals are most likely to be insulin resistant and not insulin deficient (49).

MAINTENANCE OF WEIGHT LOSS

Successful weight loss is defined as intentionally losing 10% or more of baseline body weight (37). Successful weight maintenance is defined as sustaining a weight reduction of at least 10% or more for more than 1 year (50). Lifestyle therapy (ie, diet and exercise) results in about a 10% weight loss over the first 6 months. Some experts have concluded that about 40% of the initial weight loss is regained after the first year, and weight returns to near baseline within 4 years (51). Similar to lifestyle therapies, drug treatment (combined with lifestyle therapy) typically results in at least a 10% weight loss over the first 6 months (52). Weight regain, however, is more gradual, but occurs quickly if the drugs are discontinued. Obesity surgery has the best maintenance profile. The average individual can expect to lose 20% to 45% of their preoperative weight during the first year (53), and 60% to 75% of such individuals maintain this weight loss long-term (54). Surgery, however, is reserved for very few individuals.

In general, only about 20% of people who successfully lose weight keep it off (50). Investigators consistently cite poor adherence to weight-loss behaviors coupled with physiological barriers, such as lowered resting metabolic rate and increased adipose lipoprotein lipase activity, as likely contributors (55). In addition, environmental cues and heightened sensitivity to energy-dense foods can make adherence to diet and exercise even more difficult.

Although they should not be the sole focus of diabetes management, weight loss and weight maintenance are very important to sustain improvements in glucose control, blood pressure, and lipids (32,56). Despite the importance of weight maintenance, it can be exceptionally difficult in the context of diabetes management. Consistent with other research (57), Guare and colleagues found that obese women with type 2 diabetes regained considerably more weight after treatment than did their counterparts who did not have diabetes (58). The reasons for this are unclear but may be related to the use of oral diabetes medications, prolonged beta-cell dysfunction, and other diabetes management activities (eg, meal timing), which complicate dieting (56,58).

Key Weight-Maintenance Behaviors

The National Weight Control Registry (NWCR), a registry of more than 3,000 individuals who have, on average, maintained a 66-lb weight loss for 5.5 years, has helped to identify some of the key behaviors associated with weight maintenance (50). Some of these real-world strategies include the following:

- *Low-energy diet:* on average, NWCR members report consuming about 1,400 kcal/day, with 24% of energy from fat, 19% from protein, and 56% from carbohydrate. Most eat breakfast daily, and fewer than 1% use a low-carbohydrate diet.
- *Regular physical activity:* NWCR members report expending about 400 kcal/day (approximately 1 hour of activity), mainly through walking.
- *Consistent self-monitoring:* NWCR members regularly observe and record their weight and lifestyle activities. Seventy-five percent weigh themselves weekly.

These lifestyle behaviors have also received considerable support from population surveys and clinical trials. A 1997 review of obesity-management studies involving individuals with type 2 diabetes concluded that a combination of moderate energy restriction (with minimal saturated fat) and intense exercise is the best available lifestyle approach for weight maintenance (32). In populations without diabetes, low-energy diets have also been recommended as the nutrition therapy of choice for long-term weight loss (59,60). In addition, a systematic review by Pronk and Wing concluded that regular physical activity, when combined with a low-energy diet, is the best predictor of weight maintenance (28).

The Role of Dietetics Professionals

Dietetics professionals can help individuals with diabetes achieve weight goals. Several weight-maintenance protocols have been examined, including extended treatment contact, added social support, relapse prevention training, problem solving, monetary incentives, meal replacements, and telephone counseling (51,61).

Extended treatment contact (ie, weekly or biweekly sessions for ≥ 40 weeks) and problem-solving training have produced some of the most encouraging results to date. Extended treatment contact clearly produces better adherence to diet and exercise behaviors (61). One investigation that combined extended treatment contact with problem solving found that participants continued to lose weight up to 1 year postbaseline (62). After 1 year, however, session participation will likely begin to decline considerably (61,62).

The most common reasons cited by unsuccessful weight maintainers include inability to reach goal weight, dissatisfaction with weight achieved, linking personal worth to weight, eating to regulate mood, no problem-solving skills, and low self-efficacy (50,61,63). Based partly on these findings, researchers (61,64) have suggested that maintenance programs emphasize clearly defined goals and expectations and weight-maintenance skills. Most individuals want to lose more weight than they can. This is driven, in part, by oversimplified societal promotions of weight loss (eg, "quick and easy") and personal beliefs that only weight loss can produce other desired endpoints (eg, improved appearance, self-respect, health). However, a large weight loss is rarely achieved, and many personal endpoints only have a weak relationship to weight. More controllable goals, such as improvements in lifestyle behaviors and cardiovascular risk factors, should be emphasized in defining success. Some individuals are unaware of the importance of using weight-maintenance skills after their initial success. The intensity between weight loss and weight maintenance can vary. Weight loss requires an energy deficit, whereas weight maintenance requires an energy balance. Individuals will likely return to old habits if they figure the work is done.

Individuals who are successful at weight maintenance believe they can control their weight but recognize the limits of their physiology and long-term tolerability of weight-maintenance behaviors. Flexible guidelines, coupled with the understanding that occasional adjustments may be needed, are essential (65).

Weight maintenance is a process that is equally important as weight loss. It cannot stop after initial success. The reality is that the overweight individual has to do the bulk of the work. Dietetics professionals can help facilitate lifestyle behavior changes by agreeing on realistic initial goals and expectations, scheduling regular follow-up contacts, using behavior therapy techniques, and, possibly, adding a training component in problem solving. Individuals attempting to lose weight can help themselves by regularly self-monitoring their weight, as well as their eating and activity habits.

It is also vital to understand how weight loss affects other important personal perceptions, such as attractiveness or self-esteem. Some individuals may need additional support from a mental health provider to cope with other, more serious issues related to obesity (eg, binge eating, body-image disorders).

The net weight loss attributable to medical nutrition therapy for obese individuals with diabetes rarely exceeds 5 kg after 1 year (56). The majority of people who attempt to lose weight do not successfully keep it off, and, in most cases, the best that behavioral technology currently has to offer is to delay weight regain. This is not cause for pessimism, however, because, as evidenced by data from the NWCR, many overweight individuals are indeed successful at weight maintenance (50). Additionally, even a modest weight loss can result in significant health benefits, such as reduced blood pressure, lower medication doses, and the prevention (or delay) of chronic diseases (37). All interested parties must continue to work closely together to develop a realistic plan that is sustainable over a lifetime.

SUMMARY

Weight loss is an important treatment component for overweight individuals with diabetes. Besides improving glucose control, sustained weight loss, even as little as 5% to 10%, can reduce blood pressure, lower medication doses, and prevent or delay the onset of other chronic diseases. As outlined in the NHLBI guidelines, there are many effective strategies to achieve this goal, including lifestyle changes (ie, diet, exercise, behavior therapy), antiobesity medications, and bariatric surgery. Although weight loss has a tendency to plateau after 6 months across treatments, long-term weight maintenance is possible when all interested parties (eg, clients, families, clinicians) continue working together to understand and prioritize weight-management goals alongside diabetes care.

REFERENCES

1. Hedley AA, Ogden CL, Johnson CL, Carroll MD, Curtin LR, Flegal KM. Prevalence of overweight and obesity among US children, adolescents, and adults, 1999–2002. *JAMA*. 2004;291:2847–2850.

2. Wing RR. Weight loss in the management of type 2 diabetes. In: Gerstein HC, Haynes RB, eds. *Evidence-Based Diabetes Care*. Hamilton, Canada: BC Decker Inc; 2000:252–276.

3. The UKPDS Study Group. UK Prospective Diabetes Study: responses of fasting plasma glucose to diet therapy in newly presenting type 2 diabetes patients. *Metabolism*. 1990;39:905–912.

4. Williamson DF, Thompson TJ, Thun M, Flanders D, Pamuk E, Byers T. Intentional weight loss and mortality among overweight individuals with diabetes. *Diabetes Care*. 2000;23:1499–1504.

5. National Heart, Lung, and Blood Institute. *Clinical Guidelines on the Identification, Evaluation, and Treatment of Overweight and Obesity in Adults*. Bethesda, Md: National Institutes of Health; 2000. NIH publication 98–4083.

6. Watts NB, Spanheimer RG, DiGirolamo M, Gebhard SS, Musey VC, Siddiq YK, Phillips LS. Prediction of glucose response to weight loss in patients with non-insulin dependent diabetes mellitus. *Arch Intern Med*. 1990;150: 803–806.

7. Wing R, Koeske R, Epstein LH, Nowalk MP, Gooding W, Becker D. Long-term effects of modest weight loss in type II diabetic patients. *Arch Intern Med*. 1987;147: 1749–1752.

8. Wolf AM, Conaway MR, Crowther JQ, Hazen KY, Nadler JL, Oneida B, Bovbjerg VE. Translating lifestyle intervention to practice in obese patients with type 2 diabetes. *Diabetes Care*. 2004;27:1570–1576.

9. Franz M, Green Pastors J, Warshaw H, Daly AE. Does "diet" fail? *Clin Diabetes*. 2000;18:162–168.

10. Beebe C. Body weight issues in preventing and treating type 2 diabetes. *Diabetes Spectrum*. 2003;16:261–266.

11. Miller WC, Koceja DM, Hamilton EJ. A meta-analysis of the past 25 years of weight loss research using diet, exercise or diet plus exercise intervention. *Int J Obes Relat Metab Disord*. 1997;21:941–947.

12. Miller WC. How effective are traditional dietary and exercise interventions for weight loss? *Med Sci Sport Exerc*. 1999;31:1129–1134.

13. Bravata DM, Sanders L, Huang J, Krumholz HM, Olkin I, Gardner CD, Bravata DM. Efficacy and safety of low-carbohydrate diets: a systematic review. *JAMA*. 2003; 348:2074–2081.

14. Freedman MR, King J, Kennedy E. Popular diets: a scientific review. *Obes Res*. 2001;9(suppl):S1–S40.

15. Samaha FF, Iqbal N, Seshadri P, Chicano KL, Daily DA, McGrory J, Williams T, Williams M, Gracely EJ, Stern L. A low-carbohydrate as compared with a low-fat diet in severe obesity. *N Engl J Med*. 2003;348:2074–2081.

16. Brehm BJ, Seeley RJ, Daniels SR, D'Alessio DA. A randomized trial comparing a very low carbohydrate diet and a calorie-restricted low fat diet on body weight and cardiovascular risk factors in healthy women. *J Clin Endocrinol Metab*. 2003;88:1617–1623.

17. Foster GD, Wyatt HR, Hill JO, McGuckin BG, Brill C, Mohammed BS, Szapary PO, Rader DJ, Edman JS, Klein S. A randomized trial of a low-carbohydrate diet for obesity. *N Engl J Med*. 2003;348:2082–2090.

18. Stern L, Iqbal N, Seshadr P, Chicano KL, Daily DA, McGrory J, Williams M, Gracely EJ, Samaha FF. The effects of low-carbohydrate versus conventional weight loss diets in severely obese adults: one year follow-up of a randomized trial. *Ann Intern Med*. 2004;140:778–785.

19. American Diabetes Association. Clinical practice recommendations 2005: standards of medical care. *Diabetes Care*. 2005;28(Suppl 1):S4–S36.

20. Kennedy ET, Bowman SA, Spence JT, Freedman M, King J. Popular diets: correlation to health, nutrition and obesity. *J Am Diet Assoc*. 2001;101:411–420.

21. Delahanty LM. Evidence-based trends for achieving weight loss and increased physical activity: applications for diabetes prevention and treatment. *Diabetes Spectrum*. 2002;15:183–189.

22. Heymsfield SB, van Mierlo CA, van der Knaap HC, Heo M, Frier HI. Weight management using a meal replacement strategy: meta and pooling analysis from six studies. *Int J Obes Relat Metab Disord*. 2003;27:537–549.

23. Metz JA, Stern JS, Kris-Etherton P, Reusser ME, Morris CD, Hatton DC, Oparil S, Haynes RB, Resnick LM, Pi-Sunyer FX, Clark S, Chester L, McMahon M, Snyder GW, McCarron DA. A randomized trial of improved weight loss with a prepared meal plan in overweight and obese patients: impact on cardiovascular risk reduction. *Arch Intern Med*. 2000;160:2150–2158.

24. Centers for Disease Control and Prevention, National Center for Chronic Disease Prevention and Health Promotion. *Physical Activity and Health: A Report of the Surgeon General*. Atlanta, Ga: US Department of Health and Human Services; 1996.

25. Zinman B, Ruderman N, Campaigne BN, Devlin JT, Schneider SH; American Diabetes Association. Physical activity/exercise and diabetes. *Diabetes Care*. 2004; 27(suppl 1):S58–S62.

26. Albright A, Franz M, Hornsby G, Kriska A, Marrero D, Ullrich I, Verity LS. American College of Sports Medicine position stand. Exercise and type 2 diabetes. *Med Sci Sports Exerc*. 2000;32:1345–1360.

27. Boule NG, Haddad E, Kenny GP, Wells GA, Sigal RJ. Effects of exercise on glycemic control and body mass in type 2 diabetes mellitus: a meta-analysis of controlled clinical trials. *JAMA*. 2001;286:1218–1227.

28. Pronk NP, Wing RR. Physical activity and long-term maintenance of weight loss. *Obes Res*. 1994;2:587–599.

29. Jakicic JM, Clark K, Coleman E, Donnelly JE, Foreyt J, Melanson E, Volek J, Volpe SL; American College of Sports Medicine. American College of Sports Medicine position stand. Appropriate intervention strategies for weight loss and prevention of weight regain for adults. *Med Sci Sports Exerc*. 2001;33:2145–2156.

30. Institute of Medicine. *Dietary Reference Intakes for Energy, Carbohydrate, Fiber, Fat, Fatty Acids, Cholesterol, Protein, and Amino Acids (Macronutrients)*. Washington, DC: National Academy Press; 2002.

31. Maggio CA, Pi-Sunyer FX. Obesity and type 2 diabetes. *Endocrinol Metab Clin North Am*. 2003;32:805–822.

32. Maggio CA, Pi-Sunyer FX. The prevention and treatment of obesity: application to type 2 diabetes. *Diabetes Care*. 1997;20:1744–1766.

33. Wing RR. Behavioral treatment of obesity: its application to type II diabetes. *Diabetes Care*. 1993;16:193–199.

34. Watson DL, Tharp RG. *Self-Directed Behavior: Self-Modification for Personal Adjustment*. 8th ed. Belmont, Calif: Thomson/Wadsworth; 2002.

35. Norris SL, Zhang X, Avenell A, Gregg E, Schmid CH, Kim C, Lau J. Efficacy of pharmacotherapy for weight loss in adults with type 2 diabetes mellitus: a meta-analysis. *Arch Intern Med*. 2004;164:1395–1404.

36. National Task Force on the Prevention and Treatment of Obesity. Long-term pharmacotherapy in the management of obesity. *JAMA*. 1996;276:1907–1915.

37. National Heart, Lung, and Blood Institute. Clinical guidelines on the identification, evaluation, and treatment of overweight and obesity in adults: the evidence report. *Obes Res*. 1998;6(Suppl 2):51S–209S.

38. Kral JG. Selection of patients for anti-obesity surgery. *Int J Obes*. 2001;25(suppl):S107-S112.

39. Position statement of the American Dietetic Association: weight management. *J Am Diet Assoc*. 2002;102: 1145–1155.

40. Brolin RE. Bariatric surgery and long-term control of morbid obesity. *JAMA*. 2002;288:2793–276.

41. Brolin RE, Robertson LB, Kenler HA, Cody RP. Weight loss and dietary intake after vertical banded gastroplasty

and roux-en-Y gastric bypass. *Ann Surg.* 1994;220: 782–790.

42. Elliot K. Nutritional considerations after bariatric surgery. *Crit Care Nurs.* 2003;26:133–138.

43. American Society for Bariatric Surgery. Rationale for the surgical treatment of morbid obesity. Available at: http://www.asbs.org. Accessed July 31, 2004.

44. Klein S, Wadden T, Sugerman HJ. AGA technical review on obesity [erratum in *Gastroenterology.* 2002;123:1752]. *Gastroenterology.* 2002;123:882–932.

45. Deitel M. The development of the surgical treatment of morbid obesity. *J Am Coll Nutr.* 2002;21:365–371.

46. Eisenberg D, Bell RL. The impact of bariatric surgery on severely obese patients with diabetes. *Diabetes Spectrum.* 2003;16:240–245.

47. Pories WJ. Who would have thought it? An operation proves to be the most effective therapy for adult-onset diabetes mellitus. *Ann Surg.* 1995;222:339–350.

48. Kushner R. Managing the obese patient after bariatric surgery. *JPEN J Parenter Enteral Nutr.* 2000;24:126–132.

49. Schauer PR. Effect of laproscopic roux-en-Y gastric bypass on type 2 diabetes mellitus. *Ann Surg.* 2003;238:467–485.

50. Wing RR, Hill JO. Successful weight loss maintenance. *Annu Rev Nutr.* 2001;21:323–341.

51. Jeffery RW, Drewnowski A, Epstein LH, Stunkard AJ, Wilson GT, Wing RR, Hill DR. Long-term maintenance of weight loss: current status. *Health Psychol.* 2000; 19(suppl 1):5–16.

52. Bray GA. Drug treatment of obesity. In: Wadden TA, Stunkard AJ, eds. *Handbook of Obesity Treatment.* 3rd ed. New York, NY: Guilford Press; 2002:317–338.

53. Latifi R, Kellum JM, DeMaria EJ, Sugerman HJ. Surgical treatment of obesity. In: Wadden TA, Stunkard AJ, eds. *Handbook of Obesity Treatment.* 3rd ed. New York, NY: Guilford Press; 2002:339–356.

54. Deitel M. Overview of operations for morbid obesity. *World J Surg.* 1998;22:913–918.

55. Perri MG, Corsica JA. Improving maintenance of weight lost in behavioral treatment of obesity. In: Wadden TA, Stunkard AJ, eds. *Handbook of Obesity Treatment.* 3rd ed. New York, NY: Guilford Press; 2002:357–379.

56. Hensrud DD. Dietary treatment and long-term weight loss and maintenance in type 2 diabetes. *Obes Res.* 2001;9(Suppl 4):348S–353S.

57. Khan MA, St Peter JV, Breen GA, Hartley GG, Vessey JT. Diabetes disease stage predicts weight loss outcomes with long-term appetite suppressants. *Obes Res.* 2000; 8:43–48.

58. Guare JC, Wing RR, Grant A. Comparison of obese NIDDM and nondiabetic women: short- and long-term weight loss. *Obes Res.* 1995;3:329–335.

59. Shick SM, Wing RR, Klem ML, McGuire MT, Hill JO, Seagle H. Persons successful at long-term weight loss and maintenance continue to consume a low-energy, low-fat diet. *J Am Diet Assoc.* 1998;98:408–413.

60. McGuire MT, Wing RR, Klem ML, Hill JO. Behavioral strategies of individuals who have maintained long-term weight losses. *Obes Res.* 1999;7:334–341.

61. Perri MG. The maintenance of treatment effects in the long-term management of obesity. *Clin Psychol Sci Pract.* 1998;5:526–543.

62. Perri MG, Nezu AM, McKelvey WF, Shermer RL, Renjilian DA, Viegener BJ. Relapse prevention training and problem-solving therapy in the long-term management of obesity. *J Consult Clin Psychol.* 2001;69:722–726.

63. Byrne S, Cooper Z, Fairburn C. Weight maintenance and relapse in obesity: a qualitative study. *Int J Obes Relat Metab Disord.* 2003;27:955–962.

64. Cooper Z, Fairburn CG. A new cognitive behavioural approach to the treatment of obesity. *Behav Res Ther.* 2001;39:499–511.

65. Sbrocco T, Nedegaard RC, Stone JM, Lewis EL. Behavioral choice treatment promotes continuing weight loss: preliminary results of a cognitive-behavioral decision-based treatment for obesity. *J Consult Clin Psychol.* 1999; 67:260–266.

ADDITIONAL RESOURCES

Cooper Z, Fairburn CG, Hawker D. *Cognitive-Behavioral Treatment of Obesity.* New York, NY: Guilford Press; 2003.

Diabetes Care and Education Dietetic Practice Group: Diabetes and the obesity epidemic. *On the Cutting Edge.* 2003;14(6):1–44.

Foster G, Nonas C, eds. *Managing Obesity: A Clinical Guide.* Chicago, Ill: American Dietetic Association; 2004.

Wadden TA, Stunkard AJ, eds. *Handbook of Obesity Treatment.* 3rd ed. New York, NY: Guilford Press; 2002.

Wylie-Rosett J, Segal-Isaacson CJ. *Leaders Guide: The Complete Weight Loss Workbook.* Alexandria, Va: American Diabetes Association; 1997.

22

Cardiovascular Disease, Dyslipidemia, and Hypertension in Diabetes

Wahida Karmally, DrPH, RD, CDE, and Megan Jahnes, RD

CHAPTER OVERVIEW

- Diabetes is an independent risk factor for cardiovascular disease (CVD) in both men and women (1–3). CVD is the major cause of death in people with diabetes (4).
- Metabolic risk factors that occur commonly in individuals with insulin resistance are atherogenic dyslipidemia, hypertension, and glucose intolerance (5,6).
- Individualized nutrition therapy is integral in the attainment of blood glucose, lipid, and blood pressure goals, and in the prevention and treatment of CVD in people with diabetes (7).
- Interventions may include modest weight loss; glycemic control; reduction of sodium, saturated and *trans* fat, and dietary cholesterol intake; increased viscous fiber intake; use of products containing plant stanols/sterols; and physical activity (8).

CARDIOVASCULAR DISEASE RISK FACTORS

Major risk factors for CVD include (7):

- High levels (> 160 mg/dL) of low-density lipoprotein (LDL) cholesterol
- Cigarette smoking

- Hypertension (blood pressure > 140/90 mm Hg or on antihypertensive medication)
- Low levels (< 40 mg/dL) of high-density lipoprotein (HDL) cholesterol. Note that having an HDL cholesterol level above 60 mg/dL counts as a "negative" risk factor; its presence removes one risk factor from the total count.
- Family history of premature coronary heart disease (CHD) (CHD in male first-degree relative younger than 55 years; CHD in female first-degree relative younger than 65 years)
- Age (men ≥ 45 years; women ≥ 55 years)
- Diabetes

In the National Cholesterol Education Program (NCEP) Adult Treatment Panel III (ATP III), diabetes is regarded as a CVD risk equivalent (7). Type 2 diabetes is associated with a three- to fourfold increase in the incidence and prevalence of CVD (4) and is now an established CVD risk factor (1–3). Insulin resistance usually precedes the onset of type 2 diabetes and often coexists with other CVD risk factors, such as dyslipidemia, obesity, hypertension, and prothrombotic factors (3,4). This cluster of CVD risk factors is often referred to as "metabolic syndrome" (7,9). In contrast, most individuals with type 1 diabetes do not have underlying abnormalities in plasma lipids and lipoproteins (3).

Metabolic syndrome is characterized by abdominal obesity, insulin resistance, hyperglycemia, dyslipidemia (elevated triglycerides [TG], small dense LDL particles, and low HDL levels), hypertension, and increased thrombotic risk (7,9) (see Chapter 4 for more information on metabolic syndrome). A common abnormal lipid pattern seen in subjects with insulin resistance, metabolic syndrome, and type 2 diabetes is an elevation of very-low-density lipoprotein (VLDL) cholesterol, a reduction in HDL cholesterol, and an LDL fraction that contains a greater proportion of the highly atherogenic, small, dense LDL particles (4).

Most individuals with type 1 diabetes do not have underlying dyslipidemias, and blood lipid levels are determined by availability of insulin and glycemic control. In cases where glycemic control is good, blood lipid levels are generally normal (8). People with type 1 diabetes who are overweight or centrally obese may exhibit patterns of dyslipidemia that are similar to those of individuals with type 2 diabetes. Improved glycemic control may be especially important in preventing CVD for these individuals (8).

ROLE OF MEDICAL NUTRITION THERAPY IN MODERATING CVD RISK IN DIABETES

MNT provided by registered dietitians is integral to the attainment of blood glucose, lipid, and blood pressure goals, and to the prevention and treatment of CVD in people with diabetes. The NCEP (7) and the Joint National Committee on Detection, Evaluation, and Treatment of High Blood Pressure (10) recommend the use of lifestyle modification as definitive or adjunctive therapy for hyperlipidemia and hypertension. Lifestyle modifications defined in ATP III include a dietary pattern designed to lower glucose, manage blood pressure, and alter lipid patterns as well as regular physical activity (7), and are unique and important tools for reducing CVD in people with diabetes.

Many strategies for prevention and treatment of CVD are also applicable for prevention and treatment of metabolic syndrome. Potential interventions and goals are outlined in Table 22.1 (7).

THERAPEUTIC LIFESTYLE CHANGE RECOMMENDATIONS

ATP III recommends a multifaceted lifestyle approach to reduce risk for CVD. This approach is designated Therapeutic Lifestyle Changes (TLC). Dietetics professionals should note that other risk factors, such as poor glycemic control, hypertension, and smoking, need to be addressed in addition to TLC recommendations.

Saturated Fatty Acids

TLC recommends that saturated fats comprise less than 7% of total energy intake (7). Dietetics professionals should note that saturated fatty acids (SFAs) can increase LDL cholesterol levels (11). SFAs and *trans* fats should be replaced with monounsaturated fats (12). See Table 22.2 for a comparison of cholesterol and saturated fats in meat, fish, and poultry.

Polyunsaturated Fatty Acids

No more than 10% of energy intake should come from polyunsaturated fats (7). Sources of polyunsaturated fats, such as safflower oil, sunflower oil, and unspecified vegetable oils should be limited. They should be replaced with monounsaturated fat, such as olive oil (7).

Monounsaturated Fatty Acids

According to TLC recommendations, monounsaturated fats should comprise no more than 20% of total energy intake (7). When substituted for saturated fats, monounsaturated fats can decrease LDL cholesterol and TG levels, without concurrent decreases in HDL cholesterol levels (12). Monounsaturated fat sources include olive oil, canola oil, avocadoes, almonds, pecans, and peanuts (13).

Total Fat

Total fat intake can range from 25% to 35% of energy intake if saturated and *trans* fats are kept to a minimum. ATP III allows a higher intake of total fat (35%), as primarily unsaturated fats, and lower carbohydrate (50%) to lower TG and raise HDL cholesterol levels in persons with metabolic syndrome. After 6 weeks, if the LDL cholesterol goal has not been achieved, additional therapeutic options for lowering LDL cholesterol, such as plant stanols or sterols (2 g/day) and viscous fiber (10 to 25 g/day), can be initiated (7).

Suggestions for decreasing fat include choosing leaner cuts of meat, such as tenderloin, eye of the round, top loin and top round for beef; tenderloin, sirloin, top loin, and lean ham for pork; and leg-shank for lamb. These cuts of cooked meat, in 3-oz portions, contain less than 10 g of fat and less than 4.5 g of saturated fat.

TABLE 22.1 Moderating Cardiovascular Disease Risk in Diabetes

Risk Factor	Nutrition Interventions	Goals
Blood glucose	• Modest weight loss • Physical activity • Carbohydrate control: eat meals/snacks at appropriate times; choose foods and amounts per meal pattern; count carbohydrates • Match medication/insulin plan to lifestyle	• A1C < 7% • Preprandial plasma glucose 90–130 mg/dL • Postprandial plasma glucose < 180 mg/dL
Blood lipids	• Initiate TLC diet • Reduce saturated and *trans* fat to < 7% of energy intake • Reduce dietary cholesterol to < 200 mg/day • Increase viscous (soluble) fiber to 10–25 g/day • Add plant stanols or sterols (2 g/day) • Modest weight loss • Physical activity	• LDL cholesterol < 100 mg/dL • Triglycerides < 150 mg/dL • HDL cholesterol > 40 mg/dL
Blood pressure	• Modest weight loss • Reduce sodium to < 2,400 mg/day • Reduce alcohol intake to no more than 1–2 alcohol equivalent/day • DASH diet	• < 130/80 mm Hg
Body weight	• Energy intake to meet weight loss goals • Physical activity • Behavior modification strategies	• BMI 18.5–24.9
Lifestyle	• Physical activity (adapt for presence of complications) • Smoking cessation	• Accumulate 30 to 60 min/day most days of the week.

Abbreviations: BMI, body mass index; DASH, Dietary Approaches to Stop Hypertension; HDL, high-density lipoprotein; LDL, low-density lipoprotein; TLC, Therapeutic Lifestyle Changes.
Source: Data are from reference 7.

Carbohydrate

TLC recommends 50% to 60% of total energy intake as carbohydrate (7). Whole grains, whole fruits, and vegetables should be emphasized. Carbohydrate intake should be adjusted to achieve blood glucose, TG, and HDL cholesterol goals.

Protein

Approximately 15% of total energy intake should come from protein (7). Dietetics professionals should encourage individuals to choose low-fat protein sources and to increase protein intake for satiety and calorie control. If individuals have decreased renal function, protein intake should be decreased accordingly (see Chapter 23).

Cholesterol

According to TLC, the recommendation for cholesterol intake should be less than 200 mg/day (7). It has been reported that 100 mg of dietary cholesterol per 1,000 kcal can raise LDL cholesterol as much as 10 mg/dL (14,15). Individuals should be encouraged to keep lean meat intake to 5 to 6 oz per day and to consume no more than two egg yolks per week. See Table 22.2 for cholesterol found in meat, fish, and poultry selections.

TABLE 22.2 Cholesterol and Saturated Fat in Meat, Fish, and Poultry

Food Item*	Cholesterol, mg	Saturated Fat, g
Beef brain	1,747	2.48
Chicken liver	537	1.56
Beef liver	331	1.62
Squid	227	0.36
Veal cutlet	93	1.96
Lamb chop (with visible fat)	78	10.86
Chicken breast (no skin)	72	1.08
Beef (tenderloin)	65	3.05
Shrimp	166	0.25
Clams	57	0.16
Lobster	61	0.09
Venison	95	1.06
Ostrich	61	0.72
Eggs (~ 2 large)	365	2.81

*Portion size is 3 oz, cooked.
Nutrient calculations were performed using the NDS software (food software version 4.05_33, NCC, University of Minnesota, Minneapolis, Minn).

TABLE 22.3 High-Fiber Foods

Food	Serving Size	Total Fiber, g	Soluble Fiber, g
Apple	1 medium	3.4	1.0
Broccoli (cooked)	½ cup	2.3	1.2
Barley (cooked)	1 cup	8.5	1.9
Brussels sprouts (cooked)	½ cup	3.2	1.9
Legumes: pinto, kidney, lima beans (cooked)	¾ cup	7.4–11.0	2.0–4.3
Oat bran (dry)	1 oz	4.4	2.0
Orange	1 medium	3.1	1.8
Pear	1 medium	4.0	2.2
Psyllium (ground seeds)	1 Tbsp	6.0	5.0
Rolled oats (dry)	1 oz	3.0	1.4

Nutrient calculations were performed using the NDS software (food software version 4.05_33, NCC, University of Minnesota, Minneapolis, Minn).

Total Energy Intake

An individual's total energy intake should be balanced with energy expenditure to maintain desirable body weight (7). In type 2 diabetes, weight loss can improve glycemic control, reduce insulin resistance, decrease TG, increase HDL cholesterol levels, and lower blood pressure (8,16).

Fiber

Fiber intake should be 25 to 35 g, of which 10 to 25 g/day should be viscous (soluble) fiber (7). Five to 10 g/day of viscous fiber can decrease LDL cholesterol levels by 5% (17,18). A comparison of high-fiber foods can be found in Table 22.3.

Plant Stanols and Sterols

TLC recommends 2 g of plant stanols or sterols per day (7). Stanol and sterol esters compete with dietary and biliary cholesterol for absorption in the intestine. Con-

sumption of 3.4 g/day showed reduction of cholesterol levels by 20 mg/dL (11). Box 22.1 shows ways to use stanol and sterol spreads.

A MODEL FOR IMPLEMENTING THERAPEUTIC LIFESTYLE CHANGES

To implement TLC, the dietetics professional may wish to schedule three initial visits with the individual over a period of 12 weeks.

Visit 1: Begin Lifestyle Therapies

At the first visit, the dietetics professional should assess the individual's current eating patterns using standard dietary methods, such as 24-hour recalls and food frequency questionnaires, or by simplified assessment tools, such as "Rate Your Plate" (19), which focuses on the foods that contribute the most fat, saturated fat, and cholesterol to the American diet. Key education topics include the following:

- Reducing saturated fat and cholesterol intake
- Decreasing energy intake if the individual needs to reduce weight (daily intake should be 250 to 500 kcal less than energy needed to maintain weight)
- Portion control
- Moderate physical activity as part of the daily routine

BOX 22.1

Tips for Using Stanols and Sterol Spreads

- Spread on whole grain toast, muffins, bagels, or English muffins, instead of using butter or margarine.
- Make a cinnamon spread by blending ½ cup spread with ½ teaspoon ground cinnamon and store in the refrigerator for use on warm waffles, toast, or pancakes.
- Add to hot cereals.
- Use instead of butter for sautéing vegetables.
- Top-baked or mashed potatoes with spread.
- Combine ½ cup spread, ½ tsp basil, ½ tsp oregano, and ½ tsp garlic powder; mix well and store in the refrigerator; spread on whole wheat bread and broil until golden.
- Use in place of butter when baking casseroles, cakes, cookies, rolls, or breads.

ADDITIONAL CONSIDERATIONS

Trans Fats

The Food and Drug Administration (FDA) has not set a daily value (DV) for *trans* fats, and there are no *trans* fat recommendations in the current TLC guidelines. *Trans* fat information can be found on many food labels, although the FDA will not require it until January 1, 2006 (20). *Trans* fat intake should be kept to a minimum, because *trans* fats have been found to lower HDL cholesterol levels and to raise LDL cholesterol (21). The major dietary sources of *trans* fats are partially hydrogenated oils in processed foods, such as solid margarine, vegetable shortening, cookies, cakes, candies, fried foods, and snack foods (see Table 22.4).

n-3 Fatty Acids

A growing body of research suggests that diets high in n-3 fatty acids, including alpha-linolenic acid (ALA), eicosapentaenoic (EPA) and docosahexanoic (DHA) acids, may offer some degree of protection against CVD

Visit 2: Evaluate LDL Response

At the second visit, which should occur in week 6, the individual's current serum cholesterol levels should be reviewed. If the LDL cholesterol goal is not achieved, LDL-lowering treatment should be intensified. Key education topics include the following:

- Reducing saturated fat and cholesterol and weight management
- The possibility of adding plant stanols and sterols (2 g/day) to meal plan
- Increasing soluble fiber intake (see Table 22.3)

Visit 3: Evaluate LDL Response

If an individual's LDL goal is not achieved by the third visit (week 12), he or she should be referred to the medical care provider to consider drug treatment. Current nutrition interventions should be continued. Weight management and physical activity should be intensified.

Subsequent Visits

To monitor adherence to TLC, subsequent visits between the individual and the dietetics professional should be scheduled every 4 to 6 months.

TABLE 22.4 Total Fat and *Trans* Fatty Acids in Selected Foods

Food Source	Amount	Total Fat, g	Trans Fat, g
Bread (commercial)	1 slice	1–2	0.1–0.6
French fries	¾ cup	8–10	1.8–2.5
Potato chips	1 oz.	10	0.02
Cupcakes	1	5–10	0.3–2
Cookies	2–3	5–9	1.3–2.6
Crackers	½ cup	4–7	1–1.5
Margarine (stick)	1 pat	3–8	0.5–1.5
Margarine (tub)	1 pat	3–8	0.4–0.8
Shortening	2 Tbsp	8.5	1.4
Milk (whole)	1 cup	8.2	0.3
Milk (nonfat)	1 cup	0.4	0
Ground beef (25% fat)	3 oz	19	0.9

Nutrient calculations were performed using the NDS software (food software version 4.05_33, NCC, University of Minnesota, Minneapolis, Minn). Calculations were performed with averages to determine ranges. Numbers have been rounded to the nearest tenth of a gram.

BOX 22.2

Tips for Using Flaxseed

- Grind before use. Refrigerated ground flaxseed can be stored up to 1 month.
- Add 1 tablespoon to regular breakfast cereal. (Store-bought brands often contain flaxseed that is not ground.)
- Add 1 teaspoon to mayonnaise or mustard and spread onto sandwich bread.
- Mix 1 tablespoon into an 8-ounce container of yogurt for a snack.
- Add 1 tablespoon to sauces, rice, pastas, or mixed dishes.
- Mix 1 teaspoon into salad dressings or sprinkle directly onto salads.
- Bake into cookies, muffins, breads, and other baked goods. Flaxseed does not significantly change the taste or texture of the product.

(22,23). Nutrition Recommendations for Canadians state that n-3 fatty acids should contribute at least 0.5% of daily energy intake (24). The American Heart Association makes the following recommendations: (*a*) people with documented CHD should consume approximately 1 g/day of EPA and DHA; and (*b*) physicians may provide 2 to 4 g/day for the treatment of high TG levels. Use of supplemental fish oil at levels greater than 3 g/day should be supervised by a physician, because high intakes may result in excessive bleeding in some people (25).

The best sources of EPA and DHA are cold-water fish, such as salmon, haddock, mackerel, swordfish, lake trout, arctic char, and fatty tuna. EPA and DHA can also be made from ALA, an n-3 fatty acid found in plant sources such as flaxseed, canola oil, soybean oil, and walnuts. One tablespoon of flaxseed contains 1.5 g of ALA, which is equivalent to the amount of EPA and DHA in 3 oz of salmon. Tips for incorporating flaxseed into one's diet are presented in Box 22.2.

Antioxidants

Antioxidants, such as vitamin E, vitamin C, and beta-carotene, are the body's defense against free-radical damage. In large observational studies, such as the Nurses' Health Study and the first National Health and Nutrition Examination Survey (NHANES I), higher dietary antioxi-dant intakes are associated with lower risk for CVD (26,27). When individual antioxidants, given in supplement form, have been tested in randomized clinical trials, results have been inconsistent. In people with diabetes, vitamin E supplements have not been shown to decrease CVD mortality (28). Because there is not sufficient evidence for their efficacy or safety, pharmacological doses of antioxidants are not recommended (29). It is currently recommended that people meet antioxidant needs through a balanced diet that includes a variety of different-colored fruits and vegetables. For both men and women, the recommended dietary allowance (RDA) for vitamin E is 15 mg/day. The RDA for vitamin C (ascorbic acid) is 75 mg/day for women, and 90 mg/day for men; smokers should consume an additional 35 mg/day (30).

Hypertension

Hypertension (blood pressure > 140/90 mm Hg) contributes to the development of chronic health complications that are common among people with diabetes. Control of hypertension has been demonstrated conclusively to reduce the rate and progression of diabetic nephropathy and to reduce complications of hypertensive nephropathy, CVD, and cerebrovascular disease (31).

The blood pressure goal for people with diabetes or chronic kidney disease is less than 130/80 mm Hg. Studies have shown that many individuals will need one or more medications to achieve these goals (10). Guidelines for lifestyle prevention and management of hypertension are summarized in Box 22.3 (10).

Dietary Approaches to Stop Hypertension Diet

The Dietary Approaches to Stop Hypertension (DASH) diet—a diet high in fruits, vegetables, and low-fat dairy (good sources of magnesium, calcium, potassium, and fiber), and low in total fat, saturated fat, cholesterol, and sweets—reduces blood pressure (32,33). In normotensive subjects, the DASH diet was associated with an average decrease of 6 mm Hg systolic pressure and 3 mm Hg diastolic pressure. In hypertensive subjects, systolic blood pressure decreased an average of 11 mm Hg, and diastolic pressure decreased 6 mm Hg.

Sodium

High sodium intake has been implicated as one of the major lifestyle factors affecting hypertension (10). The original DASH study did not evaluate the effect of sodium on blood pressure; all three diets contained approximately 3,000 mg/day. A follow-up study found

Lifestyle Modification for the Prevention and Management of Hypertension

- Maintain normal body weight for adults (BMI 18.5–24.9).
- Reduce dietary sodium intake to no more than 100 mmol/day or about 6 g/day of sodium chloride or 2.4 g/day of sodium.
- Engage in regular aerobic physical activity, such as brisk walking (> 30 min/day, most days of the week).
- Limit alcohol consumption to no more than 1 oz (30 mL) of ethanol (eg, 24 oz [720 mL] of beer, 10 oz [300 mL] of wine, or 2 oz [60 mL] of 100-proof whiskey per day in most men and no more than 0.5 oz (15 mL) of ethanol per day in women and lighter-weight men.
- Maintain adequate intake of dietary potassium (> 90 mmol [3,500 mg]/day) by consuming adequate daily intake of fruits and vegetables.
- Consume a diet that is rich in fruits and vegetables and in low-fat dairy products, with a reduced content of saturated and total fat (Dietary Approaches to Stop Hypertension [DASH] eating plan.).

Source: Data are from reference 10.

BOX 22.4

Herb and Spice Replacements for Salt

- For beef recipes, try aleppo pepper, basil, bay, chili, cilantro, curry, cumin, garlic, marjoram, mustard, oregano, parsley, pepper, rosemary, sage, savory, tarragon, or thyme.
- For chicken recipes, try aleppo pepper, allspice, basil, bay, cinnamon, chili, curry, dill, fennel, garlic, ginger, lemongrass, mustard, paprika, pepper, rosemary, saffron, sage, savory, star anise, sumac, tarragon, or thyme.
- For fish, try anise, basil, bay, cayenne, celery seed, chives, curry, dill, fennel, garlic, ginger, lemon peel, mustard, oregano, parsley, rosemary, thyme, saffron, sage, savory, star anise, tarragon, or marjoram.
- For vegetables, try chili, chives, curry, dill, marjoram, parsley, savory, or thyme.

that the mean effect of a moderate sodium restriction plus the DASH eating pattern decreased blood pressure in hypertensive subjects approximately 5 mm Hg systolic and 2 mm Hg diastolic, compared with decreases of approximately 3 mm Hg systolic and 1 mm Hg diastolic in normotensive individuals (32). The lower the sodium intake, the more blood pressure was lowered. Sodium intake can be lowered by using a variety of herbs and spices to flavor foods (see Box 22.4).

Alcohol

High alcohol consumption is contraindicated for persons with hypertension. Men should consume no more than two drinks per day, and women (or small men) should have no more than 1 drink per day (10). A drink is defined as 5 oz of wine (100 kcal), 12 oz of beer (150 kcal), or 1.5 oz of 80-proof whiskey (100 kcal).

Weight Management

Weight control is a powerful tool for the prevention and treatment of CVD, diabetes, dyslipidemia, and hypertension. Although individuals may have hopes for a large amount of weight loss, risk for the above chronic diseases can be reduced with a 5% to 10% weight loss (16). Approaches for weight-loss treatment should include dietary modification, behavioral treatment, and physical activity (see Chapters 3, 7 and 21).

Physical Activity

Regular physical activity is beneficial for reducing the risk of chronic disease states, such as CVD, hyperlipidemia, hypertension, and type 2 diabetes, and can facilitate weight loss and weight maintenance (34). The Surgeon General's report (34) defined moderate physical activity as the intensity and frequency of exercise required to burn approximately 150 kcal/day, or 1,000 kcal/week. A 150-lb female could achieve moderate physical activity by briskly walking 30 minutes each day, salsa dancing for 25 minutes, or riding a bicycle for 20 minutes. Each activity would use about 150 kcal.

Smoking Cessation

In The Health Benefits of Smoking Cessation (35), the Surgeon General stated that smokers have twice the risk of dying from CHD as do nonsmokers. The risk for former smokers falls by one half after 1 year of abstinence, and by 15 years they are no longer at high risk.

Menu	Carbohydrate choices	Effect on Nutritional Status
Breakfast: 1 cup oatmeal 1 Tbsp raisins ⅛ cup almonds 8 oz nonfat milk	3½	• Oatmeal and other whole grains provide increased fiber. • At least 3 servings of whole grains are recommended per day. • Oats are a source of B-glucan (soluble fiber). • Nuts are a good source of protein, fiber, unsaturated fatty acids, vitamins, and minerals, but are also high in calories, so intake should be monitored.
Snack: 1 homemade flaxseed muffin 8 oz nonfat, sugar-free yogurt	2	• n-3 fatty acid intake can be increased by using ground flaxseed in baked goods, sauces, casseroles, stir-fried dishes, or dressings. • Low-fat dairy products provide minerals, such as potassium, calcium, and magnesium.
Lunch: 1 dinner roll, whole wheat 2 tsp margarine, *trans* fat–free Green salad (2 cups dark mixed greens, ⅛ cup tuna, water pack, ½ cup chickpeas, ½ cup red pepper and onion, 2 Tbsp vinegar/olive oil)	3½	• Whole grains can replace high-fat potato chips, tortillas, and fries. • Decrease saturated and *trans* fats by using *trans* fat–free margarine or stanol/sterol ester spreads instead of butter and by using olive oil or canola oil instead of regular dressings. • Lean protein sources—such as chicken, tuna, turkey, and extra-lean meat (up to 5 oz/day), legumes including soy, nuts, nonfat cheese, and egg whites—can replace higher-fat lunchtime proteins. Limit egg yolks to 2 per week.
Snack: Apple, 1 small 2 Tbsp peanut butter 4 oz nonfat milk	1½	• Low-fat milk, nonfat milk, and low-fat or nonfat yogurt provide less saturated fat than whole-milk versions. Two to three servings help meet calcium and vitamin D requirements.
Dinner: 2 oz chicken breast, grilled Pasta primavera (1⅛ cup pasta, 1 cup tomato and eggplant, 2 tsp olive oil, 1 Tbsp parmesan cheese, herbs and spices [as desired])	4½	• Moderate portions of lean chicken breast replace high-fat/cholesterol red meat. Remove the skin before eating. • Choose salmon, sardines, herring, or other fatty fish to increase n-3 fatty acid intake. • Add flavor with herbs and spices, instead of salt, in accordance with DASH dietary recommendations.
Snack: 1 cup fruit salad	2	• As recommended in the DASH diet plan, consume a variety of fruits and vegetables (8–10 servings) each day, because each has unique nutrients.

Nutrient Information
Energy, 2,018 kcal
Total fat, 71 g
     Energy from fat, 635 kcal (32% total kcal)
     Saturated fat, 12 g (5.6% total kcal)
     Monounsaturated fatty acids, 38 g (17% total kcal)
     Polyunsaturated fatty acids, 16 g (7% total kcal)
     α-Linolenic acid, 2.09 g (0.78% total kcal)
     Cholesterol, 82 g
Carbohydrate, 252 g (50% total kcal)
     Dietary fiber, 35 g
     Soluble fiber, 11 g
Protein, 107 g (21% total kcal)

Sodium, 2,080 mg	Vitamin A, 867 µg
Vitamin C, 137 mg	Potassium, 3,823 mg
Calcium, 1,272 mg	Iron, 15 mg

FIGURE 22.1 Integrating medical nutrition therapy guidelines for cardiovascular disease treatment into diabetes meal planning. Meals and snacks should reflect patient preferences and meal times should vary according to medication/insulin schedule. Nutrient calculations were performed using the NDS software (food software version 4.05_33, NCC, University of Minnesota, Minneapolis, Minn).

People may be reluctant to quit smoking because they are afraid of associated weight gain. The average person gains 4.5 to 7 pounds after quitting (36). One third of the weight gain can be attributed to a decrease in resting metabolic rate, which results in an energy expenditure decrease of approximately 100 kcal/day (32–35). The rest of the weight gain is attributed to increased energy intake (37–41). Although smoking cessation is difficult, it should be stressed that the small weight gain is less risky than continued smoking (35).

Dietary education for prevention of weight gain or possible weight reduction should be combined with behavior modification techniques for avoidance of overeating and continued avoidance of smoking. Encouragement of increased physical activity will also be helpful for increasing resting metabolic rate.

APPLYING MNT RECOMMENDATIONS

Integrating nutrition interventions into the usual eating habits and preferred lifestyle of persons with diabetes and CVD is essential for long-term success. Dietetics professionals need to support people in making changes by tailoring the information they provide to the individuals and to their chosen lifestyles (42). The dietetics professional also plays an important role in communicating the individual's usual eating and activity habits to the health care team, so that medical interventions can also be tailored to individual needs. Figure 22.1 presents the conversion of clinical recommendations into healthful food guidelines.

SUMMARY

Type 2 diabetes is an established risk factor for CVD. MNT is critical in attaining blood glucose, lipid, and blood pressure goals and in the prevention and treatment of CVD in people with diabetes. ATP III guidelines recommend a lifestyle approach known as Therapeutic Lifestyle Changes to reduce CVD risk. Implementing TLC could require an average of three visits with a dietetics professional.

Hypertension contributes to the development of chronic health complications that are common among people with diabetes. A dietary pattern high in fruits, vegetables, and low-fat dairy, and low in total fat, saturated fat, cholesterol, and sweets (ie, the DASH diet) has been shown to reduce blood pressure.

REFERENCES

1. Wilson PW, D'Agostino RB, Levy D, Belanger AM, Silbershatz H, Kannel WB. Prediction of coronary heart disease using risk factor categories. *Circulation.* 1998;97: 1837–1847.
2. Wilson PW. Diabetes mellitus and coronary heart disease. *Am J Kidney Dis.* 1998;32(suppl):S89–S100.
3. McGill HC Jr, McMahan CA. Determinants of atherosclerosis in the young: Pathobiological Determinants of Atherosclerosis in Youth (PDAY) Research Group. *Am J Cardiol.* 1998;82(suppl):30T–36T.
4. Grundy SM. Approach to lipoprotein management in 2001 National Cholesterol Guidelines. *Am J Cardiol.* 2002;90(8 Suppl 1):S11–S21.
5. Hopkins PN, Hunt SC, Wu LL, Williams GH, Williams RR. Hypertension, dyslipidemia, and insulin resistance: links in a chain or spokes on a wheel? *Curr Opin Lipidol.* 1996;7:241–253.
6. Gray RS, Fabsitz RR, Cowan LD, Lee ET, Howard BV, Savage PJ. Risk factor clustering in the insulin resistance syndrome: the Strong Heart Study. *Am J Epidemiol.* 1998;148:869–878.
7. National Cholesterol Education Program. Third Report of the Expert Panel on Detection, Evaluation, and Treatment of High Blood Cholesterol in Adults (Adult Treatment Panel III). Available at: http://www.nhlbi.nih.gov/guidelines. Accessed September 12, 2002.
8. American Diabetes Association. Nutrition principles and recommendations in diabetes. *Diabetes Care.* 2004; 27(suppl 1):S36–S42.
9. Grundy SM. Approach to lipoprotein management in 2001 National Cholesterol Guidelines. *Am J Cardiol.* 2002;90(8 Suppl 1):11–21.
10. Chobanian AV, Bakris GL, Black HR, Cushman WC, Green LA, Izzo JL Jr, Jones DW, Materson BJ, Oparil S, Wright JT Jr, Roccella EJ; Joint National Committee on Prevention, Detection, Evaluation, and Treatment of High Blood Pressure. National Heart, Lung, and Blood Institute; National High Blood Pressure Education Program Coordinating Committee. Seventh report of the Joint National Committee on Prevention, Detection, Evaluation, and Treatment of High Blood Pressure. *Hypertension.* 2003;42:1206–1252.
11. Hegsted DM, Ausman LM, Johnson JA, Dallal GE. Dietary fat and serum lipids: an evaluation of the experimental data [erratum in *Am J Clin Nutr.* 1993;58:245]. *Am J Clin Nutr.* 1993;57:875–883.
12. Kris-Etherton PM. Monounsaturated fatty acids and risk of cardiovascular disease. *Circulation.* 1999;100: 1253–1258.

13. US Department of Agriculture, Agricultural Research Service. 2003. USDA National Nutrient Database for Standard Reference, Release 16. Available at: http://www.nal.usda.gov/fnic/foodcomp. Accessed: March 4, 2004.

14. Grundy SM, Barrett-Connor E, Rudel LL, Miettinen T, Spector AA. Workshop on the impact of dietary cholesterol on plasma lipoproteins and atherogenesis. *Arteriosclerosis.* 1988;8:95–101.

15. National Research Council. Diet and health: implications for reducing chronic disease risk. Washington, DC: National Academy Press, 1989:171–201.

16. National Heart, Lung, and Blood Institute. Clinical Guidelines on the Identification, Evaluation, and Treatment of Overweight and Obesity in Adults. Bethesda, Md: National Institutes of Health; 1998. NIH publication 98-4083. Available at: http://www.nhlbi.nih.gov/guidelines/obesity/ob_gdlns.pdf. Accessed December 22, 2004.

17. Anderson JW, Hanna TJ. Impact of nondigestible carbohydrates on serum lipoproteins and risk for cardiovascular disease. *J Nutr.* 1999;129(7 Suppl):1457S–1466S.

18. Food and Drug Administration. Food labeling: health claims; soluble fiber from certain foods and coronary heart disease: final rule. 63 *Federal Register* 8103–8121 (1998).

19. Gans KM, Hixson ML, Eaton CB, Thomas ML. Rate your plate: a dietary assessment and education tool for blood cholesterol control. *Nutr Clin Care.* 2000;3:163–169.

20. Office of Nutritional Products. Labeling and dietary supplements: questions and answers about *trans* fat nutritional labeling. July 09, 2003. Available at: http://www.cfsan.fda.gov/~dms/qutrans2.html. Accessed January 26, 2004.

21. Krauss RM, Eckel RH, Howard B, Appel LJ, Daniels SR, Deckelbaum RJ, Erdman JW Jr, Kris-Etherton P, Goldberg IJ, Kotchen TA, Lichtenstein AH, Mitch WE, Mullis R, Robinson K, Wylie-Rosett J, St Jeor S, Suttie J, Tribble DL, Bazzarre TL. Revision 2000: a statement for healthcare professionals from the Nutrition Committee of the American Heart Association. *J Nutr.* 2001;131:132–146.

22. Lopez PM, Ortega RM. Omega-3 fatty acids in the prevention and control of cardiovascular disease. *Eur J Clin Nutr.* 2003;57(Suppl 1):S22–S25.

23. Gruppo Italiano per lo Studio della Sopravvivenza nell'Infarto miocardico: Dietary supplementation with n-3 polyunsaturated fatty acids and vitamin E after myocardial infarction: results from the GISSI-Prevenzione trial. *Lancet.* 1999;354:447–455.

24. National Institute of Nutrition. Nutritional significance of n-6 and n-3 essential fatty acids. Available at: http://www.nin.ca/public_html/Publications/NinReview/fall99.html. Accessed January 23, 2004.

25. American Heart Association. Fish and omega-3 fatty acids. Available at: http://www.americanheart.org/presenter.jhtml?identifier=4632. Accessed September 20, 2004.

26. Stampfer MJ, Hennekens CH, Manson JE, Colditz GA, Rosner B, Willett WC. Vitamin E consumption and the risk of coronary heart disease in women. *N Engl J Med.* 1993;328:1444–1449.

27. Enstrom JE, Kanim LE, Klein MA. Vitamin C intake and mortality among a sample of the United States population. *Epidemiology.* 1992;3:194–202.

28. Lonn E, Yusuf S, Hoogwerf B, Pogue J, Yi Q, Zinman B, Bosch J, Dagenais G, Mann JF, Gerstein HC; HOPE Study; MICRO-HOPE Study. Effects of vitamin E on cardiovascular and microvascular outcomes in high-risk patients with diabetes: results of the HOPE study and MICRO-HOPE substudy. *Diabetes Care.* 2002;25:1919–1927.

29. Tribble DL. Antioxidant consumption and risk of coronary heart disease: emphasis on vitamin C, vitamin E, and ß-Carotene: a statement for healthcare professionals from the American Heart Association. *Circulation.* 1999;99:591–595.

30. Institute of Medicine. *Dietary Reference Intakes for Vitamin C, Vitamin E, Selenium, and Carotenoids.* Washington, DC: National Academy of Sciences Press; 2000.

31. Sowers JR, Epstein M. Diabetes mellitus and associated hypertension, vascular disease, and nephropathy: an update. *Hypertension.* 1995;26:869–879.

32. Sacks FM, Svetkey LP, Vollmer WM, Appel LJ, Bray GA, Harsha D, Obarzanek E, Conlin PR, Miller ER 3rd, Simons-Morton DG, Karanja N, Lin PH; DASH-Sodium Collaborative Research Group. Effects on blood pressure of reduced dietary sodium and the Dietary Approaches to Stop Hypertension (DASH) diet. DASH-Sodium Collaborative Research Group. *N Engl J Med.* 2001;344:3–10.

33. Vollmer WM, Sacks FM, Ard J, Appel LJ, Bray GA, Simons-Morton DG, Conlin PR, Svetkey LP, Erlinger TP, Moore TJ, Karanja N; DASH-Sodium Trial Collaborative Research Group. Effects of diet and sodium intake on blood pressure: subgroup analysis of the DASH-sodium trial. *Ann Intern Med.* 2001;135:1019–1028.

34. *Physical Activity and Health: A Report of the Surgeon General.* Atlanta, Ga: National Center for Chronic Disease Prevention and Health Promotion; 1996.

35. The Surgeon General's 1990 Report on the Health Benefits of Smoking Cessation Executive Summary Preface. October 5, 1990. Available at: http://www.cdc.gov/mmwr/preview/mmwrhtml/00001800.htm. Accessed January 24, 2004.

36. Gerace TA, Hollis J, Ockene JK, Svendsen K. Smoking cessation and change in diastolic blood pressure, body

weight, and plasma lipids. MRFIT Research Group. *Prev Med.* 1991;20:602–620.

37. Klesges RC, Meyers AW, Klesges LM, La Vasque ME. Smoking, body weight, and their effects on smoking behavior: a comprehensive review of the literature. *Psychol Bull.* 1989;106:204–230.

38. Williamson DF, Madans J, Anda RF, Kleinman JC, Giovino GA, Byers T. Smoking cessation and severity of weight gain in a national cohort. *N Engl J Med.* 1991; 324:739–745.

39. Perkins KA, Epstein LH, Marks BL, Stiller RL, Jacob RG. The effect of nicotine on energy expenditure during light physical activity. *N Engl J Med.* 1989;320:898–903.

40. Stamford BA, Matter S, Fell RD, Papanek P. Effects of smoking cessation on weight gain, metabolic rate, caloric consumption, and blood lipids. *Am J Clin Nutr.* 1986; 43:486–494.

41. Gilbert RM, Pope MA. Early effects of quitting smoking. *Psychopharmacology* (Berl). 1982;78:121–127.

42. Prochaska JO, Velier WF. The transtheoretical model of health behavior change. *Am J Health Promotion.* 1997; 12:38–48.

ADDITIONAL RESOURCES

American Heart Association. Cholesterol. Available at: http://www.americanheart.org/cholesterol. Accessed October 6, 2004.

National Heart, Lung and Blood Institute. Live healthier, live longer. Available at: http://rover.nhlbi.nih.gov/chd. Accessed October 6, 2004. (Expanded interactive site, a useful adjunct to the counseling session.)

You Can Quit Smoking Consumer Guide. June 2000. Available at: http://www.surgeongeneral.gov/tobacco/consquits.htm. Accessed October 6, 2004.

23

Chronic Kidney Disease—Nondialysis

Lois Hill, MS, RD, CSR, and Catherine M. Goeddeke-Merickel, MS, RD

CHAPTER OVERVIEW

- Approximately 44% of individuals diagnosed with chronic kidney disease (CKD) have some form of diabetes (1).
- When individuals with diabetes follow intensive treatment for glycemic control, A1C can be reduced to near normal, and reduction in microalbuminuria and diabetic nephropathy can be achieved (2–4).
- Blood glucose control and effective treatment of hypertension and proteinuria have been shown to be effective in delaying the onset and progression of CKD in individuals with both type 1 and type 2 diabetes (4).
- Because individuals with CKD often have a compromised nutritional status and protein-energy malnutrition (PEM) (5), maintaining and improving nutritional status while maintaining glycemic control are often the primary goals for MNT.
- A modified protein diet is recommended to reduce nitrogenous wastes in the body that may exacerbate further kidney damage (5). Energy intake and other nutrition recommendations (eg, potassium, phosphorous, and sodium) must also be considered for individuals with CKD.

RENAL DISEASE IN PEOPLE WITH DIABETES

Renal disease is a significant clinical concern in people with both type 1 and type 2 diabetes, and steps should be taken early to prevent its development or progression. Risk of nephropathy varies among ethnic groups, with African Americans, Native Americans, and people of Hispanic heritage having much higher rates for type 2 diabetes (6). Forty-four percent of all new cases of end-stage renal disease (ESRD) in the United States result from diabetic nephropathy (1).

Individuals with type 1 diabetes and overt nephropathy (> 300 mg/day albuminuria) have a greater rate of progression to ESRD than do those with type 2 diabetes. ESRD develops in 50% of individuals with type 1 diabetes within 10 years and in more than 75% of these individuals within 20 years. On the other hand, 20% to 40% of individuals with type 2 diabetes and microalbuminuria progress to overt nephropathy, but only 20% progress to ESRD by the 20th year (7).

STAGES OF CHRONIC KIDNEY DISEASE

The National Kidney Foundation (NKF) outlined the stages of CKD in the 2002 Update NKF Kidney Disease

Outcomes Quality Initiative (K/DOQI) Clinical Practice Guidelines for CKD (8). CKD was defined as:

- Glomerular filtration rate (GFR) below 60 mL/min/1.73 m² for more than 3 months with or without kidney damage; or
- Kidney damage for more than 3 months, with or without decreased GFR, manifest by either pathological abnormalities or markers of kidney damage, including abnormalities in the composition of the blood or urine, or abnormalities in imaging tests (8).

The NKF K/DOQI Clinical Practice Guidelines classifies five stages of CKD by the degree of renal damage and the remaining kidney function, as assessed by GFR. Table 23.1 (8) summarizes the five stages of CKD, associated GFR levels, suggested clinical actions, potential metabolic consequences, and prevalence in adults 20 years and older.

Key markers of impaired renal function include (a) proteinuria (the presence of abnormal protein levels in the urine), which is an early and sensitive marker of kidney impairment in many types of CKD (8), and (b) microalbuminuria (defined as 30 to 300 mg/day loss of albumin in the urine). Microalbuminuria refers to the abnormal excretion of small molecular weight protein and requires a more sensitive laboratory testing method for assessment.

GFR CALCULATIONS

GFR is usually accepted as the best overall index of kidney function in health and disease. There are several equations for estimating GFR in adults; these equations are based on serum creatinine. The two formulas most often used are the Modification of Diet in Renal Disease (MDRD) formula and the Cockcroft-Gault equation. The MDRD formula is the "standard of measurement," which incorporates the serum creatinine, serum albumin, and serum urea nitrogen, along with age, gender, and race (7). The NKF's Kidney Learning System MDRD GFR calculator is available on-line (9). The Cockcroft-Gault equation (10,11) uses serum creatinine as the only laboratory parameter, along with age, gender, and weight. See Box 23.1 (8) for equations that can be used to predict GFR in adults based on serum creatinine.

BOX 23.1

Equations to Predict Glomerular Filtration Rate in Adults Based on Serum Creatinine

Modification of Diet in Renal Disease (MDRD) formula

$$186 \times S_{cr}^{-1.154} \times A^{-0.23} \times (0.742 \text{ if female}) \times (1.21 \text{ if African American})$$

Cockcroft-Gault equation

$$\text{Men: } C_{cr} = \frac{(140 - A) \times (Wt)}{72 \times S_{cr}}$$

$$\text{Women: } C_{cr} = \frac{0.85 \times (140 - A) \times (Wt)}{72 \times S_{cr}}$$

Abbreviations: A, age (years); C_{cr}, creatinine clearance (mL/min); S_{cr}, serum creatinine (mg/dL); Wt, weight (kg).

Source: Data are from reference 8.

ASSESSMENT OF NUTRITIONAL STATUS IN CKD

People with CKD often have compromised nutritional status and protein-energy malnutrition (PEM) (5). The K/DOQI Clinical Practice Guidelines for Nutrition outlines the recommended frequency of monitoring and assessment of clinical indicators in people with CKD (5). The primary goal for MNT in the early stages of CKD is to prevent PEM, which increases the risk of poor clinical outcomes and morbidity and mortality. As a result, it is necessary to monitor and assess the individual with both diabetes and CKD routinely. Box 23.2 (5,8) outlines the nutrition assessment and monitoring parameters for PEM in CKD.

Subjective Global Assessment (SGA)

Subjective Global Assessment (SGA) is a comprehensive evaluation that includes both objective and subjective aspects of a medical history and physical exam to assess nutritional status. SGA rates clients as well nourished, mild to moderately malnourished, or severely malnourished. The recommended SGA uses a seven-point scale, with the 1 and 2 ratings defined as severely malnourished, the 3 through 5 ratings defined as mild to moderately

TABLE 23.1 Stages of Chronic Kidney Disease

Stage	Description	GFR, mL/min/1.73 m²	Clinical Action	Metabolic Consequences	Prevalence in Adults Age ≥ 20 y (%)
At increased risk		> 90 with CKD risk factors*	• Screening • CKD risk reduction		> 20 million (> 12)
1	Kidney damage with normal or increased GFR	≥ 90	• Diagnosis and treatment • Treatment of comorbid conditions • Slow progression, CVD risk reduction		5.9 million (3.3)
2	Mild reduction in GFR	60–89†	• Actions from preceding stages • Estimating progression	• Concentration of parathyroid hormone starts to rise (GFR 60–80 mL/min/1.73 m²)	5.3 million (3)
3	Moderate reduction in GFR	30–59	• Actions from preceding stages • Evaluating and treating complications	• Decrease in calcium absorption (GFR < 50 mL/min/1.73 m²) • Lipoprotein activity falls • Malnutrition • Onset of left ventricular hypertrophy • Onset of anemia (erythropoietin deficiency)	7.6 million (4.3)
4	Severe reduction in GFR	15–29	• Actions from preceding stages • Preparation for kidney replacement therapy	• Triglyceride concentrations start to rise • Hyperphosphatemia • Metabolic acidosis • Tendency toward hyperkalemia	400,000 (0.2)
5	Kidney failure	< 15 or dialysis	• Actions from preceding stages • Replacement (if uremia present)	• Azotemia develops	300,000 (0.1)

Abbreviations: CKD, chronic kidney disease; CVD, cardiovascular disease; GFR, glomerular filtration rate.
*Individuals with CKD risk factors include those with diabetes, high blood pressure, or a family history of chronic kidney disease; older adults; African-Americans, American Indians, Hispanics, Asians and Pacific Islanders.
†May be normal for age.
Source: Adapted from: National Kidney Foundation. Kidney Disease Outcomes Quality Initiative clinical practice guidelines for chronic kidney disease: evaluation, classification, and stratification. *Am J Kidney Dis.* 2002;39(suppl):S1–S264, with permission from National Kidney Foundation.

malnourished, and the 6 and 7 ratings defined as well nourished (12). NetNutrition (13), a comprehensive Web-based tool to assist clinicians with the implementation of the K/DOQI Clinical Practice Guidelines, has more information on SGA. To use this tool, one must register as a user first.

Assessment Using the ADA MNT Protocol

The ADA MNT protocol (4) includes an initial assessment, a reassessment 3 to 4 weeks later, and a third session 3 to 4 weeks after the second, and follow-up as needed. See Figure 23.1 (p. 268) (4) for MNT Intervention Protocol for CKD. Assessment forms used in the

BOX 23.2

Nutrition Assessment and Monitoring Parameters for Protein-Energy Malnutrition in Chronic Kidney Disease

NKF K/DOQI Guideline 23:
GFR < 20 mL/min/1.73 m^2

- Measure serum albumin every 1–3 months.
- Measure edema-free actual body weight, percent standard body weight, OR use SGA every 1–3 months.
- Conduct nutritional intake interviews, assess nutrient intake diaries and/or nPNA every 3–4 months.

NKF K/DOQI Guideline 24:
GFR < 25 mL/min/1.73 m^2

- Assess dietary protein intake.
- Recommend 0.6–0.75 g protein/kg body weight/day. Emphasize use of high biologic value protein with a goal of 50%.

NKF K/DOQI Guideline 25:
GFR < 25 mL/min/1.73 m^2

- Assess dietary energy intake.
- Recommend 30–35 kcal/kg body weight/day for individuals 60 years of age and older.
- Recommend 35 kcal/kg body weight/day for individuals younger than 60 years.

Abbreviations: GFR, Glomerular filtration rate; NKF K/DOQI, National Kidney Foundation Kidney Disease Outcomes Quality Initiative; nPNA, normalized protein nitrogen appearance; SGA, subjective global assessment.

Source: Data are from references 5 and 8.

initial and follow-up assessments should be formatted to provide a comprehensive yet quick and accurate snapshot of the client for the health care team. It is important that the assessment identifies not only nutritional status parameters but also perceived and actual problems and drug-drug or drug-nutrient interactions.

Medicare payment is based on dietetics professionals using the ADA protocol. K/DOQI Guidelines specify that for clients with more advanced GFR (< 15 mL/min), more frequent monitoring may be necessary, which may require a physician order for change in condition for Medicare payment (5).

Laboratory Values

Nutrition assessment may include biochemical parameters, anthropometrics, comprehensive assessment forms, and drug-drug and drug-nutrient interactions. Assessment of the nutritional status and progress of renal clients using laboratory values requires the clinician to recognize that acceptable values and ranges for renal clients may differ from standard "lab normal." Two excellent resources are available to health professionals for assessing clients. The first is Satellite Healthcare's NetNutrition (13). Once in the NetNutrition Web site, select the category "nutrition assessment" and then select "laboratory" for a complete list of laboratory tests and values pertinent for the renal population. The second resource is the NKF publication, *The Pocket Guide to Nutrition Assessment of the Patient with Chronic Kidney Disease,* 3rd edition (12).

Serum Protein

Serum proteins (albumin, total protein) are routinely measured as indicators of nutritional status. Special care should be taken when interpreting them in CKD, because all can be affected by the hydration status of the individual. Serum transferrin levels are affected by iron status (12).

Albumin is the preferred indicator for assessment of nutritional status in people with CKD, because it correlates well with clinical outcomes (5). Because prealbumin or transthyretin levels are affected by GFR (prealbumin levels increase with decreased renal clearance), it is a less accurate measure of nutritional status in CKD (14).

Anthropometrics

As a tool used for nutrition assessment and evaluation, anthropometrics is time intensive and requires a precise and consistent technique to obtain valid measurements. Anthropometrics generally used to assess this population are body weight, height, frame size, skinfold thickness, midarm muscle circumference, percent of usual body weight, percent of standard body weight, and BMI (5).

BMI is used to measure acceptable weight for height or level of body fat. The calculation is body weight in kilograms divided by height in meters squared (kg/m^2). An acceptable range for BMI is 22 to 25; less than 20 may indicate increased nutrition risk, and more than 26 may indicate risk factors for obesity (5).

Referral/Consult Information (< 30 days prior to encounter 1)	
RD to obtain pertinent clinical data from referral source or client medical record/information system:	
✓ Laboratory values (creatinine, GFR, serum albumin, Hgb, bicarbonate, potassium, phosphorus, calcium, urine albumin, PTH, cholesterol, fasting TG, A1C if diabetic)	✓ Presenting signs and symptoms (eg, poor appetite, altered taste, recent weight loss, GI symptoms)
✓ Physician goals or medical plans	✓ Medications (dose, frequency)
✓ Primary cause of chronic kidney disease	✓ Prescribed vitamins/minerals
✓ Medical history (co-morbidities, e.g., diabetes)	✓ Physical activity clearance or limitations

↓

Encounter 1: 60–90 minutes

RD to obtain clinical data from client medical record/information system and client interview:

☐ **Nutrition-focused assessment**: Evaluation of height, weight, usual weight, BMI, GFR, laboratory values, other clinical data (e.g., blood pressure, ADLs, IADLs, SGA), client's knowledge of kidney disease, readiness to learn; comprehensive diet history including meal pattern and current dietary intake of calories, protein, type of fat, sodium (potassium, phosphorus, calcium as appropriate for stage of CKD and GFR), vitamin/mineral supplements, herbal supplements and over the counter medications (OTC), physical activity pattern, and psychosocial and economic issues impacting nutrition therapy. Consider co-morbid conditions and need for additional modifications in the nutrition care plan, e.g., diabetes.

☐ **Intervention and self-management training**: Provide rationale for nutrition therapy to slow the progression of kidney disease and to maintain normal blood pressure and blood glucose. Nutrition therapy should include an individualized nutrition prescription appropriate to the stage of CKD and GFR to maintain optimal laboratory indices, a meal plan and self-monitoring strategies (e.g., food and medication records to be kept). The nutrition prescription may include g protein/day, type of fat, sodium, % carbohydrates (if diabetic), nutritional supplements, specific amounts of potassium, phosphorus, calcium, phosphate binders and vitamin D supplementation. Mutually established goals and outcomes for eating, following medication protocol, recording food and medication intake, participating in physical activity, and self-blood glucose monitoring (if diabetic).

☐ **Plan for reassessment and follow-up:** Establish timeline for follow-up and provide client with contact information. Identify *expected outcomes* to determine response to care (e.g., ↓ blood pressure, maintain weight, glycemic control if diabetic).

☐ **Communication:** Provide documentation to physician and other relevant health care team members according to organization's policy.

3 to 4 weeks between encounters ↓

Encounter 2: 45–60 minutes

RD to obtain clinical data from client medical record/information system and client/caregiver interview:

☐ **Nutrition-focused assessment**: Reassess weight, BMI, laboratory values, other clinical data (e.g., blood pressure, blood glucose records, and medication changes). Obtain brief diet history and assess client's adherence/comprehension to nutrition prescription (e.g., intake of calories, fat, type of fat, sodium, key nutrients appropriate for stage of CKD and GFR, e.g., protein, potassium, phosphorus, calcium, and physical activity goals—refer to food/medication records). Reinforce or modify mutually established goals/outcomes for eating and keeping food and medication records.

☐ **Intervention and self-management training**: Provide new nutrition information (e.g., food label reading, food preparation methods). Reinforce or modify individualized nutrition prescription, meal plan, self-monitoring and behavior strategies. Reinforce or modify mutually established goals/outcomes for eating, behavior changes, self-monitoring, and physical activity.

☐ **Plan for reassessment and follow-up:** Establish timeline for follow-up and provide client with contact information. Identify *expected outcomes* to determine response to care (e.g., ↓ blood pressure, ↓ A1C, ↑ intake of protein and energy).

☐ **Communication:** Provide documentation to physician and other relevant health care team members according to organization's policy.

FIGURE 23.1 Medical nutrition therapy process for chronic kidney disease (non-dialysis). Reprinted with permission from *American Dietetic Association Medical Nutrition Therapy Evidence-Based Guide for Practice: Chronic Kidney Disease (non-dialysis) Medical Nutrition Protocol* [CD-ROM]. Chicago, Ill: American Dietetic Association; 2002.

3 to 4 weeks between encounters

Encounter 3: 30–45 minutes
RD to obtain clinical data from client medical record/information system and client/caregiver interview:
☐ **Nutrition-focused assessment**: Reassess weight, BMI, SGA, laboratory values and medication changes. Obtain brief diet history and assess client's adherence to any diet modifications (kcal, protein, sodium, potassium, phosphorus), review labs and discuss other clinical data (e.g., blood pressure, A1C if diabetic) and comprehension to nutrition prescription (e.g., intake of calories, protein, sodium, potassium, phosphorus, calcium), and physical activity goals (review food/medication records).
☐ **Intervention and self-management training**: Reinforce or modify mutually established goals/outcomes for eating, self-monitoring (food/medication records), physical activity. Review lab results (serum and urine albumin, serum potassium and phosphorus) and modify diet prescription as appropriate. Review food and medication records and reinforce/modify mutually established goals/outcomes for eating, behavior changes, self-monitoring with food/medication records. Provide new nutrition information (e.g, recipe modification for specific nutrients that need modifying e.g., sodium and dining out strategies). Reinforce or modify individualized nutrition prescription, meal plan, self-monitoring and behavior strategies.
☐ **Plan for reassessment and follow-up:** Establish timeline for follow-up and provide client with contact information. Identify *expected outcomes* to determine response to care (e.g., ↑ serum albumin, ↓ blood pressure, ↓ urine albumin, ↓ A1C, ↑ dietary intake of protein and energy, ↓ serum phosphorus).
☐ **Communication:** Provide documentation to physician and other relevant health care team members according to organization's policy.

6 to 8 weeks between encounters

Encounters 4, 5, 6 : 30–45 minutes
RD to obtain clinical data from client medical record/information system and client/caregiver interview:
☐ **Nutrition-focused assessment**: Reassess weight, BMI, SGA, laboratory values and medication changes. Obtain brief diet history and assess client's adherence to any diet modifications (kcal, protein, kind of fat, potassium, phosphorus), review labs and discuss other clinical data (e.g., blood pressure, A1C if diabetic) and comprehension to nutrition prescription (e.g., intake of calories, protein, sodium, potassium, phosphorus, calcium), and physical activity goals (review food/medication records).
☐ **Intervention and self-management training**: Reinforce or modify mutually established goals/outcomes for eating, self-monitoring (food/medication records), physical activity. Review lab results (serum and urine albumin, serum potassium and phosphorus) and modify diet prescription as appropriate. Review food and medication records and reinforce/modify mutually established goals/outcomes for eating, behavior changes, self-monitoring with food/medication records. Provide new nutrition information based on changes in kidney function, medications, diet prescription. Reinforce or modify individualized nutrition prescription, meal plan, self-monitoring and behavior strategies.
☐ **Plan for reassessment and follow-up:** Establish timeline for follow-up and provide client with contact information. Identify *expected outcomes* to determine response to care (e.g., ↑ serum albumin, ↓ blood pressure, ↓ urine albumin, ↓ A1C, ↑ dietary intake of protein and energy, ↓ serum phosphorus, normalize serum potassium).
☐ **Communication:** Provide documentation to physician and other relevant health care team members according to organization's policy.

FIGURE 23.1   (*Continued*)

NUTRITION RECOMMENDATIONS IN CKD

A modified dietary protein intake is recommended to reduce the amount of nitrogenous wastes in the body that may exacerbate further kidney damage (5). Clinical studies suggest that protein intakes of 0.6 g/kg day or less may reduce the damaging impact of hyperphosphatemia, metabolic acidosis, and other electrolyte disorders, although evidence is not yet conclusive that lower protein intakes will decrease the rate of progression of kidney disease (5,15,16). Although it is important to lower dietary protein intake to prevent further kidney damage, the clinician must ensure that the client is receiving adequate protein, to avoid compromising nutritional status. Thus, a higher energy intake is recommended for clients prescribed with lower dietary protein intakes.

In addition to the protein and energy requirements, there are numerous nutrient recommendations that must be considered for the client with both diabetes and renal disease. Refer to Table 23.2 (5,7,12) for nutrient requirements.

The K/DOQI Clinical Practice Guidelines for Nutrition in Chronic Renal Failure is an excellent resource for the intervention and education of renal clients with diabetes (5). The complete set of NKF K/DOQI Clinical Practice Guidelines may be accessed on-line (16).

BLOOD GLUCOSE CONTROL IN CKD

Glycemic control and effective treatment of hypertension and proteinuria have been shown to delay the onset and progression of CKD in clients with both type 1 and type 2 diabetes (4). Dietetics professionals must stress the importance of optimizing blood glucose level, to help prevent further complications. These complications may be macrovascular (coronary artery disease, cardiovascular disease, and peripheral vascular disease) or microvascular (retinopathy, neuropathy, and nephropathy). Typically, blood glucose levels can be assessed over time by measurement of A1C. In CKD, this value may be lowered, because of the shortened lifespan of erythrocytes (17). Thus, this possibility must be taken into consideration when assessing and monitoring A1C in clients with CKD.

TABLE 23.2 Daily Nutrition Recommendations for Chronic Kidney Disease

Nutrient	Recommendation
Energy, kcal/kg	≥ 60 years of age: 30–35 < 60 years of age: 35 Obese: 20–30/ABW Underweight or catabolic: 45/ABW
Carbohydrate, % total kcal	50–65
Fiber, g	20–40*
Fat, % total kcal	≤ 3
Saturated fat, % total kcal	< 10
Cholesterol, mg	< 300
Protein, g/kg	0.6–0.75†
Sodium, g	1–3 to no added salt
Potassium	Correlated to lab values
Phosphorus	Correlated to lab values
Calcium, mg	< 2000‡
Other vitamins and minerals	RDA for B complex and vitamin C; individualize for vitamin D, iron, zinc, and other disease states such as anemia
Fluid	Usually no restriction unless signs of edema

Abbreviations: ABW, adjusted body weight; RDA, recommended dietary allowance.
*Optimal dose, source, and long-term clinical benefits have not been established.
†Recommendation is for nondialysis patients with GFR < 25 mL/min/1.73m^2 (CKD Stage 4). At least 50% of protein intake should be from high biological value protein.
‡Include dietary calcium intake, calcium-based phosphate binders, and calcium supplements.
Source: Data are from references 5, 7, and 12.

Early detection and intervention—the keys to optimizing quality of life for this population—help to delay progression of kidney disease and the onset of renal replacement therapy. Monitoring and assessment of routine laboratory measurements are necessary for early detection and treatment of CKD and diabetes.

RESOURCES FOR PROVIDING OPTIMAL MNT INTERVENTION

The American Dietetic Association Renal Dietitians Practice Group (ADA RPG) and the National Kidney Foundation Council on Renal Nutrition (NKF CRN) have published numerous resources to guide both the new clinician and the experienced clinician in optimal MNT intervention in CKD and diabetes. The main focus of these resources, along with the NKF K/DOQI Clinical Practice Guidelines, is to improve and optimize client care and ultimately client outcomes.

Clinician Resources

Renal dietetics professionals representing the ADA RPG and the NKF CRN published the first edition of the National Renal Diet (NRD) (18) in 1993 as a joint effort. This edition of the NRD was field tested by a group of volunteer, field-based dietetics professionals (19). The NRD series consisted of six different client booklets, which covered pre-ESRD, hemodialysis, and peritoneal dialysis for individuals with or without diabetes. The first edition of the NRD offered the first national standardized guidelines for MNT intervention and client education in CKD.

In 2002, the RPG published second editions of client workbooks, *A Healthy Food Guide for People With Kidney Disease* (20) and *A Healthy Food Guide for People on Dialysis* (21), and the *National Renal Diet: Professional Guide* (22). The *National Renal Diet: Professional Guide* provides an overview of client education materials, reviews how to use the two client workbooks, outlines diabetes management in clients with CKD, and provides a chapter on the client education process.

Client Resources

A Healthy Food Guide for People With Kidney Disease (20) may be used in the counseling of clients with diabetes that are newly diagnosed with CKD. The guide is targeted to a 5th to 6th grade education level, to enhance adherence and understanding at all levels of education. This guide has the following sections with tear-out pages, which allows for individualization of the client MNT prescription and education plan:

- Getting started on a modified low-protein nutrition prescription
- High- or low-protein choices
- Fruit choices
- Caloric and flavoring choices
- Diabetes and CKD
- Vegetarian choices
- Low-protein food guide pyramid

The food pyramid section also includes menu-planning tear-out pages, which can be used to facilitate client interaction and knowledge retention. The use of symbols throughout this guide, such as a bone for high-phosphorus foods, a saltshaker for high-sodium foods, and a heart for foods that are higher in potassium, also helps to increase client adherence. The fruits and vegetables are grouped by potassium content into low, medium, and high lists. An appendix includes lists of high-, medium-, and low-potassium fruits and vegetables. It is advised that dietetics professionals recommend specific foods as part of the MNT prescription for both renal disease and diabetes. Nutrient composition of foods may vary depending on size, variety, growing conditions, processing, packaging, and preparation.

Within *A Healthy Food Guide for People With Kidney Disease*, the needs of the client with renal disease and diabetes are incorporated in the section titled "Diabetes Management in Patients with Chronic Kidney Disease." This section discusses the following topics for the individual with diabetes and renal disease:

- General guidelines for regular and consistent meals/snacks
- Insulin and oral diabetes medication guidelines
- Optimal serum glucose and A1C levels
- Optimal lipid levels
- Adequate energy intake to maintain reasonable body weight and spare protein
- Acceptable laboratory test parameters and fluid status
- Prevention of short- and long-term complications of diabetes
- Delay of the need for renal replacement therapy or transplantation

The inclusion of a vegetarian protein section in this resource offers options for the growing vegetarian population. The interactive workbook format helps the client practice learned skills in areas such as menu planning.

The dietetics professional works with the client to determine serving sizes and to incorporate a variety of food choices that fit the lifestyle of the client. A user-friendly feature is that each chapter of the guide contains an information box that explains the rationale for each section. For example, "why do I need protein?" explains the importance of appropriate protein intake and the rationale for limiting protein in CKD. The low-protein food guide pyramid is a comprehensive guide that may be used as a stand-alone tool or with the other sections for the initial and reassessment sessions.

Eating Simply With Renal Disease (23) is the simplified version of the NRD developed by the ADA RPG. It is a colorful, low-literacy pamphlet that provides basic information about calories, protein, sodium, fluids, and diabetes. The pamphlet includes green light "go" foods and yellow light "caution" foods for potassium and phosphorus.

MNT INTERVENTION PROTOCOLS AND MNT REIMBURSEMENT

In 2002, the ADA developed MNT intervention protocols for timely assessment and monitoring of CKD (4). These protocols have been reviewed and accepted by Centers for Medicare and Medicaid Services (CMS). *A Healthy Food Guide for People With Kidney Disease*, 2nd edition (20), can be adapted and used within the following ADA-MNT intervention protocol time frames. MNT intervention protocol time frames are as follows (4):

- Initial assessment/intervention: 60 to 90 minutes
- Second session/reassessment: 45 to 60 minutes (3 to 4 weeks after initial assessment)
- Third session/reassessment: 30 to 45 minutes (3 to 4 weeks after session 2)
- Additional sessions as needed

The CMS approved reimbursement for MNT for both CKD and diabetes mellitus (24). It is important to note the number of billable hours that are covered for MNT services in the first year and in subsequent years. In the first year, 3 hours are covered; in subsequent years, 2 hours are covered. One exception is when a physician documents a change in the client's status, which may allow for 2 additional billable hours. The dietetics professional must be a registered Medicare provider and may only bill for face-to-face time with the client. This means that preparation and posteducation documentation time is not billable. The accepted method for calculating billable time is recording it in 15-minute increments with no rounding up. See Chapter 2 or visit the ADA Web site (25) for Medicare MNT resources.

CKD CASE STUDY

The following case study provides an example of a potential client who has both renal disease and diabetes and who completes three interventions and assessments.

JB is a 58-year-old African American male with type 2 diabetes. JB has been referred for CKD diagnosis (GFR 23 mL/min/1.73 m^2). JB measures 173 cm tall (68 inches). His body weight is 70 kg (154 lb), and he has a small frame.

JB's blood pressure is 167/72 mm Hg; JB measures his blood pressure routinely. JB's medications include valsartan (80 mg daily), insulin glargine (30 units), rapid-acting insulin before meals (8 units), and a renal vitamin and mineral.

Laboratory data show the following: blood urea nitrogen, 37 mg/dL; creatinine, 3.6 mg/dL; potassium, 4.3 mEq/L; calcium: 9.9 mg/dL; phosphorus, 5.5 mg/dL; albumin, 4.3 g/dL; blood glucose, 194 mg/dL; cholesterol, 154 mg/dL; hemoglobin, 11.2 g/dL; transferrin saturation, 31%; ferritin, 564 ng/mL.

Nutrition referral for renal disease and diabetes is 0.6 to 0.75 g protein/kg/day, consistent carbohydrate, and a low-sodium, low-phosphorus diet. Using the NFK K/DOQI Nutrition Clinical Practice Guideline Recommendations (5), calculated daily nutrient needs for JB are as follows: 2,450 kcal (35 kcal/kg/day); 42 to 53 g protein (0.6–0.75 g protein/kg/day); 1 to 3 g sodium; 840 mg phosphorus (body weight in kg × 12 mg/kg). There are no fat, potassium, calcium, or fluid limits.

First Session

Teaching Points

At the first session, it is important to review with the client the overall prescribed MNT plan and goals of disease state management for diabetes and CKD. This would include the prevention and accumulation of harmful toxins, preserving kidney function, minimizing urinary protein losses, optimizing blood pressure control, optimizing blood glucose control, maximizing bone health, etc. For the dietetics professional, it is imperative to understand that ongoing client monitoring and individualization of the MNT prescription to avoid PEM is an essential component of nutrition care for the CKD client.

Reviewing MNT Plan and Setting Goals

During the first meeting with JB, a nutrition history is recorded. JB's nutrition history shows that he prefers not to eat salt, sugar, or concentrated sweets; he reports good appetite (body weight stable); and he eats three meals daily plus a snack at night. Each meal contains an animal protein source.

Protein intake is assessed and reviewed with the client. The dietetics professional reviews the protein list and suggests selecting three servings from the list to meet 50% of the daily protein requirement for JB. JB likes dairy products, so two servings of the high-protein, high-phosphorus foods are selected for daily consumption. His intake of high-sodium, high-protein sources is minimal, so he agreed to limit these foods to once weekly.

Next, the lower-protein foods (vegetables, starches, and added salt and phosphorus foods) are reviewed. The remaining 50% of his protein will be obtained from these lower-protein foods. JB elected to eat two to three servings of vegetables daily and eight to nine servings of grain foods daily. High-phosphorus and high-sodium foods are reviewed with JB. He agrees to limit these foods to twice weekly. Three servings of fruits are added. The sample meal plan is developed and written with JB.

SGA is performed with a score of 7. Functional status is reviewed. The dietetics professional reviews the following behavioral and clinical goals with JB, to be achieved and checked at the next intervention:

- Follow sample meal plan.
- Limit high-phosphorous and high-sodium foods to twice weekly.
- Monitor and maintain albumin level less than 4.0 g/dL.
- Monitor and maintain serum potassium between 3.5 and 5.5 mEq/L, phosphorus between 2.7 and 4.6 mg/dL, pre-meal blood glucose between 90 and 130 mg/dL, and A1C less than 7%; weight maintenance at current level; blood pressure goal of less than 130/80 mm Hg.

The dietetics professional sends documentation to the physician, along with a request for follow-up laboratory data. A return appointment is made for 4 weeks. Nutrient drug interactions are reviewed; valsartan, an angiotensin II receptor antagonist, can increase potassium.

Second Session

Teaching Points

During the second session, it is important to discuss volume status (edema), body weight, and labs (blood and urine), and to review symptoms (problems and complaints) and medication names and doses.

Reviewing Nutrition History and Reassessing Goals

As part of the second session, nutrition intake records are reviewed. JB's body weight has remained stable. His premeal blood glucose range is 100 to 140 mg/dL; his blood pressure is 140/70 mm Hg. JB reported being hungry. Energy intake is calculated to be approximately 1,700 kcal/day. His albumin level (3.9 g/dL) has decreased, so additional calories in the form of "healthier fats" are added. The dietitian suggests that JB add three "healthier fat" servings from this list and periodically some concentrated sweets, counting them within his carbohydrate choices. He is agreeable to this recommendation. Counseling is also provided on food label reading and recipe modification. SGA is completed with a score of 7. Functional status is reviewed.

The dietetics professional reviews goals to be achieved and checked at next intervention. The following goals were set with JB:

- Add three "healthier fat" servings.
- Continue to eat no more than 2 to 3 g sodium daily.
- Maintain current weight.
- Increase albumin level to greater than 4.0 g/dL.
- Maintain potassium between 3.5 and 5.5 mEq/L, phosphorus between 2.7 and 4.6 mg/dL, premeal blood glucose between 90 and 130 mg/dL, and A1C less than 7%.
- Decrease blood pressure to less than 130/80 mm Hg.

The dietetics professional sends documentation to referring provider, along with a request for follow-up laboratory data. The third session is scheduled 3 to 4 weeks after session 2.

Third Session

Teaching Points

During the third session, it is important to discuss volume status (edema), body weight, and laboratory values (blood and urine), and to review symptoms (problems/complaints), blood pressure, and medication names and doses.

Reviewing Nutrition History and Emphasizing Key Points

Since the initial session, the physician ordered a low-potassium nutrition prescription (potassium, 5.8 mEq/L). JB was on a blood pressure medication (valsartan) that resulted in increased potassium level. JB's body weight is stable and his premeal blood glucose level remains between 100 to 140 mg/dL. Nutrition intake records are reviewed to determine daily potassium intake (75 mEq or 2,925 mg daily). A lower-protein foods list is reviewed for appropriate vegetables to select and for high-potassium vegetables to avoid. The dietetics professional reinforces limiting vegetable servings to two to three daily and emphasizes appropriate portion sizes. Fruit choices are reviewed, to ensure that lower potassium fruits are selected and that high-potassium fruits are avoided. Limiting intake to three servings of fruits daily and choosing appropriate serving sizes are emphasized. Follow-up is completed on label reading and food preparation. SGA score remains stable at 7. Functional status is reviewed and remains unchanged.

After the third session, the dietetics professional asks the physician to order a repeat potassium level to assess the effects of the intervention. A follow-up appointment will be scheduled if JB's potassium level remains elevated.

SUMMARY

Integrated MNT is essential in the treatment of diabetes with CKD. The MDRD study proved the value of a self-management nutrition intervention by the dietetics professional for CKD (14). The Diabetes Control and Complications Trial also validated the role of the dietetics professional and how improved blood glucose control is possible when individuals with diabetes learn self-management skills (2). It is imperative to implement and use MNT in the early stages of CKD, to prevent PEM (5). To do this, ongoing and timely monitoring and individualization of the MNT prescription is essential. Experience shows that the most motivated clients are those who want to delay the disease state progression and initiation of renal replacement therapy. It is the ultimate challenge for the dietetics professional to use education materials and resources to motivate and instill a life-long desire for clients to achieve optimal self-care and monitoring of both diabetes and CKD. The dietetics professional and the client are an integral part of the medical care team. It requires efforts from all to be successful with nutrition intervention in CKD and diabetes.

REFERENCES

1. United States Renal Data System: USRDS 2002. Annual Data Report: Atlas of End-Stage Renal Disease in the United States. *Am J Kidney Dis.* 2002;41(4 suppl 2): S50–S51.

2. DCCT Research Group. The effect of intensive treatment on the development and progression of long-term complications in insulin-dependent diabetes mellitus. *New Engl J Med.* 1993;329:927–986.

3. UKPDS Group. Tight blood pressure control and risk of macrovascular and microvascular complications in type 2 diabetes. *BMJ.* 1998;317:703–713.

4. *American Dietetic Association Medical Nutrition Therapy Evidence-Based Guide for Practice: Chronic Kidney Disease (non-dialysis) Medical Nutrition Protocol* [CD-ROM]. Chicago, Ill: American Dietetic Association; 2002.

5. National Kidney Foundation. K/DOQI clinical practice guidelines for nutrition in chronic renal failure. *Am J Kidney Dis.* 2000;35(6 suppl 2):S56–S61.

6. Molitch ME, DeFronzo RA, Franz MJ, Keane WF, Mogensen CE, Parving HH, Steffes MW; American Diabetes Association. Nephropathy in diabetes. *Diabetes Care.* 2004;27(suppl 1):S79–S83.

7. Byham-Gray L, Wiesen K. *A Clinical Guide to Nutrition Care in Kidney Disease.* Chicago, Ill: American Dietetic Association; 2004.

8. National Kidney Foundation. Kidney Disease Outcomes Quality Initiative clinical practice guidelines for chronic kidney disease: evaluation, classification, and stratification. *Am J Kidney Dis.* 2002;39(suppl):S1–S264.

9. National Kidney Foundation. Kidney learning system GFR calculator. Available at: http://www.kidney.org/kls/professionals/gfr_calculator.cfm. Accessed October 25, 2004.

10. Cockcroft DW, Gault MH. Prediction of creatinine clearance from serum creatinine. *Nephron.* 1976;16:31–41.

11. Gault MH, Longerich LL, Harnett JD, Wesolowski C. Predicting glomerular function from adjusted serum creatinine. *Nephron.* 1992;62:249–256.

12. Council on Renal Nutrition of the National Kidney Foundation. *The Pocket Guide to Nutrition Assessment of the Patient with Chronic Kidney Disease.* 3rd ed. New York, NY: National Kidney Foundation; 2002.

13. Satellite Dialysis Web site. Available at: http://www.satellitehealth.com/dialysis/default.asp. Accessed October 25, 2004.

14. Mitch WE, Klahr S. *Handbook of Nutrition and the Kidney*. 4th ed. Philadelphia, Pa: Lippincott Williams and Wilkins; 2002:64–65.

15. Klahr S, Levey AS, Beck GJ, Caggiula AW, Hunsicker L, Kusek JW, Striker G. The effects of dietary protein restriction and blood pressure control on the progression of chronic renal disease. *New Engl J Med*. 1994;330:877–884.

16. National Kidney Foundation Published K/DOQI Guidelines Web site. Available at: http://www.kidney.org/professionals/kdoqi/guidelines.cfm. Accessed October 25, 2004.

17. *Mosby's Diagnostic and Laboratory Test Reference*. 6th ed. St. Louis, Mo: Mosby; 2003:472–474.

18. Renal Dietitians Dietetic Practice Group of the American Dietetic Association and National Kidney Foundation Council on Renal Nutrition. *National Renal Diet*. Chicago, Ill: American Dietetic Association; 1993.

19. Meeting the challenge of the renal diet. *J Am Diet Assoc*. 1993;93:637–639.

20. Renal Dietitians Dietetic Practice Group of the American Dietetic Association. *A Healthy Food Guide for People With Kidney Disease*. 2nd ed. Chicago, Ill: American Dietetic Association; 2002.

21. Renal Dietitians Dietetic Practice Group of the American Dietetic Association. *A Healthy Food Guide for People on Dialysis*. 2nd ed. Chicago, Ill: American Dietetic Association; 2002.

22. Renal Dietitians Dietetic Practice Group of the American Dietetic Association. *National Renal Diet: Professional Guide*. 2nd ed. Chicago, Ill: American Dietetic Association; 2002.

23. Renal Dietitians Dietetic Practice Group of the American Dietetic Association. *Eating Simply With Renal Disease* (pamphlet). Berkley, Mass: Kidney Thinking Company; 2002.

24. Medicare Program; Revisions to Payment Policies and Five-Year Review of and Adjustments to the Relative Value Units Under the Physician Fee Schedule for Calendar Year 2002; Final Rule. 66 *Federal Register* 55245–55294 (2001) (codified at 42 CFR 45 et al).

25. American Dietetic Association Web site. Available at: http://www.eatright.org. Accessed October 28, 2004.

ADDITIONAL RESOURCES

Wiggins K. *Guidelines for Nutrition Care of Renal Patients*. 3rd ed. Chicago, Ill: American Dietetic Association; 2002.

Wiggins K. *Renal Care: Resources and Applications*. Chicago, Ill: American Dietetic Association; 2004.

Appendixes

Organizations and Resources

Janelle Waslaski, RD, CDE

NUTRITION INFORMATION AND HEALTH ASSESSMENT TOOLS

Body Mass Index (BMI) Charts and Calculators

Centers for Disease Control and Prevention
http://www.cdc.gov/nccdphp/dnpa/bmi/calc-bmi.htm

Calorie Control Council
http://www.caloriecontrol.org/bmi.html

Shape Up America
http://www.shapeup.org

Dietary Reference Intakes

Food and Nutrition Information Center
http://www.nal.usda.gov/fnic/etext/000105.html

Glycemic Index and Glycemic Load

Diabetes Mall
http://www.diabetesnet.com/diabetes_food_diet/glycemic_index.php

Glycemic Research Institute
http://www.glycemicfoodlist.com

Home of the Glycemic Index (University of Sydney)
http://www.glycemicindex.com

International Food Information Council Foundation
http://ific.org/publications/qa/glycemicqa.cfm

Joslin Diabetes Center
http://www.joslin.harvard.edu/education/library/glycemic_index.shtml

Nutrition Practice Guidelines

Nutrition Practice Guidelines for Gestational Diabetes Mellitus (CD-ROM)
American Dietetic Association
http://www.eatright.org
800/877-1600, ext. 5000

Nutrition Practice Guidelines for Type 1 and Type 2 Diabetes Mellitus (CD-ROM)
American Dietetic Association
http://www.eatright.org
800/877-1600, ext. 5000

Pediatric Growth Charts

Centers for Disease Control and Prevention
http://www.cdc.gov/growthcharts

COMPLICATIONS AND COMORBIDITIES OF DIABETES

Amputations

American Amputee Foundation
PO Box 250218
Hillcrest Station
Little Rock, AR 72225
501/666-2523

Provides information, referrals, counseling, and support for amputees and their families.

National Amputation Foundation
40 Church St
Malverne, NY 11565
516/887-3600
http://www.nationalamputation.org

Sponsors of Amp-to-Amp program in which a new amputee is visited by an amputee who has successfully resumed normal life activities. Also provides support group lists by state and offers pamphlets of special interest to the amputee.

Cardiac

American Heart Association (AHA)
7272 Greenville Ave
Dallas, TX 75231
800/242-8721
http://www.americanheart.org

AHA's mission is to reduce disability and death from cardiovascular disease and stroke. It is involved in advocacy, fund-raising, patient education, public awareness, and research.

American Stroke Association
7272 Greenville Ave
Dallas TX 75231
888/478-7653
http://www.strokeassociation.org

A division of the AHA that focuses on reducing risk, disability, and death from stroke, through research, education, fund-raising, and advocacy.

National Cholesterol Education Program (NCEP)
NHLBI Health Information Network
PO Box 30105
Bethesda, MD 20824–0105
301/592-8573
http://www.nhlbi.nih.gov/about/ncep

NCEP aims to educate professionals and the public about the benefits of lowering cholesterol levels as a means of reducing the risk for coronary heart disease. NCEP raises cholesterol awareness through a cooperative effort among groups that include practitioners, public health professionals, community and voluntary organizations (including the AHA), state and local government officials, and health care administrators.

National Heart, Lung, Blood Institute (NHLBI)
PO Box 30105
Bethesda, MD 20824-0105
301/592-8573
http://www.nhlbi.nih.gov

NHLBI is a national program focusing on diseases of the heart, blood vessels, lungs, and blood. It plans, conducts, fosters, and supports an integrated and coordinated program of basic research, clinical investigations and trials, observational studies, and demonstration and education projects. NHLBI provides health information for patients and professionals, including clinical practice guidelines.

Obesity

American Obesity Association (AOA)
1250 24th St, NW, Suite 300
Washington, DC 20037
202/776-7711
http://www.obesity.org

AOA is focused on changing public policy and perceptions about obesity. Provides comprehensive information on education, research, prevention, treatment, consumer protection, and discrimination, to policy makers, media, professionals, and patients.

American Society for Bariatric Surgery (ASBS)
7328 W University Ave, Suite F
Gainesville, FL 32607
352/331-4900
http://www.asbs.org

ASBS provides education and support programs for surgeons and allied health professionals, with the goal to advance the art and science of bariatric surgery through continued encouragement of its members.

North American Association for the Study of Obesity (NAASO)

8630 Fenton St, Suite 918
Silver Springs, MD 20910
301/563-6526
http://www.naaso.com

NAASO is an interdisciplinary society whose purpose is to develop, extend, and disseminate knowledge in the field of obesity. Encourages research on the causes and treatment of obesity, and keeps the medical community and public informed of new advances.

Shape Up America

c/o WebFront Solutions Corporation
15009 Native Dancer Rd
North Potomac, MD 20878
240/631-6533
http://www.shapeup.org

Nonprofit organization dedicated to achieving healthy weight for life. Provides patient and professional educational materials, including interactive tools, to calculate body mass index (BMI) and to plot BMI percentiles on CDC growth charts.

Weight Control Information Network (WIN)

1 WIN Way
Bethesda, MD 20892-3665
202/828-1025 or 877/946-4627
http://www.niddk.nih.gov/health/nutrit/win.htm

WIN is a national information service of the National Institute of Diabetes and Digestive and Kidney Diseases. Provides health professionals and consumers with science-based information on obesity, weight control, and nutrition.

Podiatric

American Podiatric Medical Association (AMPA)

9312 Old Georgetown Rd
Bethesda, MD 20814
301/571-9200 or 800/ASK-APMA
http://www.apma.org

AMPA is an organization focused on education, research, and specialty interest areas. Provides general foot health information to patients and on-line access to the *Journal of American Podiatric Medical Association* to health professionals.

Pedorthic Footwear Association (PFA)

7150 Columbia Gateway Dr, Suite G
Columbia, MD 21046-1151
410/381-7278
http://www.pedorthics.org

PFA is a not-for-profit organization representing professionals involved in the field of pedorthics, to alleviate foot problems caused by disease, congenital condition, overuse, or injury. Their mission is to increase knowledge and understanding of pedorthics and its practice, to encourage development of new pedorthic tools and techniques, and to foster the professional development of pedorthic practitioners.

Renal

National Kidney and Urologic Disease Information Clearinghouse (NKUDIC)

3 Information Way
Bethesda, MD 20892–3580
800/891-5390 or 301/654-4415
http://kidney.niddk.nih.gov

Provides an information dissemination service of the National Institute of Diabetes and Digestive and Kidney Diseases, to increase knowledge and understanding about diseases of the kidneys and the urologic system, for professionals and the general public. Provides a variety of resources for patients and health professionals.

Rehabilitation

Resources for Rehabilitation (RFR)

22 Bonad Rd
Winchester, MA 01890
781/368-9094
http://www.rfr.org

Source for publications that provide information about the most prevalent conditions that cause disability. Focuses on enabling people with disabilities and chronic conditions to remain independent.

Visual Impairment

American Academy of Ophthalmology (AAO)
PO Box 7424
San Francisco, CA 94120-7424
415/561-8500
http://www.aao.org

AAO's mission is to advance the lifelong learning and professional interests of ophthalmologists, to ensure that the public can obtain the best possible eye care. Provides educational resources for patients and professionals.

American Council of the Blind (ACB)
1155 15th St, NW, Suite 1004
Washington, DC 20005
202/467-5081 or 800/424-8666
http://www.acb.org

ACB strives to improve the well-being of the blind and visually impaired. Provides services including toll-free information and referral services, in addition to a free monthly magazine produced in Braille, large print, cassette, and IBM-compatible computer disc.

American Foundation of the Blind (AFB)
11 Penn Plaza, Suite 300
New York, NY 10001
212/502-7600
http://www.afb.org

AFB promotes wide-ranging, systemic change by addressing the most critical issues facing the growing blind and visually impaired population—employment, independent living, literacy, and technology. Publishes textbooks and teaching materials, in addition to talking books.

American Printing House for the Blind (APH)
1839 Frankfort Ave
PO Box 6085
Louisville, KY 40206-0085
502/895-2405
http://www.aph.org

APH's mission is to promote the independence of blind and visually impaired persons, by providing specialized materials, products, and services needed for education and life.

National Association for Visually Handicapped (NAVH)
22 W 21st St, 6th Floor
New York, NY 10010
212/889-3141 or 212/255-2804
http://www.navh.org

NAVH is a nonprofit health agency solely dedicated to providing assistance to those with partial vision loss. Services include large-print library, low-vision aids, and public and professional education.

National Federation of the Blind (NFB)
1800 Johnson St
Baltimore, MD 21230
410/659-9314
http://www.nfb.org

NFB's main purpose is to help blind persons achieve self-confidence and self-respect and to act as a vehicle for collective self-expression by the blind. Provides public education about blindness; information and referral services; scholarships; literature and publications about blindness; aides, appliances, and other adaptive equipment for the blind; advocacy services and protection of civil rights; development and evaluation of technology; and support for blind persons and their families.

EDUCATIONAL RESOURCES

American Diabetes Association (Publishing)
1701 North Beauregard St
Alexandria, VA 22311
800/232-6733
http://store.diabetes.org

Publishes patient and professional educational resources, including books and pamphlets.

American Dietetic Association (ADA) (Publishing)
120 South Riverside Plaza, Suite 2000
Chicago, IL 60606-6995
800/877-1600
http://www.eatright.org

ADA and the Diabetes Care and Education Dietetic Practice Group publish many nutrition and diabetes education materials, including exchange lists for meal planning, cookbooks, pamphlets, and brochures.

Channing L. Bete Co.
One Community Place
South Deerfield, MA 01373-0200
800/477-4776
http://www.channing-bete.com

Offers products and programs focusing on areas such as smoking prevention and cessation, substance abuse and violence prevention, and school success. Also provides promotion, publishing, and distribution services to corporate partners, including the American Heart Association.

Combined Health Information Database (CHID)
7830 Old Georgetown Rd
Bethesda, MD 20814
http://chid.nih.gov

CHID is a bibliographic database produced by health-related agencies of the federal government. This database provides titles, abstracts, and availability information for health information and health education resources.

Diabetes Research and Training Centers (DRTC)
1 Information Way
Bethesda, MD 20892-3560
800/860-8747 or 301/654-3327
http://diabetes.niddk.nih.gov/dm/pubs/drtc

Program established by the Diabetes Research and Education Act in response to a recommendation by the National Commission on Diabetes. Six DRTCs are supported by the National Institute of Diabetes and Digestive and Kidney Diseases and offer a range of educational materials, including videotapes, curricula, and program guides for health professionals.

Food and Nutrition Information Center (FNIC)
National Agricultural Library, Room 105
10301 Baltimore Ave
Beltsville, MD 20705-2351
301/504-5719
http://www.nal.usda.gov/fnic

FNIC at the National Agricultural Library provides a directory to credible, accurate, and practical resources for consumers, nutrition and health professionals, educators, and government personnel. Offers printable format educational materials, government reports, research papers, and more.

Hoechst Marion Roussel
10236 Marion Park Drive
Kansas City, MO 64134
800/552–3656

Produces a variety of patient education materials on diabetes.

Indian Health Service (IHS)
801 Thompson Ave, Suite 400
Rockville, MD 20852-1627
505/248-4182
http://www.ihs.gov

The goal of the IHS is to improve the health level of Native Americans and Alaska natives. It has created low reading level educational materials directed toward populations served by IHS.

International Diabetes Center (IDC)
3800 Park Nicollet Blvd
Minneapolis, MN 55416-2699
952/993-3393 or 888/825-6315
http://www.parknicollet.com/Diabetes

IDC provides education, conducts clinical research, and offers team management and outreach programs, to ensure improved quality of life for all people with diabetes. IDC publishes many educational materials for individuals with diabetes.

Joslin Diabetes Center
One Joslin Place
Boston, MA 02215
617/732-2400
http://www.joslin.harvard.edu

Joslin's mission is to improve the lives of people with diabetes and its complications through innovative care, education, and research that will lead to prevention and cure of the disease. Offers a wide variety of patient services, including on-line library and classes. Also provides professional education services, including clinical guidelines.

Krames Communications
780 Township Line Rd
Yardley, PA 19067
800/333-3032
http://www.krames.com

Produces a comprehensive product line to promote healthy lifestyles, improve productivity, educate patients and consumers, enhance the efficiency of health care services, and reduce health care costs.

National Account Service Company (NASCO)
Nutrition Teaching Aids

901 Janesville Ave
PO Box 901
Fort Atkinson, WI 53538-0901
800/558-9595
http://www.enasco.com

Produces teaching aids for dietitians in hospitals, schools, foodservice, weight-loss programs, and industry. Products include food replicas, videos, cookbooks, scales, and more.

National Eye Institute (NEI)

2020 Vision Place
Bethesda, MD 20892-3655
301/496-5248
http://www.nei.nih.gov

NEI's goal is to protect and prolong the vision of the American people through research that helps prevent and treat eye disease. Produces patient education materials related to eye disease and its treatment.

National Health Video (NHV)

11312 Santa Monica Blvd #5
Los Angeles, CA 90025
800/543-6803 or 310/268-2809
http://www.nhv.com

Produces and distributes patient education videotapes on nutrition, diabetes, substance abuse, alcohol, and smoking cessation. Most of the titles are also available in Spanish.

National Minority Health Resource Center (NMHRC)

PO Box 37337
Washington, DC 20013-7337
800/444-6472
http://www.omhrc.gov/omhrc

NMHRC serves as a national resource and referral service on minority health issues. Collects and distributes information on a wide variety of health topics.

Nutrition Counseling Education Services

1904 East 123rd Street
Olathe, KS 66061
877/623-7266
http://www.ncescatalog.com

Distributes nutrition education resources, including books, manuals, videos, and teaching tools. Call or e-mail for a catalog.

DIABETES PROGRAMS AND CREDENTIALS

Board Certified Advanced Diabetes Management (BC-ADM)

American Association of Diabetes Educators (AADE)
100 W Monroe St, Suite 400
Chicago, IL 60603
800/338-3633
http://www.aadenet.org/ProfessionalEd/credentialing.html

The scope of advanced clinical practice includes management skills, such as medication adjustment, nutrition therapy, exercise planning, counseling for behavior management, and psychosocial issues. Specific criteria must be met to sit for the exam.

Certified Diabetes Educator (CDE)

National Certification Board for Diabetes Educators (NCBDE)
330 East Algonquin Road, Suite 4
Arlington Heights, IL 60005
847/228-9795
http://www.ncbde.org

Certification is a voluntary testing program used to assess qualified health care professionals' knowledge in diabetes education. The CDE credential demonstrates that the certified health professional possesses distinct and specialized knowledge, thereby promoting quality care for persons with diabetes. Specific criteria must be met to sit for the examination.

Education Recognition Program

American Diabetes Association (ADbA)
1701 N Beauregard St
Alexandria, VA 22311
800/342-2383
http://www.diabetes.org/for-health-professionals-and-scientists/recognition/edrecognition.jsp

The Education Recognition Program assesses whether applicants meet the National Standards for Diabetes Self-Management Education. The Standards are designed to be flexible enough to apply to any health care setting, from physicians' offices and HMOs, to clinics and hospitals.

DIABETES AND NUTRITION ORGANIZATIONS

American Association of Diabetes Educators (AADE)
100 W Monroe St, Suite 400
Chicago, IL 60603
800/338-3633
http://www.aadenet.org

AADE is a multidisciplinary professional membership organization dedicated to advancing the practice of diabetes self-management training and care as integral components of health care for persons with diabetes, and lifestyle management for the prevention of diabetes.

American Diabetes Association (ADbA)
1701 N Beauregard St
Alexandria, VA 22311
800/342-2383
http://www.diabetes.org

ADbA's mission is to prevent/cure diabetes and to improve the lives of all people affected by diabetes. It's involved in research, public awareness, advocacy, fund-raising, diabetes treatment guidelines, and publishing education materials.

American Dietetic Association (ADA)
120 South Riverside Plaza, Suite 2000
Chicago, IL 60606-6995
800/877-1600
http://www.eatright.org

ADA is the nation's largest organization of food and nutrition professionals, with a commitment to helping people enjoy healthy lives by focusing on five critical health areas facing all Americans: obesity and overweight, aging, complementary care and dietary supplements, safe and nutritious food supply, and human genome and genetics.

Diabetes Care and Education (DCE) Dietetic Practice Group
American Dietetic Association
120 South Riverside Plaza, Suite 2000
Chicago, IL 60606-6995
800/877-1600
http://www.dce.org

DCE promotes quality diabetes care and education by making positive contributions to people with diabetes and their families, providing an environment for professional growth to members, and promoting clinical and educational research.

Diabetes Exercise and Sports Association (DESA)
8001 Montcastle Dr
Nashville, TN 37221
800/898-4322
http://www.diabetes-exercise.org

DESA exists to enhance the quality of life for people with diabetes through exercise and physical fitness (formerly called the International Diabetes Athletes Association).

Diabetes Research Institute Foundation (DRI)
3440 Hollywood Blvd
Hollywood, FL 33021
800/321-3437 or 954/964-4040
http://www.drinet.org

DRI is an international center dedicated exclusively to the cure and treatment of diabetes and improving the lives of children. It has had landmark advances in several areas of diabetes research and patient care, including gestational diabetes, transplant immunology, and islet cell isolation and transplantation.

Juvenile Diabetes Foundation International
120 Wall St
New York, NY 10005-4001
800/533-2873
http://www.jdf.org/

Founded by parents of children with juvenile diabetes, JDRF works to find a cure for diabetes and its complications through the support of research.

National Certification Board for Diabetes Educators (NCBDE)

330 East Algonquin Rd, Suite 4
Arlington Heights, IL 60005
847/228-9795
http://www.ncbde.org

The purpose of the NCBDE certification program is to conduct certification activities in a manner that upholds standards for competent practice in diabetes education.

National Diabetes Education Program (NDEP)

One Diabetes Way
Bethesda, MD 20814-9692
301/496-3583
http://www.ndep.nih.gov

NDEP is a federally funded program that includes more than 200 partners at the federal, state, and local levels, working together to reduce the morbidity and mortality associated with diabetes.

National Diabetes Information Clearinghouse (NDIC)

1 Information Way
Bethesda, MD 20892-3560
800/860-8747 or 301/654-3327
http://diabetes.niddk.nih.gov

NDIC is an information dissemination service of the National Institute of Diabetes and Digestive and Kidney Diseases (NIDDK), established to increase knowledge and understanding about diabetes among patients, health care professionals, and the general public.

National Institute of Diabetes and Digestive and Kidney Diseases (NIDDK)

Center Dr, MSC 2560
Bethesda, MD 20892-2560
301/496-4000
http://www.niddk.nih.gov

The NIDDK is part of the National Institutes of Health. It conducts and supports biomedical research, and disseminates research findings and health information to the public.

OTHER NATIONAL ORGANIZATIONS

Centers for Disease Control and Prevention (CDC)

1600 Clifton Rd
Atlanta, GA 30333
800/311-3435
http://www.cdc.gov

CDC is a federal agency for protecting the health and safety of people (at home and abroad), providing credible information to enhance health decisions, and promoting health through strong partnerships. CDC serves as the national focus for developing and applying disease prevention and control, environmental health, and health promotion and education activities designed to improve the health of the people of the United States.

National Association of Social Workers (NASW)

750 First St, NE, Suite 700
Washington, DC 20002-4241
http://www.naswdc.org

NASW works to enhance the professional growth and development of its members, to create and maintain professional standards, and to advance sound social policies.

National Eye Care Project

PO Box 429098
San Francisco CA 94142-9098
800/222-3937

Cosponsored by the Foundation of the American Academy of Ophthalmology, the National Eye Care Project provides medical and surgical eye care to low-income US citizens or legal residents who are age 65 or older.

Use of Foods and Beverages With Nonnutritive Sweeteners, Sugar Alcohols, and Fat Replacers

Hope S. Warshaw, MMSc, RD, BC-ADM, CDE

The use of food and beverages containing nonnutritive sweeteners, sugar alcohols, and fat replacers can assist individuals in taking steps toward achieving their nutrition goals (1). Table B.1 is a quick reference for counting carbohydrate in foods and beverages con-

TABLE B.1 Counting Carbohydrates for Foods and Beverages Containing Nonnutritive Sweeteners, Sugar Alcohols, and Fat Replacers	
Total Carbohydrate, g	Count As
0–5	Do not count
6–10	½ carbohydrate serving; ½ starch, fruit or milk serving; or the actual grams of carbohydrate
11–20	1 carbohydrate serving; 1 starch, fruit or milk serving; or the actual grams of carbohydrate
21–25	1½ carbohydrate servings; 1½ starch, fruit or milk servings; or the actual grams of carbohydrate
26–35	2 carbohydrate servings; 2 starch, fruit or milk servings; or the actual grams of carbohydrate

taining nonnutritive sweeteners, sugar alcohols, and fat replacers.

When one or more of the ingredients is a sugar alcohol, the following guidelines should be used (2):

- If all the carbohydrate comes from sugar alcohols and the carbohydrate is less than 10 g, consider it a free food and do not count.
- If all the carbohydrate comes from sugar alcohols and the sugar alcohols are more than 10 g, then subtract one half the grams of sugar alcohols from the total carbohydrate and count the remaining grams of carbohydrate into the eating plan.
- If there are several sources of carbohydrate, including sugar alcohols, then subtract one half the grams of sugar alcohols from the total carbohydrate and count the remaining grams of carbohydrate into the eating plan.

NONNUTRITIVE SWEETENERS

Safety and Uses

Nonnutritive sweeteners, used to replace granulated sugar or another tabletop sweetener, are also referred to as no-calorie, low-calorie, or high-intensity sweeteners, or sugar substitutes. The goal of using these products is to reduce sugar and calorie intake. All five are noncariogenic and do

287

TABLE B.2   Selected Nonnutritive Sweeteners

Nonnutritive Sweetener (Brand Names*)	Acceptable Daily Intake, mg/kg body weight	Description
Acesulfame-K (Sunett, Sweet One)	15	200 times sweeter than sucrose; sweetening power not reduced with heating
Aspartame (Nutrasweet, Equal, Sugar Twin)	50	160–220 times sweeter than sucrose; sweetening power is reduced with heating
Neotame	18	8,000 times sweeter than sucrose; sweetening power not reduced with heating
Saccharin (Sweet 'n Low, Necta Sweet)	5	200–700 times sweeter than sucrose; sweetening power not reduced with heating
Sucralose (Splenda)	5	600 times sweeter than sucrose; sweetening power not reduced with heating

*Manufacturers: Sunett, Nutrinova Inc, Somerset, NJ 08873, http://www.nutrinova.com; Sweet One, Stadt Corporation, Brooklyn, NY 11205, http://www.sweetone.com; NutraSweet and Equal, Nutrasweet Company, Chicago, IL 60654, http://www.nutrasweet.com; Sugar Twin, Alberto-Culver Company, Melrose Park, IL 60160, http://www.sugartwin.com; Neotame, Nutrasweet Company, Chicago, IL 60654, http://www.neotame.com; Sweet 'n Low, Cumberland Packing Corp., Brooklyn, New York, 11205, http://www.sweetnlow.com; Necta Sweet, NSI Sweeteners, Deerfield, IL 60015, http://www.flavourcreations.com/NectaSweet.html; Splenda, McNeil Nutritionals, Fort Washington, PA 19034, http://www.splenda.com. Additional information about aspartame available at: http://www.aspartame.org; additional information about saccharin available at: http://www.saccharin.org.

Source: Data are from references 6 and 7 and from manufacturers.

not elicit a glycemic response. They are considered safe for use by people with diabetes, including children and pregnant women (3–5). For a comparison of nonnutritive sweeteners, see Table B.2.

In approving these sweeteners, the Food and Drug Administration (FDA) set an Acceptable Daily Intake level (ADI), which is defined as the amount of a food additive that can be safely consumed on a daily basis over a person's lifetime without risk. The ADI includes a 100-fold safety factor. It has been shown that the actual intake of nonnutritive sweeteners is much less than the ADI (5).

Nonnutritive sweeteners are commonly blended in foods and beverages. They may also be blended with sugar alcohols. There are some synergistic effects between some nonnutritive sweeteners, so sweetener blends are used to produce a taste profile that cannot be obtained with a single sweetener (8).

Teaching Points

Key points to teach in relation to nonnutritive sweeteners include the following:

- Explain the meaning of nutrition claims on product labels, such as "sugar-free," "reduced sugars," and "no sugar added."
- Encourage individuals with diabetes to check the ingredient list, to verify the sweetening agent and the nutrition information.
- Explain that the nutrition claim "sugar-free" does not necessarily mean calorie- or carbohydrate-free.

- Show individuals with diabetes how to fit foods sweetened with nonnutritive sweeteners into the meal plan, according to Table B.1.

SUGAR ALCOHOLS

Uses

Sugar alcohols, also referred to as polyols, are a group of low-digestible carbohydrates that provide a range from 0 to 3 kcal/g (approximate average is 2 kcal/g). They are neither sugars nor alcohols. Their primary use by the food industry is to replace sugars and/or fat, yielding products that are lower in calories, sugar, and/or fat. Sugar alcohols are also used to add bulk and/or texture, retain moisture, promote crystallizing, and decrease calories. Products containing sugar alcohols in place of sugar are often labeled "sugar-free." Several sugar alcohols have "ol" endings, such as sorbitol, mannitol, and xylitol. Others are isomalt and hydrogenated starch hydrolysate. Sugar alcohols are generally approved by FDA through the GRAS (Generally Recognized As Safe) process. The FDA has regulatory guidelines for the labeling of food with sugar alcohols.

The American Diabetes Association's nutrition position statement explains that "sugar alcohols produce a lower post-prandial glucose response than fructose, sucrose, or glucose and have lower available energy values. However, there is no evidence that the amounts likely to be consumed in a meal or day result in a significant reduction in total daily energy intake or improvement in long-term glycemia" (4). There is also a caution about their potential laxative effect, especially in children.

Teaching Points

Key points to teach in relation to sugar alcohols include the following:

- Encourage individuals with diabetes to check the ingredient list, to verify the sweetening ingredients and the nutrition information.
- Explain that the nutrition claim "sugar-free" can mean sweetened with nonnutritive sweeteners and/or sugar alcohols, and that it doesn't necessarily mean calorie- or carbohydrate-free.
- Explain that sugar alcohols do impact blood glucose control.
- Show individuals with diabetes how to fit foods sweetened with sugar alcohols into the meal plan, according to Table B.1.

FAT REPLACERS

Uses

Fat replacers are a group of ingredients that mimic the properties of fat and are used by food manufacturers to lower the fat content, and sometimes calorie content, of foods. They are most often carbohydrate-based ingredients (such as modified food starch, polydextrose, or guar gum), although some are protein- or fat-based. Most fat replacers have been approved for use by the FDA through the GRAS process. People with diabetes often are not aware that many of the lower fat or fat-free foods are higher in carbohydrate than the regular product.

Teaching Points

Key concepts to teach in relation to fat replacers include the following:

- Explain the meaning of the nutrition claims on product labels, such as fat-free, reduced-fat, low-fat, and less fat.
- Explain that the lower fat nutrition claims don't usually mean calorie- or carbohydrate-free. In fact, the carbohydrate content can be increased.
- Encourage individuals with diabetes to try a variety of reduced-fat and fat-free products, to find ones that are acceptable and enjoyable.
- Show individuals with diabetes how to fit foods containing fat replacers into the meal plan, according to Table B.1.

REFERENCES

1. *Nutrition and Your Health: Dietary Guidelines for Americans.* 5th ed. Washington, DC: US Depts of Agriculture and Health and Human Services; 2000. Home and Garden Bulletin 232.

2. Warshaw HS, Powers MA. A search for answers about foods with polyols (sugar alcohols). *Diabetes Educator.* 1999;25:307–321.

3. Gannon MC, Nuttall FQ. Protein and diabetes. In: Franz MJ, Bantle JP, eds. *American Diabetes Association Guide to Medical Nutrition Therapy for Diabetes.* Alexandria, Va: American Diabetes Association; 1999:107–125.

4. American Diabetes Association. Position statement: evidence-based nutrition principles and recommendations for the treatment and prevention of diabetes and related complications. *J Am Diet Assoc.* 2002;102:109–118.

5. Franz MJ, Bantle JP, Beebe CA, Brunzell JD, Chiasson JL, Garg A, Holzmeister LA, Hoogwerf B, Mayer-Davis E, Mooradian AD, Purnell JQ, Wheeler M. Evidence-based nutrition principles and recommendations for the treatment and prevention of diabetes and related complications. *Diabetes Care*. 2002;25:148–198.

6. US Food and Drug Administration. FDA food additive approval for neotame. Available at: http://www.neotame.com/pdf/neotame_fda_US.pdf. Accessed July 27, 2004.

7. American Dietetic Association. Position of the American Dietetic Association: use of nutritive and nonnutritive sweeteners. *J Am Diet Assoc*. 2004;104:255–275.

8. Powers MA. Sugar alternatives and fat replacers. In: Franz MJ, Bantle JP, eds. *American Diabetes Association Guide to Medical Nutrition Therapy for Diabetes*. Alexandria, Va: American Diabetes Association; 1999:148–164.

ADDITIONAL RESOURCES

Calorie Control Council. Available at: http://www.carloriecontrol.org. Accessed September 20, 2004.

Freeman J, Hayes C. "Low carbohydrate" food facts and fallacies. *Diabetes Spectrum*. 2004;17:137–140.

International Food Information Council. Available at: http://www.ific.org. Accessed September 20, 2004.

Powers MA, Warshaw HS. Low-calorie sweeteners and fat replacers: the ingredients, use in foods and diabetes management. In: Powers MA, ed. *Handbook of Diabetes Medical Nutrition Therapy*. Gaithersburg, Md: Aspen Publishers; 1996:437–457.

Sigman-Grant M. Can you have your low-fat cake and eat it too? The role of fat-modified products. *J Am Diet Assoc*. 1997;97(suppl):S76-S81.

Warshaw HS. FAQs about polyols. *Today's Dietitian*. April 2004:37–44.

Appendix C

Use of Herbs, Supplements, and Alternative Therapies

Janis Roszler, RD, CDE

Individuals with diabetes may be even more likely than the general public to use herbs, supplements, or alternative therapies. Fewer than 40% of persons using alternative diabetes treatments inform their health care providers (1).

When teaching herb and supplement use, dietetics professionals should encourage individuals with diabetes to do the following:

- Notify their health care providers of all prescribed and over-the-counter herbs, supplements, and other alternative formulations/treatments used, so that possible side effects and interactions with other medications can be evaluated.

- Use only one new product at a time, to monitor for adverse effects.
- Stop taking the new product immediately if any reactions occur, and contact the health care provider.
- Monitor blood glucose frequently.
- Discuss with the health care provider discontinuing herbs and supplements before surgery because some can cause complications.

Table C.1 reviews herbs and supplements used to manage diabetes and related complications (2–10). This information is based on what data are currently available; in some cases, research is limited.

TABLE C.1 Herbs and Supplements Used to Manage Diabetes and Related Complications

Herb/Supplement (Reference)	Use in Diabetes	Recommended Dosage	Notes and Possible Adverse Effects
Alpha-lipoic acid (ALA) (2)	Used in Germany for peripheral neuropathy. May prevent or slow development of atherosclerosis.	300 mg/day in divided doses for treatment of diabetic neuropathy.	May lower blood glucose levels.
Capsaicin (cayenne pepper) (3)	Cream reduces neuropathy pain.	Limit use to 2 days; only use again after 2 weeks.	Avoid contact with eyes. External use can lead to blister and ulcer formation.
Chromium (4)	May improve insulin cell sensitivity. Positive effects observed in type 1 and type 2 diabetes.	Typical dose is 50–200 μg/day.	Generally well tolerated when typical dose is used.
Cinnamon (5)	Used to improve blood glucose and lipids in type 2 diabetes.	1–6 g/day.	Contraindicated during pregnancy.
Coenzyme Q10 (2)	May improve beta-cell function and glycemic control in type 2 diabetes. Does not appear to aid glycemic control in type 1 diabetes.	Effective dose is considered 50–200 mg/day. Best taken with food.	Possible diarrhea, nausea, and gastric distress.
Bitter melon (bitter gourd, karela, bitter cucumber) (6)	Has hypoglycemic effect in type 1 and type 2 diabetes.	500 mg capsule of 2.5% extract 3 times/day, 1 small melon/day, or 2 oz fresh juice/day.	High doses may cause intestinal pain or diarrhea.
Evening primrose oil—source of gamma linolenic acid (GLA) (2)	Used to treat diabetic neuropathy and elevated triglyceride levels.	360–480 mg/day.	Discontinue before surgery. Can cause inhibition of lymphocyte function. Possible headache, bloating, and diarrhea.
Fenugreek (6)	Believed to decrease blood glucose, to improve glucose tolerance, and possibly to decrease cholesterol levels.	Typical dose is 1 tablespoon mashed seeds in 1 cup hot water at least once a day. May require higher dose for hypoglycemic effect.	May cause stomach upset and diarrhea.
Garlic (3)	Has lipid-lowering effect.	Supplements: 600–900 mg of garlic powder/day (standardized to 1.3% of alliin content).	Garlic breath and gastrointestinal irritation. Caution with anticoagulants—may increase bleeding time.
Ginseng (American and Korean, panax ginseng) (3)	Hypoglycemic effect in type 2 diabetes.	Typical dose is 100–200 mg.*	Nervousness, insomnia, and headache. Possible hypoglycemia.
Gymnema sylvestre (6)	May regenerate insulin-secreting cells in pancreas and may stimulate insulin secretion. Has hypoglycemic effect in type 1 and type 2 diabetes.	1–2 Tbsp fresh leaves, 1–2 tsp liquid extract, 2–3 g dried leaves, or 2–4 g powdered leaves daily.	Can cause significant drop in blood glucose levels—monitor closely.

(continued)

TABLE C.1 (Continued)

Herb/Supplement (Reference)	Use in Diabetes	Recommended Dosage	Notes and Possible Adverse Effects
Magnesium (6)	Deficiency associated with pathogenesis of diabetes mellitus. Possibly protective against atherosclerosis.	Typical dose is 100–350 mg/day.	Possible diarrhea, nausea, and abdominal cramping.
Nicotinamide (4)	May protect beta cell function by improving resistance to autoimmune destruction. May prevent diabetes.	Males age ≥ 14 y: 16 mg NE[†]/day. Females age ≥ 14 y: 14 mg NE[†]/day.	Possible skin flushing and gastrointestinal disturbances. Contraindicated in liver disease, gout, peptic ulcer disease, and allergies.
Psyllium (3)	Reduces postprandial blood glucose and lowers serum cholesterol levels.	Use as directed on label.	May delay absorption of drugs taken simultaneously.
Vanadium (4)	May decrease insulin requirements in type 1 diabetes; may increase tissue sensitivity in type 2 diabetes.	10–30 μg/day may be sufficient for most people.	Diarrhea, abdominal cramping, and flatulence. Caution with anticoagulants. Greenish tongue discoloration has been reported with vanadium use.
Vitamin C (2)	May have positive effect on coronary artery disease in type 1 and type 2 diabetes; may help prevent cataracts.	250–2000 mg/day.	Oral doses < 3 g/d should not cause adverse reactions in healthy adults. Larger doses may cause nausea, abdominal cramps, diarrhea, and flatulent distention.
Vitamin E (4)	May lead to a lower A1C level; may decrease risk of coronary artery disease.	200–800 IU/day is considered safe for any person with risk factors for diabetes or heart disease.	High doses of single antioxidant may upset antioxidant/ pro-oxidant balance.

*Many products for sale are adulterated and contain little or no ginseng. Check for reliable brands at ConsumerLab.com (10).
†Niacin equivalents.
Source: Data are from references 2 through 9.

REFERENCES

1. Eisenberg DM, Davis RB, Ettner SL, Appel S, Wilkey S, Van Rompay M, Kessler RC. Trends in alternative medicine use in the United States, 1990–1997: results of a follow-up national survey. *JAMA.* 1998;280:1569–1575.

2. Hendler S, Rorvik D. *PDR for Nutritional Supplements.* Montvale, NJ: Thomson Healthcare; 2001.

3. Thomson Healthcare. *PDR for Herbal Medicines.* 2nd ed. Montvale, NJ: Medical Economics Company; 2000.

4. Dattilo A. Micronutrients in diabetes: chromium. *On the Cutting Edge.* 2001;22(4):19–22

5. Geil P. The buzz on B3: the role of nicotinamide in the prevention and treatment of diabetes. *On the Cutting Edge.* 2001;22(4):23–24.

6. Montgomery S, Rosati K. Vitamin E: an adjunct to diabetes management. *On the Cutting Edge.* 2001;22(4):25–27.

7. Shane-McWhorter L. Vanadium, alpha-lipoic acid, and gamma-linolenic acid: unique agents for lowering blood glucose and/or treating complications of diabetes. *On the Cutting Edge.* 2001;22(4):28–31.

8. Khan A, Safdar M, Ali Khan MM, Khattak KN, Anderson RA. Cinnamon improves glucose and lipids of people with type 2 diabetes. *Diabetes Care.* 2003;26:3215–3218.

9. Duke JA. *The Green Pharmacy Herbal Handbook: Your Comprehensive Reference to the Best Herbs for Healing.* New York, NY: Rodale Books; 2000.

10. Consumer Lab.com. Available at: http://www.consumerlab.com. Accessed October 7, 2004.

ADDITIONAL RESOURCES

Altdiabetes.com. Available at: http://www.altdiabetes.com. Accessed January 6, 2005 (sells supplements and provides links to research articles).

Balch PA, Balch JF. *Prescription for Nutritional Healing: A Practical A-Z Reference to Drug-Free Remedies Using Vitamins, Minerals, Herbs & Food Supplements.* 3rd ed. New York, NY: Avery; 2000.

Roszler J, Trecroci D. Herbs, supplements & vitamins: what to try, what to buy. *Diabetes Interview.* 2002. Available at: http://diabeteshealth.com/read,2006,2809.html. Accessed December 30, 2004.

Sarubin-Fragakis A. *The Health Professional's Guide to Popular Dietary Supplements.* 2nd ed. Chicago, Ill: American Dietetic Association; 2002.

Problem-Solving Hyperglycemia With Insulin Pump Therapy

Jan Kincaid-Rystrom, MEd, RD, CDE

Possible Causes	Recommended Action
Infusion site	
Redness/irritation or swelling at site, exudates, or blood in tubing	Change infusion set and site.
Insertion in scarred or hypertrophied tissue	Change site and avoid scar tissue and hypertrophied areas.
Cannula not inserted properly	Replace infusion set.
Irritation from infusion set	Avoid friction areas, such as waistline. Review frequency of site changes and site rotation. Suggest alternate infusion set, tape, or skin preparation.
Infusion set/cartridge	
Loose connection between cartridge and tubing or leaking "quick release"	Check for leaks, bubbles, and insulin odor. Tighten connection. Change infusion set and site.
Damaged tubing	Replace infusion set.
Cartridge/cannula not primed	Prime completely.
Disconnected pump	Prime cartridge, then reconnect. Prime cannula.
Cannula not inserted properly	Replace infusion set.
Blood in infusion set	Change infusion set and site.
Air in infusion set	Change infusion set and site. If using set with quick disconnect, disconnect from site and prime pump to remove air bubbles in tubing.
Empty cartridge	Fill new cartridge and change infusion set.

(*continued*)

Possible Causes	Recommended Action
Insulin	
Outdated or temperature impaired	Change infusion site and set and replace cartridge with fresh insulin from a new vial.
Empty cartridge	Replace insulin cartridge and change infusion set.
Pump	
Pump malfunction	Review history of insulin delivery. Replace batteries as needed. Confirm alarms and take action as outlined in User Guide. Contact pump company.
Pump in "suspend delivery" mode	Check pump function and take out of "suspend" mode.
Basal rate incorrectly programmed	Review basal programming.
Individual management	
Incorrect or missed bolus dose	Review bolus history in pump. Review insulin:carohydrate ratio, carbohydrate counting, and programming bolus. An "extended" or "split bolus" may be needed for appropriate coverage of high protein/high fat meals, long meals, continuous snacking, or gastroparesis. Consult with health care team.
Incorrect basal program	Check basal programming. Conduct basal test.
Stress or illness	Review insulin sensitivity ratio for correction boluses. Follow sick-day management guidelines from health care team.
Activity level increased or decreased	Review use of temporary basal rate change to increase or decrease insulin delivery. Monitor blood glucose frequently.
Pregnancy	Hormone changes may result in increased insulin requirements.
Menstrual cycles	Blood glucose levels are often higher 10 days before the period and lower the first day or two of the period. Adjust basal rate (or use alternate basal program) as needed.
Other	
Weight change	Change in weight will enhance or impede insulin sensitivity. May require recalculation of basal and/or bolus doses.
Medication change	Certain medications, such as steroids, may interfere with blood glucose levels. Inform health care team of all medications and any changes.

INDEX

*Page numbers with *b* indicate a box; page numbers with *f* indicate a figure, and page numbers with *t* indicate a table.